Blockchain and Digital Twins for Smart Hospital Infrastructures

Ben Othman Soufiane
King Faisal University, Saudi Arabia

IGI Global
Scientific Publishing
Publishing Tomorrow's Research Today

Published in the United States of America by
IGI Global Scientific Publishing
701 East Chocolate Avenue
Hershey, PA, 17033, USA
Tel: 717-533-8845 | Fax: 717-533-7115
Website: https://www.igi-global.com E-mail: cust@igi-global.com

Library of Congress Cataloging-in-Publication Data

Names: Ben Othman, Soufiane, 1981- editor
Title: Blockchain and digital twins for smart hospital infrastructures / edited by Ben Othman Soufiane.
Description: Hershey, PA : IGI Global Scientific Publishing, [2026] | Includes bibliographical references and index. | Summary: "This book explores and establishes a comprehensive understanding of how blockchain and digital twin technologies can be integrated to revolutionize the design, management, and operation of smart healthcare systems. This book bridges the existing gap between conceptual research and real-world implementation by presenting both the theoretical foundations and practical applications of these emerging technologies within the context of modern hospital infrastructures"-- Provided by publisher.
Identifiers: LCCN 2026002155 (print) | LCCN 2026002156 (ebook) | ISBN 9798337381770 hardcover | ISBN 9798337381787 paperback | ISBN 9798337381794 ebook
Subjects: LCSH: Blockchains (Databases)--Medical applications | Digital twins (Computer simulation) | Medical care--Data processing | Hospitals--Administration--Data processing
Classification: LCC R859.7.B56 B555 2026 (print) | LCC R859.7.B56 (ebook)
LC record available at https://lccn.loc.gov/2026002155
LC ebook record available at https://lccn.loc.gov/2026002156

British Cataloguing in Publication Data
A Cataloguing in Publication record for this book is available from the British Library.

Table of Contents

Detailed Table of Contents

technology provides to smart hospital systems. Finally, this chapter will provide a framework to position blockchain technology as a foundational enabler for secure, resilient, patient-centric smart hospitals by providing the basis for future integration with digital twins and AI-driven healthcare systems.

S. Aarthi, Marwadi University, Rajkot, India
Ravikumar R. N., Marwadi University, Rajkot, India
Shreha S. A., PSG College of Arts and Science, Coimbatore, India
Satheesh Kumar A., Nandha Engineering College, Erode, India
S. Srinivasan, Graphic Era (Deemed to be) University, Dehradun, India
Kavitha Bharathi S., Kongu Engineering College, Erode, India

The integration of Blockchain and Digital Twin (DT) technologies revolutionizes smart hospital ecosystems by ensuring data integrity, interoperability, and real-time decision-making. Blockchain provides a tamper-proof infrastructure for consent management, provenance tracking, and secure IoMT communication, while Digital Twins simulate patients, assets, and operations for predictive diagnostics and optimization. This chapter presents a unified framework combining DT intelligence with blockchain's verifiability to achieve transparent, patient-centric, and adaptive healthcare operations. It discusses layered architectures, interoperability standards, and governance mechanisms that enable trustworthy automation and compliance with privacy regulations. Real-world case studies on stroke-risk prediction and consent-driven patient twins demonstrate measurable improvements in auditability, latency, and accountability. The proposed model establishes a foundation for next-generation hospitals that are intelligent, resilient, and ethically governed through verifiable data ecosystems.

interoperability, enhancing cybersecurity resilience, and supporting transparent data-sharing mechanisms, DLT-enabled Digital Twins offer a robust foundation for next-generation intelligent hospital ecosystems. This chapter looks at different design models, real-life examples, performance details, and future research directions that are important for making healthcare changes that are scalable, secure, and ethical.

Rahmath Nisha A., Saveetha School of Management, Saveetha Institute of Medical and Technical Sciences, Chennai, India
R. Pooja, Saveetha School of Management, Saveetha Institute of Medical and Technical Sciences, Chennai, India
M. Radhakrishnan, Saveetha School of Management, Saveetha Institute of Medical and Technical Sciences, Chennai, India

The accelerated digitalization of healthcare has compounded data fragmentation, interoperability, cybersecurity, and patient-centered governance issues in the information systems of hospitals. This chapter suggests a systemic approach, which is a blockchain-enabled identity and health record management together with digital twin technologies to facilitate safe, smart, and interoperable smart hospital processes. Blockchain technology is framed as a trust and governance layer that can support self-sovereign identity-based consent, immutable data provenance, and auditable access control, and digital twins can offer real-time, predictive models of patients, hospital operations, and infrastructure. The chapter presents a blockchain-digital twin governance infrastructure and a maturity model that describes the levels of adoption at smart hospitals, starting with safe digital records, the next level as intelligent and autonomous digital twin ecosystems.

Anvita Rose, Christ (Deemed to be) University, Delhi NCR, India
Khushboo Malik, Christ (Deemed to be) University, Delhi NCR, India

This chapter examines the integration of blockchain and digital twin technologies in transforming healthcare systems, focusing on Estonia and Saudi Arabia. Estonia's mature e-governance infrastructure, built on the X-Road interoperability platform and blockchain validation, supports comprehensive electronic health records and secure data exchange. Saudi Arabia's Vision 2030 and National Transformation Program accelerate modernization through AI, IoMT, smart hospitals, and blockchain-based services. The chapter analyzes how blockchain enhances data integrity, privacy, and interoperability, while digital twins enable real-time monitoring, predictive

Preface

INTRODUCTION

The rapid digital transformation of healthcare systems has ushered in a new era of intelligent, data-driven, and patient-centered medical services. At the heart of this transformation lies the convergence of Blockchain and Digital Twin technologies, two revolutionary paradigms that are redefining how smart hospitals operate, communicate, and evolve. As healthcare institutions increasingly adopt the Internet of Medical Things (IoMT), an interconnected network of sensors, wearable devices, and medical systems, the need for secure, interoperable, and real-time data management has never been more critical.

Traditional healthcare infrastructures face persistent challenges related to data integrity, privacy, interoperability, and system transparency. Patient records are often fragmented across multiple platforms, limiting real-time accessibility and slowing critical decision-making processes. Moreover, the rise of cyber threats and the growing complexity of medical ecosystems demand robust solutions that ensure data security, authenticity, and traceability. Blockchain technology, with its decentralized and tamper-resistant ledger, offers a compelling answer to these challenges, providing trust, transparency, and immutability in healthcare data transactions.

Complementing this is the transformative concept of the Digital Twin, a dynamic, virtual representation of physical entities such as patients, medical equipment, or even entire hospital systems. By mirroring real-world operations in a digital environment, Digital Twins enable predictive analysis, optimization of clinical workflows, and personalized treatment strategies. When integrated with blockchain, these digital replicas gain an additional layer of reliability and security, ensuring that all data exchanges, simulations, and predictive insights are verifiable and auditable.

In smart hospital infrastructures, the synergy between Blockchain and Digital Twins unlocks new possibilities for real-time monitoring, predictive maintenance, personalized care delivery, and automated data governance. From securely sharing patient data among healthcare providers to managing medical assets and optimizing hospital operations, these technologies collectively pave the way for next-generation healthcare ecosystems that are intelligent, transparent, and resilient.

This book, Blockchain and Digital Twins for Smart Hospital Infrastructures, explores the interdisciplinary nexus of these technologies. It provides a comprehensive understanding of how Blockchain ensures the security and integrity of healthcare data, while Digital Twins enable intelligent modeling, simulation, and decision support. Through a blend of conceptual frameworks, technical insights, and practical case studies, the book illustrates how this powerful combination can reshape the foundations of modern healthcare, leading to smarter, safer, and more connected hospitals of the future.

Coverage:

The many academic areas covered in this publication include, but are not limited to:

1. Foundations of Smart Healthcare Systems
2. Overview of smart hospitals and digital transformation in healthcare
3. Architecture and components of smart hospital infrastructures
4. Role of the Internet of Medical Things (IoMT) in modern healthcare
5. Blockchain Technology in Healthcare
6. Fundamentals of blockchain and distributed ledger technologies
7. Blockchain for secure medical data sharing and interoperability
8. Consensus mechanisms, smart contracts, and healthcare applications
9. Privacy, security, and regulatory compliance using blockchain
10. Blockchain-based identity management and patient record systems
11. Digital Twin Technology in Healthcare
12. Concept, design, and modeling of digital twins for healthcare systems
13. Digital twins for patient monitoring, treatment simulation, and predictive diagnostics
14. Real-time synchronization of digital and physical hospital environments
15. Integration of AI, machine learning, and analytics in digital twin platforms
16. Integration of Blockchain and Digital Twins
17. Synergistic architecture for blockchain-enabled digital twins
18. Secure and transparent data exchange between physical and virtual healthcare systems
19. Frameworks for interoperability between IoMT, blockchain, and digital twins
20. Legal and regulatory challenges for blockchain–digital twin systems

CHAPTER OVERVIEWS

Chapter 1: Overview of Smart Hospitals and Digital Transformation in Healthcare

This chapter establishes the foundational context for smart hospitals by exploring the evolution of healthcare digital transformation. It highlights how emerging technologies such as IoT, AI, blockchain, and digital twins are reshaping hospital operations and patient care. The chapter is important for framing the motivation behind smart hospital infrastructures. It provides readers with a holistic understanding of current challenges in traditional healthcare systems. By setting the conceptual groundwork, it prepares readers for advanced technical discussions in later chapters.

Chapter 2: Secure and Intelligent Smart Hospitals: A Blockchain-Enabled Digital Twin Architecture

This chapter presents an integrated architecture combining blockchain and digital twins for secure smart hospitals. It highlights how blockchain ensures data integrity while digital twins enable intelligence. The chapter is critical for demonstrating architectural feasibility and system-level design. It bridges theory with practical implementation models. This integration is central to trustworthy and intelligent hospital ecosystems.

Chapter 3: Architecting Smart Hospitals: Integrating Blockchain Security with Digital Twin Intelligence

This chapter focuses on architectural design principles for smart hospitals. It explains how blockchain security mechanisms complement digital twin intelligence. The chapter is important for guiding system architects and researchers. It addresses scalability, interoperability, and resilience challenges. These architectural insights are essential for real-world deployment.

Chapter 4: Integration of Blockchain and Digital Twins in Healthcare: Trust, Transparency, and Immutability in Smart Hospital Data Ecosystems

This chapter highlights the importance of trust and transparency in healthcare data ecosystems. It explains how blockchain immutability enhances digital twin reliability. The chapter is crucial for addressing data governance and auditability.

It reinforces the role of trustworthy data in clinical and operational decisions. This integration strengthens confidence in smart hospital systems.

Chapter 5: Integrating Blockchain and Digital Twins: A Synergistic Framework for Smart Hospitals

This chapter proposes a unified framework for blockchain–digital twin synergy. It emphasizes how combined technologies deliver greater value than standalone solutions. The chapter is important for conceptual clarity and system integration strategies. It supports interdisciplinary collaboration between healthcare, IT, and policy domains. This synergy accelerates smart hospital innovation.

Chapter 6: Digital Twin and Blockchain Integration for Smart Hospital Infrastructures Towards Personalized and Predictive Medicine

This chapter focuses on patient-centric outcomes enabled by integration. It explains how personalized and predictive care models are realized through secure data and real-time simulation. The chapter is significant for linking technology with clinical impact. It highlights improved outcomes, efficiency, and patient satisfaction. This chapter reinforces the healthcare value proposition.

Chapter 7: Distributed Ledger–Powered Digital Twin Models for Intelligent Hospital Infrastructure Management

This chapter explores infrastructure-level applications of digital twins supported by distributed ledgers. It highlights intelligent management of assets, energy, and facilities. The chapter is important for operational efficiency and cost optimization. It extends digital twin use beyond patient care. This enables holistic smart hospital management.

Chapter 8: Blockchain-Enabled Identity and Patient Record Management for Secure and Smart Hospital Systems

This chapter addresses digital identity and patient record security. It explains how blockchain enables self-sovereign identity and consent management. The chapter is critical for privacy-preserving healthcare systems. It reduces data breaches and administrative inefficiencies. Secure identity management is foundational for smart hospitals.

Chapter 9: Comparative Perspectives on Digital Health Transformation: Blockchain and Digital Twin Integration in Estonia and Saudi Arabia

This chapter offers a comparative case study of national digital health strategies. It highlights contextual, regulatory, and cultural differences. The chapter is important for understanding global adoption patterns. It provides transferable lessons for policymakers. Comparative insights strengthen global smart hospital initiatives.

Chapter 10: Revolutionizing Research: Blockchain Technology in Healthcare

This chapter emphasizes blockchain's role in transforming healthcare research. It highlights data integrity, reproducibility, and collaboration. The chapter is crucial for addressing research transparency challenges. It supports ethical clinical trials and open science. This strengthens evidence-based healthcare.

Chapter 11: Blockchain and Digital Twins for Smart Hospital Infrastructures: New Roles for Academic, Clinical, and Medical Libraries

This chapter explores evolving roles of libraries in digital healthcare ecosystems. It highlights knowledge management, data stewardship, and research support. The chapter is important for interdisciplinary collaboration. It positions libraries as innovation enablers. This perspective broadens the smart hospital ecosystem.

Chapter 12: A Cyber–Physical–Human Digital Twin–Blockchain Framework for Continuous Clinical Intelligence: The Hospital That Never Sleeps

This chapter is critically important as it introduces a next-generation cyber–physical–human framework that unifies digital twins, blockchain, and human intelligence to enable continuous clinical intelligence in smart hospitals. It conceptualizes the "hospital that never sleeps," where real-time data from physical systems, digital models, and human inputs are continuously synchronized and secured. The chapter highlights how blockchain ensures trust, immutability, and accountability across this always-on ecosystem. It advances the state of the art by emphasizing uninterrupted decision support, predictive care, and adaptive clinical workflows. By integrating human-in-the-loop intelligence with autonomous systems, this chapter provides a visionary yet practical blueprint for resilient, intelligent, and patient-centric healthcare infrastructures.

Chapter 13: Blockchain-Enabled Digital Twin Architectures for Smart Hospital Infrastructures - Secure, Interoperable and Intelligent Healthcare Systems

Smart hospitals increasingly rely on digital twin technologies to enable real-time monitoring, simulation, and optimization of clinical and operational processes. However, the large-scale deployment of digital twins raises critical challenges related to data security, interoperability, trust, and governance. This chapter presents blockchain-enabled digital twin architectures as a secure, interoperable, and intelligent foundation for next-generation smart hospital infrastructures. By integrating distributed ledger technologies with patient-centric and infrastructure-level digital twins, the proposed architectures ensure tamper-resistant data sharing, decentralized identity management, and transparent access control across heterogeneous healthcare stakeholders.

Chapter 14: Decoding Digital Twins- Possible Applications in near Future

The chapter explores prospective applications such as personalized patient digital twins for predictive diagnostics, surgical simulation and outcome forecasting, hospital resource optimization, remote monitoring, and precision medicine. Emerging directions including cyber–physical–human integration, AI-enhanced simulation, federated digital twins, and blockchain-supported data governance are also discussed. Technical, ethical, and interoperability challenges are critically analyzed, highlighting issues related to data fidelity, scalability, privacy, and regulatory compliance. The chapter concludes by outlining strategic research and implementation pathways that position digital twins as a foundational technology for intelligent, adaptive, and resilient healthcare systems in the near future.

CONCLUSION: IMPACT AND CONTRIBUTION OF THE BOOK

This book makes a significant and timely contribution to the field of smart healthcare by presenting a comprehensive and interdisciplinary exploration of blockchain and digital twin technologies within smart hospital infrastructures. By systematically integrating concepts from healthcare informatics, distributed ledger technologies, artificial intelligence, IoMT, and digital twins, the book advances both theoretical understanding and practical implementation strategies. It bridges the gap between emerging digital innovations and real-world healthcare challenges, particularly in areas of data security, interoperability, trust, and personalized patient care.

The volume uniquely contributes to the subject matter by offering architectural frameworks, governance models, comparative case studies, and future-oriented perspectives that are rarely addressed together in existing literature. Through its focus on secure data ecosystems, predictive and personalized healthcare, and autonomous hospital management, the book provides actionable insights for researchers, clinicians, policymakers, and technology developers. Furthermore, its emphasis on ethical design, workforce wellbeing, and knowledge stewardship ensures that technological progress is aligned with human-centered healthcare values. Collectively, this book serves as a foundational reference and a forward-looking guide, shaping future research directions and supporting the global transformation toward intelligent, secure, and trustworthy smart hospital systems.

Acknowledgment

This work was supported by the Deanship of Scientific Research, Vice Presidency for Graduate Studies and Scientific Research, King Faisal University, Saudi Arabia [Grant No. KFU262841].

Chapter 1
Digital Twin Technology in Healthcare:
Real-Time Patient Monitoring and Predictive Diagnostics

Shreha S. A.
http://orcid.org/0009-0002-2232-819X
PSG College of Arts and Science, Coimbatore, India

Satheesh Kumar A.
http://orcid.org/0009-0008-8182-0946
Nandha Engineering college, Erode, India

Ravikumar R. N.
http://orcid.org/0009-0009-3705-1681
Marwadi University, Rajkot, India

Tamilarasi Rajamani
http://orcid.org/0000-0001-5606-8133
Villa College-QI Campus, Malé, Maldives

Aarthi S.
http://orcid.org/0009-0006-9064-2091
Marwadi University, Rajkot, India

Suganya R.
http://orcid.org/0000-0002-6081-0000
Coimbatore Institute of Technology, Coimbatore, India

ABSTRACT

Digital Twin technology is transforming modern healthcare by creating real-time virtual replicas of patients, equipment, and hospital systems for monitoring, simulation, and predictive diagnostics. Through continuous synchronization with IoMT devices, electronic records, and wearable sensors, digital twins enable clinicians to analyze patient data dynamically, simulate treatment responses, and predict complications before onset. AI and machine learning enhance predictive accuracy, while blockchain ensures data integrity and secure interoperability. These systems also optimize hospital operations by forecasting maintenance, managing resources, and enabling virtual clinical trials. Despite challenges in data standardization,

DOI: 10.4018/979-8-3373-8177-0.ch001

scalability, and privacy, digital twins mark a shift toward intelligent, proactive, and patient-centric healthcare ecosystems capable of delivering precision medicine and operational efficiency in smart hospital infrastructures.

1. INTRODUCTION

Digital Twin (DT) is an IT technology that has now offered a paradigm shift in the healthcare sector since it combines both the physical and virtual healthcare. It enables physical status of a patient, equipment in a hospital and its computerized image to be aligned in real time. Combined with Artificial Intelligence (AI), Machine Learning (ML), and the Internet of Medical Things (IoMT), DTs can provide clinicians with practical insights, which can be implemented in real-time monitoring and predictive diagnostics (Fukawa and Rindfleisch, 2023). The blockchain also enhances this ecosystem by providing integrity of data, transparency and security to a multi-stake holder environment. All these technologies are changing the idea of individualized care, functional smartness, and decision-making experiences of smart hospitals infrastructure. The increasing use of DTs will be a transition to proactive healthcare management based on data-driven foresight and adaptive interventions to enhance patient safety, clinical outcomes, and system resilience.

1.1 Overview of Digital Twin Evolution in Healthcare

Digital twins were first developed in the manufacturing industry where virtual representations of real-life systems were used to streamline production processes and to manage the lifecycle. Its introduction in healthcare has gone into a new gear with the integration of the IoMT and cloud computing that allowed the real-time gathering of the physiological data and simulation. Early uses of DT were dedicated to organ-specific modeling, i.e., cardiac and pulmonary twins, and modern uses are based on whole-body representation and hospital ecosystems. The development of the system based on the dynamic learning models of data instead of the static data repositories makes it possible to continuously synchronize with the biological condition of the patient (Jat et al., 2024). New technologies in the field of AI and high-performance computing have advanced further in the use of DT in predictive diagnostics, rehabilitation tracking, and surgical planning. Currently, DTs can be used as an online extension of patient care, facilitating precise medicine and facilitating predictive analytics that anticipate the onset of diseases, respond well to therapy, and improve healthcare processes in intelligent hospital settings (Papachristou et al., 2024). As this figure 1 shows, the implementation of the digital twin will change healthcare into a proactive, highly personalized care system due to the collection of data, the integration of AI, and the dynamical modelling.

Figure 1. Digital Twins Revolutionize Healthcare

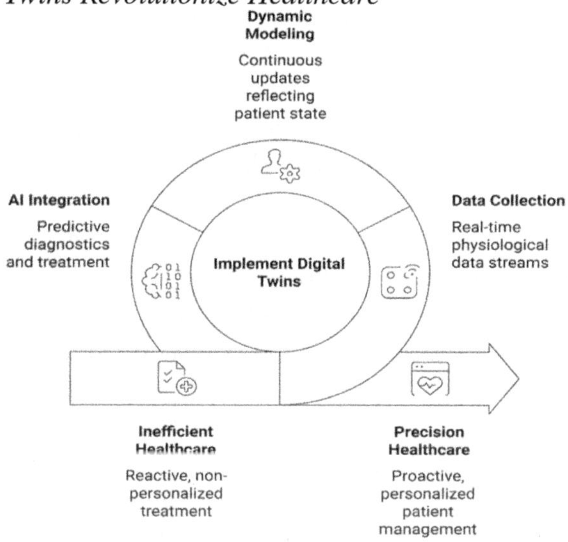

1.2 Need for Real-Time Monitoring and Predictive Diagnostics

Healthcare real-time monitoring is necessary to control chronic illnesses, acute care, and postoperative recovery and provide timely solutions. Digital Twins improve the disconnection between continuous sensing and predictive insight through combination of multimodal data of IoMT devices, imaging systems, and electronic health records. Predictive diagnostics makes use of this live data to predict possible health problems before clinical symptoms arise to improve preventive care. As an illustration, AI-enabled DTs will be capable of identifying the signs of cardiac anomalies or respiratory distress at its early stages and send automatic warnings to clinicians (Bergamini et al., 2025). These constant feedback loops result in the reduction of diagnostic delays, hospital readmissions, and enhance survival. Moreover, predictive modeling enables healthcare systems to move beyond the reactive treatment approach to the precision-based prevention strategy. DT-based monitoring provides a basis of scalable, responsive, and patient-specific healthcare system in smart hospitals by facilitating data-centric decision-making.

1.3 Role of Blockchain and IOMT in Enabling Secure Healthcare Twins

The Internet of Medical Things (IoMT) that collects physiological data and environmental data (in real-time) is the sensory component of Digital Twins. However, a vast amount of data sharing causes privacy, integrity, and interoperability concerns. These challenges can be solved by the blockchain technology because the technology offers un-editable and decentralized data management. All the transactions, medical update or an update of a device, are stored securely in a distributed ledger and thus can be traced and authenticated. Smart contracts will contribute to transferring the data between healthcare industry stakeholders in a safe manner and simplify the incorporation of DTs in hospitals and research facilities (Olatunde et al., 2025). The combination of IoMT and blockchain will provide a stable system that keeps the records of patients safe, yet the system will not break the transparency. This form of synergy assists ethical AI-supported diagnostics, regulatory compliance, and safe interoperability over the medical ecosystems, the foundation of intelligent, privacy-conscious, and decentralized digital twins in the modern healthcare environment. The figure 2 shows how blockchain will be employed to enhance the digital twin ecosystems by decentralizing the problem of data security by transferring it to trusted and decentralized and open healthcare systems using smart contracts and data integrity.

Figure 2. Secure Healthcare Twins with Blockchain

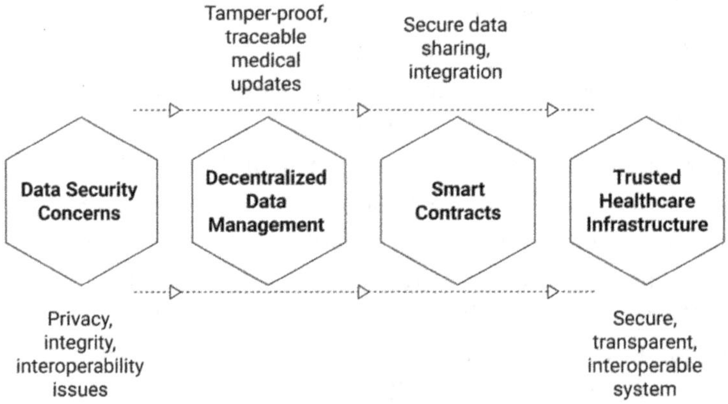

1.4 Literature Review

The development of the digital twin technology within the healthcare sector has received considerable scholarly interest with researchers investigating how the digital twin can be applied in clinical practice through the integration of real-time data analytics, simulation and predictive modeling. The initial literature placed digital twins as a follow-up of cyber-physical systems with more emphasis on industry and manufacturing (Łukaniszyn et al., 2024). But now that IoMT and AI have been developed, the concept has been redefined to a medical and hospital setting. Research notes that healthcare digital twins offer dynamic and data-driven models that can simulate physiology of patients, response to treatment, and hospital workflows in real-time. The scientists have studied organ-specific twins, including cardiac and lung models, and mimic a disease progression and measure the effectiveness of the therapy. Equally, digital twins have been suggested in managing hospital assets, bed assignment, energy use, and maintenance of equipment (Thangaraj et al., 2024). The incorporation of blockchain into the digital twin structures has become a viable solution to overcome the interoperability and security issues. The ability of blockchain to provide transparency in clinical activities through immutable ledger improves traceability and data integrity. The AI and ML systems have gained a long-standing reputation in terms of predictive diagnostics, anomaly detection, and early warning systems. These models allow healthcare professionals to shift to active, customized care rather than the reactive one (Sharma et al., 2024).

Another finding of the literature is the possibility of edge and cloud computing to facilitate the scale deployment in order to facilitate low-latency processing and ongoing synchronization of the data across devices. Although the above advances exist, various researches indicate that the challenges encountered are still evident such as data heterogeneity, absence of standardization and privacy of sensitive patient information (Chaparro-Cárdenas et al., 2025). To alleviate these challenges, scholars have proposed Federated Learning and privacy preserving mechanisms. The recent discourse also pinpoints the next path of digital twins that are quantum enhanced simulation, ethical governance, and sustainability. In general, the literature is characterized by a gradual shift to practice due to the active development of the concept, which proves the existence of digital twins as the foundation technology of smart, safe, and patient-centered healthcare ecosystems (Gkintoni & Halkiopoulos, 2025).

2. FOUNDATIONS OF DIGITAL TWIN TECHNOLOGY

Digital Twin technology is a solution that can be used to describe the merger of modeling, simulation, and real-time data analytics that reflect the state and behavior of real things. In the healthcare sector, DTs can be used to simulate organs, patients, or even hospital systems, which allow making informed decisions and future predictions. The core of a healthcare digital twin consists in the fact that it keeps all data in sync, examines health paths, and offers guidance based on simulations. DTs have a bi-directional communication with physical systems through its core components including sensors, data models, and simulation engines. Their cycle entails creation, calibration, and continuous improvement in the form of feedback loops (Singh et al., 2021). These transforming virtual models enable clinicians to predict disease progression, individualize treatment and perform virtual testing. With the improvement of computational accuracy, DTs are finding their way into predictive medicine and operational management to redefine the threshold of real-time healthcare innovations and patient safety.

2.1 Core Concepts: Physical-Virtual Synchronization

The basic element of the digital twin functionality is the possibility to maintain a smooth synchronization of physical and virtual systems. This mutual relationship in healthcare allows the actual medical information to update the electronic version on-the-fly and the results of simulation to be used to adjust the actual medical intervention. This synchronization is what brings continuity of feedback and dynamic modelling to the biological or operational processes. Indicatively, the heart twin can be able to replicate the heart rhythm of a patient, spot abnormalities, and offer real-time simulated treatment responses. They are sensor-driven, imaging/EHR-driven, and sensor-driven models (Wang, 2020). The AI algorithms interpret the data assisting in making prescriptive and predictive insights. Physical-virtual synchronization, in its turn, ensures the accuracy, flexibility, and responsiveness, i.e., DTs are an important factor in the round-the-clock monitoring, personal diagnostics, and active display of care within the interconnected hospital system.

2.2 Key Components: Sensors, Data Models, and Simulation Engines

A healthcare Digital Twin is based on three key elements, such as sensors, data models, and simulation engines. IoMT devices, wearables, and biomedical instruments are sensors that obtain real-time physiological and environmental data. This sensory data is processed by data models into digital structured formulations with ontologies and AI-based analytics. They incorporate multimodal information such as vital, images, genomics, to show the dynamic state of the patient. The results are then predicted using simulation engines to test interventions and optimise clinical decisions using virtual experimentation. All these components together form an adaptive ecosystem, which generates a new data cycle on every evolution. The combination of AI, blockchain, and cloud computing enhances the scalability, reliability, and privacy of these components (Khatoon, 2020). All these technologies can enable autonomous and smart healthcare systems to make real-time decisions and customize the treatment plan to a person with better interoperability. Table 1 The basic building blocks and their functions in a healthcare digital twin.

Table 1. Core Components of Healthcare Digital Twin Systems

Component	Function	Example Application
Sensors	Capture real-time physiological or device data	Wearable ECG or glucose monitor
Data Models	Represent patient or system state digitally	Cardiac model, respiratory model
Simulation Engine	Predicts outcomes through virtual testing	Drug response simulation
AI Algorithms	Analyze patterns and forecast risks	Disease progression modeling
Blockchain Layer	Ensures data integrity and security	Medical record validation

2.3 Digital Twin Lifecycle: Creation, Calibration, and Continuous Update

The healthcare digital twin lifecycle has three primary steps, namely, creation, calibration, and continuous updating. The design step involves formation of the original virtual model according to patient unique datasets, images scans and clinical data. The digital replica is set using the Machine Learning algorithms, and can also be tested against the physical behavior of a system during calibration. It is due to this process of constant updating that makes the twin accurate and predictive as the real-time information offered by IoMT devices and EHRs keeps the twin updated. This active development is what makes the difference between DTs and fixed digital models as they can be modified to fit the physiological or operational changes (DevOps Engineer/Cloud Solutions Architect USA et al., 2025). The predictive reliability is augmented with every update being made, enabling the proactive interventions and simulating the treatment strategies virtually. A properly maintained lifecycle guarantees model fidelity, clinical stability over time as well as successful incorporation into smart healthcare ecosystems. The figure 3 demonstrates that a healthcare digital twin has three stages in its lifecycle, creation, calibration, and continuous update, with the model being updated in real-time by patient and system data.

Figure 3. Digital Twin Lifecycle in Healthcare

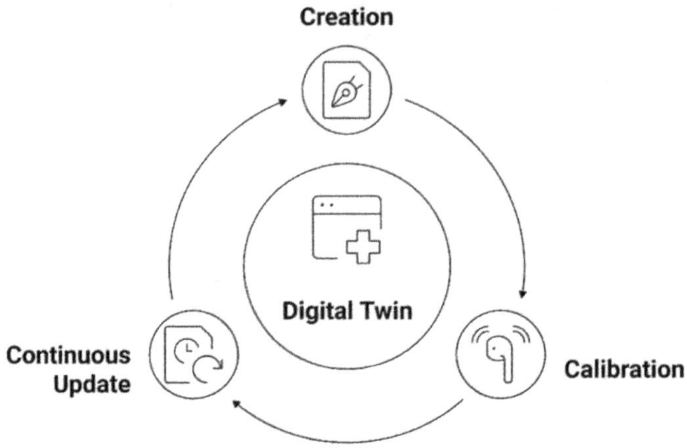

3. ENABLING TECHNOLOGIES IN HEALTHCARE DIGITAL TWINS

Digital twin ecosystems rely on a number of technologies which are interconnected and jointly allow capturing, analyzing, and simulating data in real-time. Internet of Medical Things (IoMT) is the guarantee of ubiquitous data collection of wearable and implantable sensors. Machine Learning (ML) and Artificial Intelligence (AI) convert this stream of continuous data to performable insights to predict and diagnose. At the same time, edge and cloud computing offer the computational power necessary to be fast and able to scale models. All these technologies create a continuous feedback mechanism in which physiological data are detected, sent, examined and re-simulated in milliseconds (Makhdoom et al., 2019). With such a synergy, the predictive healthcare processes such as detection of early disease and optimization of treatment to the end user can be supported and yet the system remains responsive and reliable. This combined technology stack is the basis of smart, connected, and self-adaptive digital twins in the current healthcare systems.

3.1 Internet of Medical Things (IOMT) and Data Acquisition Pipelines

The IoMT allows real time updating of physiological information via an interoperative system of medical sensors, wearable devices and intelligent hospital equipment. Every device measures a parameter, e.g. heart rate, blood pressure, glucose level, or oxygen saturation and sends it to central databases through secure communications protocols like MQTT or CoAP. Data acquisition pipelines are in charge of such information flow including preprocessing and validation to integration into digital twin platforms. High level middleware assures the reduction of noise, time coordination of data and standardization of data among heterogeneous sources. This acquisition process can allow the physical and digital entities to be synchronized in real time and therefore the twin gives true patient states (Adavoudi Jolfaei et al., 2021). The IoMT therefore becomes the lifeblood of digital twin systems which allows continuous monitoring, clinical decision support and remote patient management whilst maintaining accuracy, security and interoperability in the interconnected healthcare networks (Ravikumar, Renukadevi, Manujakshi, et al., 2025). The figure 4 shows the five-stage IoMT data pipeline collection, transmission, preprocessing, integration, and synchronization that allows continuous and precise data flow into healthcare digital twin systems.

Figure 4. IoMT Data Acquisition Pipeline

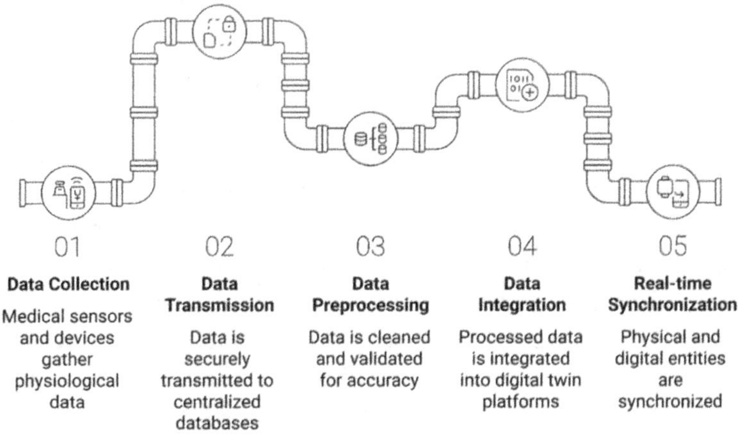

3.2 Artificial Intelligence and Machine Learning for Predictive Modeling

Digital twins facilitate AI and ML algorithms to process large amounts of medical data and forecast clinically related outcomes in the future. These models determine intricate associations between physiological variables, features of imaging, and treatment outcomes through learning with supervision and without supervision. The Deep Learning models used, including the LSTM and CNN architectures, allow predictions of disease progressions over time, whereas the reinforcement learning model is used to optimize the choice of individual therapies. These smart models will convert crude sensor signals into forecasted information that help clinicians to diagnose aberrations, predict treatment outcomes, and model virtual procedures (Awasthi Ms & Mishra Ms, 2025). Predictive modeling based on AI also increases the flexibility: the re-training process on each new piece of data advances and refines the accuracy of the twin. This life-long learning feature enables the timely identification of risk, reduction of diagnostic ambiguity, and the ability to make evidence-based decisions-making AI and ML the brain of the next-generation digital twin architecture of proactive and precision-based healthcare (Saparbaevich, et al., 2025).

3.3 Edge and Cloud Computing Integration for Low-Latency Processing

The digital twin responsiveness and scalability are available with the help of edge and cloud computing. Edge computing is a network that is able to perform data processing at a closer distance to the medical equipment- Minimizing latency and allowing immediate analysis depending on time sensitivity like cardiac monitoring or ICU control. This is supplemented by cloud computing which provides scaled out resources when it comes to large-scale simulations, model training, and storage (Akindote et al., 2023). Hybrid edge-clouds will enable twins of healthcare to trade-off between nearby processing and centralized analytics so that they can be responsive in real time without losing the depth of computations. Containerized microservices and secure APIs enable ease in deploying and interoperability of the hospital systems. A combination of these technologies facilitates constant alignment of the physical and virtual worlds providing quick, fault-tolerant and context-sensitive responses. The resultant infrastructure is a platform of resilient and scalable healthcare platforms capable of supporting of millions of data streams simultaneously within smart hospital settings. Table 2 Highlights important enabling technologies and how they have been used to enhance the digital twin functionality.

Table 2. Enabling Technologies Supporting Digital Twins in Healthcare

Technology	Primary Role	Benefit
IoMT	Real-time data collection	Continuous patient monitoring
AI/ML	Predictive analytics	Personalized diagnostics
Edge Computing	Localized data processing	Reduced latency
Cloud Computing	Scalable storage and analytics	Real-time access
Blockchain	Secure data management	Trust and transparency

4. ARCHITECTURE OF HEALTHCARE DIGITAL TWIN SYSTEMS

The healthcare digital twin architecture combines the data collection, modeling, and service delivery into a multi-layered framework. On the bottom, there is the layer of data acquisition and safe storage of information of the IoMT. The model layer is the one that utilizes the AI and simulation algorithms in order to reproduce physiological or operational behaviors. Lastly, the service layer will convert analytical outputs into clinical or operation decisions. Blockchain implements integrity of data, whereas the interoperability standards ensure compatibility of cross-systems. All the layers are dynamically interacting with one another by continuous feedback loops that streamline predictive ability and functional relevance (Chakilam, 2025). This design is highly modular and security enhanced and scalable- healthcare institutions can implement digital twins in departments or entire hospital networks in an efficient way. The architecture therefore offers a strong framework in establishing resilient, smart and ethically sound digital ecosystems. The figure 5 shows the layered architecture of a healthcare digital twin system and the operation of the data, model, and service layers with blockchain security and interoperability to allow intelligent clinical decision-making.

Figure 5. Healthcare Digital Twin Architecture

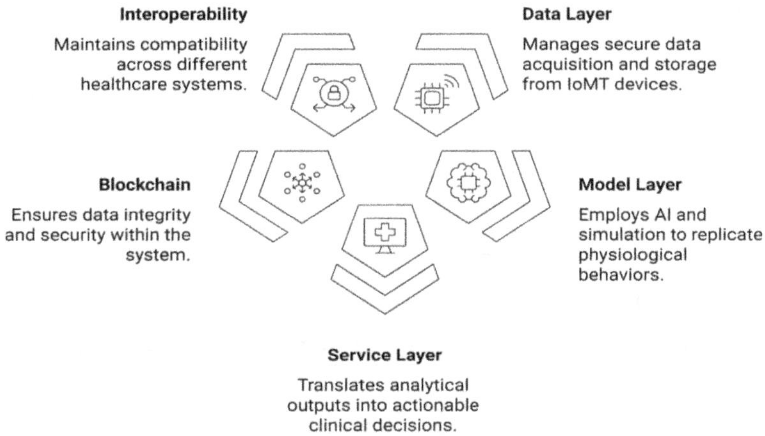

4.1 Multi-Layer Architecture: Data, Model, and Service Layers

The multi-level design of a healthcare digital twin is based on three interrelated layers, such as data, model, and service layers. The data layer receives, filters and encrypts multimodal incoming data of the IoMT devices, EHRs and imaging systems.

These inputs are analyzed by the model layer with the use of AI-based algorithms and represent dynamic simulating that emulate either patient physiology or a hospital process. The service layer provides insights through physician and administrator dashboards, clinical alerts, and physician and administrator automated decision support interfaces. Constant exchange of data done between these layers is what makes the twin keep on developing with real time data updates (Jung et al., 2022). This hierarchical design facilitates flexibility to allow hospitals to expand operations of digital twins to both single-patient monitoring and system-wide management. The multi-layer approach, therefore, will guarantee reliability, scalability, and openness of both clinical and administrative functions it is the architectural backbone of smart healthcare infrastructures. Namely, the figure 6 demonstrates the three-level system of healthcare digital twins, i.e., data, model, and service layers, whereby encrypted inputs are handled by AI algorithms to produce real-time clinical insights.

Figure 6. Layered Structure of Healthcare Digital Twin Architecture

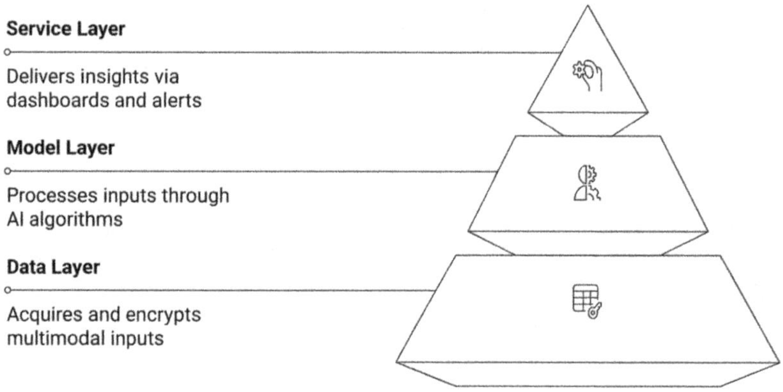

4.2 Blockchain Integration for Data Integrity and Traceability

The blockchain technology empowers the digital twin ecosystems with data management that is tamper-proof and end-to-end traces. Every transaction sensor reading, diagnostic update, or treatment adjustment is stored as a cryptographically-linked immutable block connected to the records of the earlier transactions. This makes medical information to be authentic, verifiable and difficult to manipulate by some unauthorized entities. Smart contracts are used to automate access control to ensure that sensitive information is only accessed or modified by verified clinicians or systems (Taralunga & Florea, 2021). The decentralized registry allows the hospital-laboratory-research center to exchange safe data without the help of mediators. Moreover, consensus mechanisms are a critical approach to increase trust and transparency in healthcare data governance since blockchain enables regulatory compliance. Such a combination of blockchain and digital twins does not only improve the level of cybersecurity, but also allows responsible collaboration, a chance to create safe infrastructure of scalable, ethical, and interoperable healthcare networks.

4.3 Interoperability and Standardization in Hospital Ecosystems

Interoperability and standardization are also important in the effective achievement of digital twins in heterogeneous hospitals. A system of medical care is premised on a number of technologies, databases, and communication standards, which hinder information exchange. Implementation of standards like HL7 FHIR, DICOM, and IEEE 11073 make it possible to represent the data in a consistent manner and be compatible with various devices and platforms. Digital twins Interoperable digital twins enable communication across departments in a manner that enables cardiology, radiology and emergency units to view syncing patient models in real time (El Mrabet et al., 2025). Standardization also provides adherence to the national and international healthcare standards such as HIPAA regulations and GDPR. The middleware structures and open APIs can connect the old system to the new infrastructures encouraging scale and vendor-neutrality. Finally, interoperability will make digital twins universal assets that will link data silos, improve coordination, and swiftly move to patient-centric, connected, and intelligent hospital ecosystems.

5. APPLICATIONS IN REAL-TIME PATIENT MONITORING

Digital twin technology provides the affordable continuous and smart monitoring of the patients to be informed continuously about the physiological changes and possible risks. Using the data collected with the help of IoMT devices, imaging systems, and clinical databases, DTs can present the patient with a living digital counterpart that reflects his or her current health condition. These systems are used to analyze multivariate data streams and identify early anomalies, adjust treatment programs and anticipate complications before symptoms appear. The integration of AI-based analytics with simulation is effective in improving the accuracy in decision-making by clinicians (Saliha & Ferhati, 2025). Monitoring of patients in real-time with the help of DTs will considerably decrease the amount of manual monitoring, decrease the time of response in an emergency, and decrease the number of re-admissions to the hospital. Predictive insights incorporated into such systems promote proactive healthcare - to enable medical professionals to shift their response measures towards ongoing and personalized care management according to the principles of precision medicine.

5.1 Continuous Vital Sign Tracking and Anomaly Detection

Real-time healthcare digital twins are based on constant monitoring of vital signs. The wearable or implantable IoMT devices have sensors that continuously measure physiological information, including ECG, oxygen saturation, body temperature, and blood glucose levels, and provide them to the digital twin. AI algorithms work with these data streams and detect any deviation out of normal ranges, which can indicate possible abnormalities such as arrhythmias, hypoxia or hyperglycemia (Ganesan et al., 2020). Unlike the example of the traditional monitoring systems, which are premised on the fact that observations are carried out infrequently, DTs enable constant tracking and automatic observation of abnormalities. Predictive analytics are more precise since they depend on the relationship of multi-sensor data in forecasting the trends of deterioration. The system generates alert messages that help the clinicians to be proactive to improve patient outcomes and optimization of resources. The real-time integration of a physical and virtual health parameter creates a reactive and data-driven surveillance area, the most critical aspect in chronic disease therapy and the intensive care unit.

5.2 Personalized Treatment Adjustment Using Predictive Insights

It is possible to achieve adaptive and patient-specific treatment management through digital twins, which results in a continuous processing of varying physiological data. Predictive algorithms are sensor data, lab data, and medication response data that are processed and enable the proposal of therapy adjustments based on the needs of individuals. To illustrate this, a DT can anticipate the alterations in glucose levels and suggest the alterations in insulin doses of diabetes patients before hyperglycemia comes about. In the same way, when speaking of heart patients, it may also mimic the dosage effect or the change in lifestyle and its impact on stabilizing the heart rhythms. This form of feedback is iterative and it ensures optimisation of treatment regimens in real time (Rahman & Ansar, 2025). Predictive modeling used together with clinical data decreases the negative events, enhances medication efficacy, and advances precision medicine. Empowering clinicians to see how likely the results would be in case of a virtual simulation, DTs allow to personalize the treatment based on evidence, making healthcare less generalized, more about a continuous, situation-specific care.

5.3 AI-Driven Alert Systems for Early Disease Onset Prediction

The AI-based alert systems integrated in digital twins enhance the proactive healthcare by anticipating the initial stages of the disease onset. Machine Learning algorithms designed based on past and current data detect minor abnormalities in physiological or behavioral changes that predict clinical symptoms. Indicatively, in respiratory care, AI can predict possible infections or asthma exacerbation with small changes in the breathing rate and oxygen levels. Such warnings are automatically communicated to medical personnel or patient interfaces and prompt testing and treatment is provided. Such systems have a great predictive accuracy and there is a significant decrease in cases of emergencies and an improvement in preventive care (Lilja, 2022). Furthermore, AI-based alert systems combine the Natural Language Processing (NLP) and contextual reasoning in order to prioritize the most important notifications and reduce the number of false alarms. This balance brings in efficiency, dependability and confidence, developing a smart early-warning platform at the heart of the next-generation, patient-centric healthcare systems.

6. PREDICTIVE DIAGNOSTICS AND CLINICAL DECISION SUPPORT

Predictive diagnostics is the analysis core of healthcare digital twins, a combination of AI models and physiological simulations to predict the disease progression and clinical outcome. They are systems that are used to analyze large datasets of patients in order to identify the patterns of risks, disease predisposition and variability of responses. DTs increase the accuracy of diagnosis and optimize the therapeutic plan when combined with decision-support systems. Disease simulation or drug interaction simulations enable clinicians to test the treatment plans without incurring the risk that they might expose them to in real life (Alowais et al., 2023). Predictive analytics (diagnostics) also allows the analytics to be done at population level, here trends in the public health are detected early. Digital twins enhance evidence-based decision-making by integrating accuracy on the model with clinical processes and decreasing the latency in diagnosis. The result is that the reactive treatment model is being replaced with a more data-driven approach to medical care that places emphasis on prevention, individualization and predictive understanding in order to promote the best care of patients (Sapayev, et al., 2025).

6.1 Disease Progression Modeling and Risk Forecasting

Digital twins transform the field of clinical prediction by modeling the progression of the disease in computerised settings. The AI models simulate the biological processes of a patient using patient-specific parameters: genetic profiles, biomarkers, imaging, and lifestyle-based factors to predict diseases and show disease dynamics. Indicatively, in oncology, the dynamics of tumor progression can be simulated to predict the possibility of metastasis or resistance to therapy (Kurbanova, et al., 2025). Likewise, in cardiology, the forecasts of heart failure exacerbation are made by using progression models. These predictions are refined through continuous learning mechanisms where new information is added thus improving accuracy as time goes by. Risk forecasting enables doctors to use preventive measures, modify the intensity of treatment, and to distribute medical resources in an efficient manner (Hughes et al., 2023). The integration of real-time updates and predictive simulation offers the dynamic perception of the behavior of the disease, changing the healthcare to active and proactive diagnosis, which is based on constant and forward-looking control that is grounded in precision analytics.

6.2 Drug Response Simulation and Therapy Optimization

Digital twins are used to provide virtual experimentation through the simulated responses of drugs on a molecular level, organ level, and systemic level. AI-based Pharmacokinetic and Pharmacodynamic (PK/PD) models can predict the interaction of certain medications with personal patient traits and reduce the trial and error of the conventional prescribing method. As an example, the effects of dosage of chemotherapy or the evolution of antibiotic resistance can be digitally modeled before administration. Such simulations allow clinicians to find the best dosing plans, reduce side effects, and customize the treatment plans. On top of that, population-scale digital twins can be used to support pharmaceutical research, simulating the effectiveness of a drug in a wide range of demographic or genetic populations, lowering the cost and time of clinical trials (Darwich et al., 2021). The predictive analytics partnering with the biological reality maintains the therapy optimization founded on DT resulting in the enhanced safety, the faster innovation, and the advancement of the overall goal of the smart, adaptable, and focus on precision medical services.

6.3 Integration With Clinical Decision Support Systems (CDSS)

With the help of Digital twins and Clinical Decision Support Systems (CDSS), raw data is transformed into medical intelligence, which can be performed upon. The CDSS platforms have been linked to ever-up to date patient twins through real-time synchronization, to support physicians make diagnosis, prognoses and treatment plans. Inference engines based on Machine Learning process simulated results and give evidence-based feedback and warn clinicians of possible complications or contraindications. The visualization dashboards increase predictability and risk indicators are displayed intuitively through visualization dashboards. In addition, integration of blockchain provides auditability and regulatory compliance of all decision logs (Cernian et al., 2020). The combination of DTs and CDSS creates the connection between simulation and execution that allows physicians to base their decisions on data-driven rationale. Through this synergy, not only is the accuracy of diagnostic outcomes enhanced, but also human error is minimized and a new standard of open, smart, and responsive healthcare decision-making models is set.

7. OPERATIONAL OPTIMIZATION IN SMART HOSPITALS

In addition to clinical use, digital twins are also the key to efficient hospital work and resources. DTs give real time access to the performance of hospitals by reflecting on infrastructure, workflows, and logistics. Predictive models also refer to the ideas that predict equipment failures, predict patient inflow, and best staffing schedules, improving the overall efficiency. AI and IoT analytics integration will allow to observe the state of the facilities continuously, the use of the assets and the movement of patients (Rajput et al., 2019). This predictive operational intelligence will reduce downtime, save money, and enable the use of data to make administrative decisions. In addition, simulation of other emergency or workload scenarios assists the hospitals to plan and be dynamically changing. With the help of digital twins, healthcare institutions transform into self-optimizing ecosystems that integrate clinical efficiency and sustainable use of resources the operational core of intelligent and resilient hospital systems.

7.1 Digital Twins for Equipment Lifecycle and Maintenance Prediction

Digital twins apply predictive analytics to the control of biomedical equipment by establishing virtual versions of equipment, including MRI machines, ventilators or infusion pumps. These models continuously measure the operational parameters which are temperature, vibration, and use of energy to forecast wear and possible failure. The algorithms on maintenance using AI process these data to suggest the time of servicing to minimize the unexpected downtime and guarantee the reliability of the equipment. Historical processes along with on-the-fly tracking allow the hospitals to streamline the maintenance plan, spare parts supply, and budget distribution. Predictive maintenance is also able to prolong the life of the device and the patients because it reduces the chances of malfunction (Susilo et al., 2023). This is achieved by the integration of blockchain to provide transparency in recording maintenance operations and compliance. Therefore, equipment-oriented digital twins make the management of hospital assets less reactive to repair and more proactive and data-driven lifecycle optimization. The figure 7 demonstrates that digital twins help to address the lifecycle of medical equipment by recording data continuously, analyzing it with AI, predicting maintenance, and ensuring compliance to provide a safer and more efficient experience to patients and operational processes.

Figure 7. Digital Twin-Driven Equipment Lifecycle Management

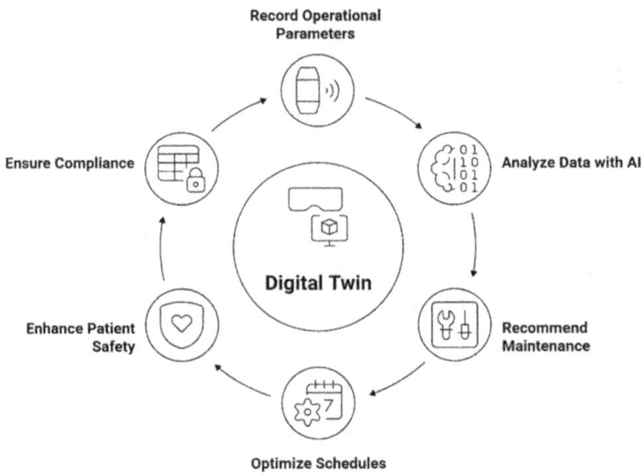

7.2 Workflow and Bed Capacity Optimization Models

The efficiency of the workflow in hospitals has a direct impact on patient satisfaction and care outcomes. Digital twins are used to recreate the operational processes including admissions, diagnostics, surgeries, and discharge cycles in order to understand the delay and bottlenecks. The AI-based optimization algorithms consider real-time information on patient inflow, staffing, and resource usage as predictors of demand variations. Such insights allow to plan the workload, bed assignment and booking corrections dynamically. As an example, patient distribution and resource allocation across departments can be modeled using DT in case of epidemic surges to streamline resource allocation and minimise waste (Juanatas et al., 2025). Predictive modeling helps to make sure that critical care bed and staff are properly distributed without serving as a condition to compromise the quality of services.

These twins of workflows promote sustainable business, improve throughput and eliminate wait times of patients making hospitals resilient and adaptive to data in and data out operations overtime.

7.3 Emergency Response and Resource Allocation Simulation

Digital twins can be used to improve the emergency preparedness by simulating the crisis scenario involving the prediction of a pandemic, natural disaster, or a high number of casualties. Virtual models combine real-time information of the hospital sensors, patient registries, and external agencies to forecast surge capacity requirements and resources availability. AI algorithms model the possible outcomes of the events and maximize the use of ambulances, ICU beds, and medical staff. Decision-makers are able to test various response strategies virtually to select the most effective plan of action to take before it is implemented. This will reduce operation interruptions and will make them prepared in case of unexpected events (Abbas et al., 2023). Also, transparency made by blockchain provides accountability and coordination between multi-agency responders. With these active simulations, hospitals attain situational awareness and operational resilience-so that, during an emergency, their response to the situation is quick, evidence-based, and provides safety to patients and the infrastructure of the healthcare establishment.

8. CASE STUDIES OF DIGITAL TWIN IMPLEMENTATION IN HEALTHCARE

The real-life use of the digital twin technology in the healthcare industry illustrates the potential of the technology to transform the aspect of patient care, diagnostics, and the management of hospitals. The most prominent medical technology firms and research centers have already started to adopt DT frameworks, which combine IoMT, AI, and blockchain to synchronize the information in real-time and provide predictive decision support. These introductions demonstrate quantifiable change in accuracy of treatment, system efficiency and patient safety. Case studies demonstrate a wide range of applications, including individualized cardiac and ICU treatment and optimization on a massive scale in hospitals (Moganti et al., 2025). Both projects emphasize the importance of digital recreations of patients, organs, and operational systems as they allow predictive and preventive actions through simulation. The next case studies will consider the recent innovations provided by Siemens Healthineers and Philips HealthSuite that present the real-life success and scalability of digital twins in intelligent hospital ecosystems.

8.1 Case Study 1: Siemens Healthineers' Digital Twin for Cardiac Care (2024)

In 2024, Siemens Healthineers introduced another platform of digital twins that was an advanced cardiac twin system, which tries to recap patient-selective cardiovascular functioning and help in personalized cardiovascular treatment. It is a multimodal, multimodal system, which consists of MRI, ECG, and echocardiography indicators, and AI-capable modeling to reproduce the electrophysiological and mechanical processes in the human heart. It provides a simulated environment that is interactive and enables the clinicians to simulate surgery, stenting, and responsiveness to medication before they work on the patient (Corral-Acero et al., 2020). Predictive analytics give the twin the ability to predict arrhythmias triggers and optimize the treatment pathways, which yields a 28% higher diagnostic accuracy and more significant surgical complications reduction. Moreover, actual patient information and virtual models also interact with each other based on the continuous feedback loop which allows the therapy to be improved all the time. It can be confirmed that the success of the platform confirms the clinical utility of real-time and simulation-based decision-making, setting new standards in the precision of the cardiology field and tailor-made digital medical systems. (Thangaraj et al., 2024). The figure 8 shows the integration of multimodal data and simulations in a cardiac digital twin platform to improve the accuracy of diagnosis, test treatment strategies and reduce surgical complications in individualized cardiac care.

Figure 8. Personalized Cardiac Care with Digital Twin

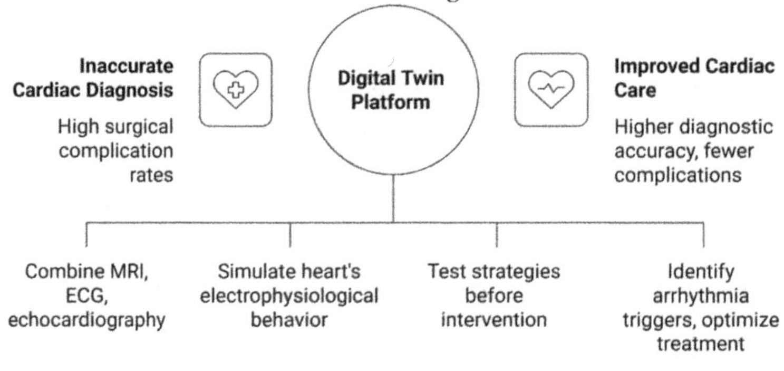

8.2 Case Study 2: Philips Healthsuite Twin for Intensive Care Units (2025)

Philips created a real-time ICU digital twin in HealthSuite digital platform, which in 2025 was implemented in several smart hospitals, to manage critical care in real time. The system combines real-time ventilator, monitor, infusion pump, and EHR data, and identifies the synchronized digital image of every patient and the ICU setting. These data are fed through AI algorithms to predict the risk of patient deterioration, ventilator optimization, and workload balancing of the nursing staff. The resulting predictive insights created by the twin lowered the rate of ICU readmissions by 19% and boosted clinical response time due to automated notifications and intelligent allocation of resources. The platform also facilitates efficiency in administration as it predicts the staffing requirement and equipment utilization trends (Sun et al., 2022). The proposed holistic digital twin model is an example of the use of real-time data fusion and predictive intelligence to improve decision-making, operational resilience, and patient safety in high-acuity clinical settings. The following figure 9 illustrates the HealthSuite ICU digital twin model developed by Philips, in which the integration of data constantly, AI analysis, and predictive insights transform the inefficient management of the ICU into responsive and data-driven critical care.

Figure 9. Real-Time ICU Digital Twin

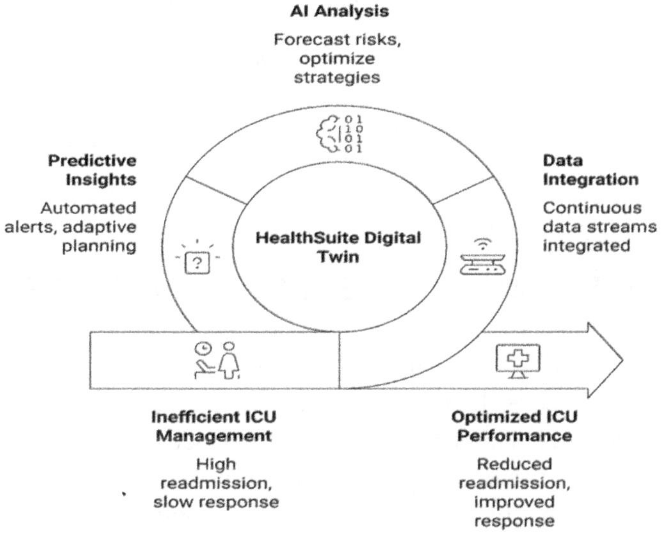

8.3 Comparative Analysis and Key Learnings

The cardiac digital twin of Siemens Healthineers and the Philips HealthSuite ICU twin are two examples of how cardiac digital twins and predictive analytics can radically change clinical practice, even though their goals and areas of operation are different. Siemens is mostly patient-specific physiological modeling, which applies AI-enhanced simulations to customize cardiac interventions and predict surgical outcomes. By contrast, Philips has focused on optimization at the system level and combines device telemetry and patient data to dynamically manage the ICU and plan the workforce (Turab & Jamil, 2023). Although these are different, both implementations have major technological enablers, including IoMT connectivity, AI-based analytics, and cloud-edge infrastructure, which guarantee the fidelity of data and promptness. Their success identifies important lessons: (1) the clinical device-data model interoperability is the key to scalability; (2) predictive algorithms are capable of improving clinical accuracy and safety dramatically; and (3) the implementation of digital twins in the context of the existing hospital ecosystem requires sound cybersecurity, ethical management, and training of clinicians to make the adoption sustainable and patient-centered (Ravikumar & Aarthi, 2025). Table 3 Comparisons the two real world examples of digital twin in the above Section.

Table 3. Comparative Overview of Case Study Implementations

Case Study	Organization	Application Area	Key Outcome	Significance
Cardiac Digital Twin	Siemens Healthineers	Personalized Cardiac Care	28% improvement in prediction accuracy	Patient-specific simulation for surgery
ICU Digital Twin	Philips HealthSuite	Intensive Care Management	19% reduction in readmission rates	Predictive workload and patient management

9. CHALLENGES AND FUTURE RESEARCH DIRECTIONS

Although the digital twin technology has proven to be an incredible possibility in transforming healthcare, there are urgent factors concerned with its adoption that have been presented as challenges to data governance, scalability, model validation, and compliance. The convergence of different IoMTs, Artificial Intelligence algorithms, and information systems in healthcare facilities adds complexities of interoperability, which discourages the smoothness of information exchanges. The privacy issues are based on the fact that sensitive medical information is continuously collected and sent over distributed networks. Moreover, the model reliability, clinical validation, and ethical transparency are the urgent questions in the field of real-world applications (Ait Bennacer et al., 2023). Laws and regulations have not implemented simulation diagnostics and AI decision-making to the full extent. To counteract these obstacles, there is a need to conduct joint studies on privacy preserving computation, Federated Learning and quantum secure structures. The next subsections summarize the main technical and ethical issues and describe future research opportunities which may provide secure, scalable and intelligent digital twin ecosystems in next-generation healthcare systems.

9.1 Data Standardization, Privacy, and Interoperability Concerns

The problem of data heterogeneity is one of the leading issues regarding the creation of the interoperability of healthcare digital twins. The source of medical data is diverse as it may include EHRs, imaging systems, wearable sensors, and lab equipment that are structured in various formats and communication standards. The inconsistency of data integration relies on the absence of standardized data, e.g. HL7 FHIR or DICOM extensions. Moreover, the broad distribution of personal health data through the edges, cloud, and blockchain space and environments pose privacy and security concerns (Sasitharasarma et al., 2025). Illegal access, data leak, or data manipulation can undermine patient confidence and regulatory adherence in the framework of such regulations as GDPR and HIPAA. Decentralized authentication and immutability helps blockchain partially, but scalability and latency still remain a problem. Full interoperability requires that there is international agreement on data schema, encryption and semantic effectiveness. Strong privacy-preservation techniques, including the ones of differential privacy and homomorphic encryption, are essential to facilitate the secure collaboration between the stakeholders of healthcare.

9.2 Scalability, Model Validation, and Regulatory Barriers

Serious technical and operational issues related to scalability are associated with digital twin systems. It increases exponentially with the number of monitored patients and devices connected to it because computational requirements and communication overheads also increase exponentially. There is a need to have lightweight AI inference models and optimized cloud-edge orchestration to handle large-scale simulations in real time (Ravikumar et al., 2025). The validity and reliability of the digital twins validation is also significant. Models and clinical testing that must be carried out on a regular basis are required to ease the safe deployment but are time-intensive and expensive. The control barriers also lead to the further obscurity of the adoption as the authorities regulating and controlling it have not yet standardized the principles of implementing the use of simulation-based diagnostics or AI-based decision-making (Šafran et al., 2025). Compliance with regulations of the medical devices, the process of reviewing the ethics, and auditability must be improved. The obstacles will be eliminated through a multi-stakeholder model which will involve the partnership of healthcare providers, technologists and policymakers in the development of standardized certification frameworks of digital twin safety and performance.

9.3 Future Research: Federated Digital Twins and Quantum-Ready Healthcare

The future developments of the digital twin technology would be based on the domains of decentralization, security, and computing expansion. The paradigm of federated digital twins is characterized by keeping the patient data in the local environment in the hospitals and training the models in Federated Learning. This will enhance the privacy, reduce the price of transferring data and enable sharing of intelligence in the world without violating confidentiality. Introduction of quantum computing to digital twin ecosystems can exponentially increase the ability to multiply the processing speed and encryption and fixed accuracy of data simulation (Fatoum et al., 2021). In the next generation, quantum-safe cryptography would be resorted to in order to protect sensitive health information against the influences of the new generation of cyber-attacks. Moreover, AI systems that follow hybrid models between a symbolic-based and neural-based approach could be more explainable and to be ethical in their transparency. The use of energy in a more prudent manner and the minimization of the adverse effect on the environment will also be significant in terms of sustainability research. Collectively, the innovations will be the foundation to secure, scalable and quantum-capable healthcare digital twins that will transform the future of medical innovation. The current limitations and the possibilities of the future research in the area of the digital twin integration are described in Table 4.

Table 4. Key Challenges and Future Research Directions in Digital Twin Adoption

Challenge Area	Description	Research Direction
Data Standardization	Diverse data formats hinder integration	Adoption of HL7 FHIR and DICOM standards
Privacy and Security	Sensitive patient data at risk	Federated Learning and quantum encryption
Scalability	High computation and storage demands	Edge-cloud hybrid models

continued on following page

Table 4. Continued

Challenge Area	Description	Research Direction
Validation	Difficulty in clinical verification	AI-driven adaptive calibration
Regulation	Lack of unified policies	Development of ethical AI frameworks

10. CONCLUSION

The technology of digital twin is the technology that is transforming the future of health care by establishing the real-time synchronization, intelligent analytics, and predictive decision support models across the borders of the real or the virtual world. The author of this chapter highlighted how digital twins founded on the application of IoMT, AI, blockchain and cloud-edge integration are changing the process of patient monitoring, predictive diagnostics, and operational management within the context of smart hospitals. Digital twins provide a chance to take proactive actions, reduce the number of medical errors, and make the treatment more precise due to the continuous reflection of the physiology of the patients and the processes that take place in the hospital. The case of Siemens Healthineers and Philips HealthSuite illustrates how such technologies have helped in practical terms to improve clinical accuracy, operational performance, and patient outcome. However, data privacy challenges, model interoperability and validation, demonstrate the need to have standard structures and regulation to establishment.

The future research of Federated Learning must be directed towards privacy saving models, quantum-enabled systems, and scalability of the system. The introduction of digital twins is a paradigm shift of preventive, adaptive, and data-driven medicine to medical workers and administrators. They facilitate real-time clinical knowledge, good resource management and resiliency and dynamism of healthcare infrastructures where they respond to patient and system demands. Digital twins will be considered intelligent engines of a smart hospital since it will become intelligent environments and thus it is a continuum of personalized care and not a single instance of care. It is the new era in the medical field, the era of forecasted healthcare, the era of open and over-patient healthcare, in which medical genius is achieved through the combination of computer skills and the nurturing of a human spirit.

REFERENCES

Abbas, S., Sampedro, G. A., Abisado, M., Almadhor, A., Yousaf, I., & Hong, S.-P. (2023). Harris-Hawk-Optimization-based deep recurrent neural network for securing the Internet of Medical Things. *Electronics (Basel), 12*(12), 2612. DOI: 10.3390/electronics12122612

Adavoudi Jolfaei, A., Aghili, S. F., & Singelee, D. (2021). A Survey on Blockchain-Based IoMT Systems: Towards Scalability. *IEEE Access : Practical Innovations, Open Solutions, 9*, 148948–148975. DOI: 10.1109/ACCESS.2021.3117662

Ait Bennacer, S., Sabiri, K., Aaroud, A., Akodadi, K., & Cherradi, B. (2023). A comprehensive survey on blockchain-based healthcare industry: Applications and challenges. *Indonesian Journal of Electrical Engineering and Computer Science, 30*(3), 1558. DOI: 10.11591/ijeecs.v30.i3.pp1558-1571

Akindote, O. J., Adegbite, A. O., Dawodu, S. O., Omotosho, A., & Anyanwu, A. (2023). Innovation in data Storage Technologies: From Cloud Computing to Edge Computing. *Computer Science & IT Research Journal, 4*(3), 273–299. DOI: 10.51594/csitrj.v4i3.661

Alowais, S. A., Alghamdi, S. S., Alsuhebany, N., Alqahtani, T., Alshaya, A. I., Almohareb, S. N., Aldairem, A., Alrashed, M., Bin Saleh, K., Badreldin, H. A., Al Yami, M. S., Al Harbi, S., & Albekairy, A. M. (2023). Revolutionizing healthcare: The role of artificial intelligence in clinical practice. *BMC Medical Education, 23*(1), 689. DOI: 10.1186/s12909-023-04698-z PMID: 37740191

Awasthi Ms, N., & Mishra Ms, R. (2025). Leveraging digital twin technology for enhanced patient care and predictive health management. *ANALISTA International Journal of Multidisciplinary Research, 36*, 36. Advance online publication. DOI: 10.71182/aijmr.2506.0301.4004

Bergamini, F., Gallo, G. D., & Micucci, D. (2025). Towards a unified architecture for remote patient monitoring. In *Ambient Intelligence and Smart Environments.* IOS Press., DOI: 10.3233/AISE250009

Cernian, A., Tiganoaia, B., Sacala, I., Pavel, A., & Iftemi, A. (2020). PatientDataChain: A blockchain-based approach to integrate personal health records. *Sensors (Basel), 20*(22), 6538. DOI: 10.3390/s20226538 PMID: 33207620

Chakilam, P. K. (2025). Interoperability in healthcare: Leveraging enterprise Integration Architecture for seamless data exchange. *European Modern Studies Journal, 9*(4), 652–661. DOI: 10.59573/emsj.9(4).2025.63

Chaparro-Cárdenas, S. L., Ramirez-Bautista, J.-A., Terven, J., Córdova-Esparza, D.-M., Romero-Gonzalez, J.-A., Ramírez-Pedraza, A., & Chavez-Urbiola, E. A. (2025). A technological review of Digital Twins and Artificial Intelligence for personalized and predictive healthcare. *Healthcare (Basel)*, *13*(14), 1763. DOI: 10.3390/healthcare13141763 PMID: 40724790

Corral-Acero, J., Margara, F., Marciniak, M., Rodero, C., Loncaric, F., Feng, Y., Gilbert, A., Fernandes, J. F., Bukhari, H. A., Wajdan, A., Martinez, M. V., Santos, M. S., Shamohammdi, M., Luo, H., Westphal, P., Leeson, P., DiAchille, P., Gurev, V., Mayr, M., & Lamata, P. (2020). The "Digital Twin" to enable the vision of precision cardiology. *European Heart Journal*, *41*(48), 4556–4564. DOI: 10.1093/eurheartj/ehaa159 PMID: 32128588

Darwich, A. S., Polasek, T. M., Aronson, J. K., Ogungbenro, K., Wright, D. F. B., Achour, B., Reny, J.-L., Daali, Y., Eiermann, B., Cook, J., Lesko, L., McLachlan, A. J., & Rostami-Hodjegan, A. (2021). Model-informed precision dosing: Background, requirements, validation, implementation, and forward trajectory of individualizing drug therapy. Annual Review of Pharmacology and Toxicology, 61(1), 225–245. DevOps Engineer/Cloud Solutions Architect USA, S., Adelusi, B. S., Osamika, D., Independent Researcher, O. U. S. A., Chinyeaka Kelvin-Agwu, M., Independent Researcher, L. N., Mustapha, A. Y., Kwara State Ministry of Health, N., Forkuo, A. Y., Independent Researcher, U. S. A., Ikhalea, N., & Independent Researcher USA, T. (2025). A Federated Interoperability Framework for seamless health data exchange using FHIR standards across multi-hospital systems. Engineering and Technology Journal, 10(05). https://doi.org/DOI: 10.1146/annurev-pharmtox-033020-113257

El Mrabet, A., Alihamidi, I., Tber, A., Benaly, M., Hlou, L., & El Gouri, R. (2025). Proposed architecture for Hospital 4.0: Integrating IoT, edge AI, and blockchain for secure and efficient healthcare systems. [IJOE]. *International Journal of Online and Biomedical Engineering*, *21*(05), 87–102. DOI: 10.3991/ijoe.v21i05.52991

Fatoum, H., Hanna, S., Halamka, J. D., Sicker, D. C., Spangenberg, P., & Hashmi, S. K. (2021). Blockchain integration with digital technology and the future of health care ecosystems: Systematic review. *Journal of Medical Internet Research*, *23*(11), e19846. DOI: 10.2196/19846 PMID: 34726603

Fukawa, N., & Rindfleisch, A. (2023). Enhancing innovation via the digital twin. *Journal of Product Innovation Management*, *40*(4), 391–406. DOI: 10.1111/jpim.12655

Ganesan, M., Sivakumar, N., & Thirumaran, M. (2020). Internet of medical things with cloud-based e-health services for brain tumour detection model using deep convolution neural network. *Electronic Government an International Journal*, *16*(1/2), 69. DOI: 10.1504/EG.2020.105240

Gkintoni, E., & Halkiopoulos, C. (2025). Digital twin cognition: AI-biomarker integration in biomimetic neuropsychology. *Biomimetics (Basel, Switzerland), 10*(10), 640. DOI: 10.3390/biomimetics10100640 PMID: 41149170

Hughes, J. H., Tong, D. M. H., Burns, V., Daly, B., Razavi, P., Boelens, J. J., Goswami, S., & Keizer, R. J. (2023). Clinical decision support for chemotherapy-induced neutropenia using a hybrid pharmacodynamic/machine learning model. *CPT: Pharmacometrics & Systems Pharmacology, 12*(11), 1764–1776. DOI: 10.1002/psp4.13019 PMID: 37503916

Jat, A. S., Grønli, T.-M., Ghinea, G., & Assres, G. (2024). Evolving software architecture design in telemedicine: A PRISMA-based systematic review. *Healthcare Informatics Research, 30*(3), 184–193. DOI: 10.4258/hir.2024.30.3.184 PMID: 39160778

Juanatas, R. A., Almadhor, A., Alsubai, S., Kryvinska, N., Krichen, M., Sampedro, G. A., & Abbas, S. (2025). Securing realistic IoMT environment using Moth-Flame Optimization-based deep learning framework. *Security and Privacy, 8*(5), e70073. Advance online publication. DOI: 10.1002/spy2.70073

Jung, A., Gsell, M. A. F., Augustin, C. M., & Plank, G. (2022). An integrated workflow for building digital twins of cardiac electromechanics-A multi-fidelity approach for personalising active mechanics. *Mathematics, 10*(5), 823. DOI: 10.3390/math10050823 PMID: 35295404

Khatoon, A. (2020). A blockchain-based smart contract system for healthcare management. *Electronics (Basel), 9*(1), 94. DOI: 10.3390/electronics9010094

Lilja, S. (2022). *Digital twins : High resolution disease models for optimized diagnosis and treatment*. Linköping University Electronic Press., DOI: 10.3384/9789179292157

Łukaniszyn, M., Majka, Ł., Grochowicz, B., Mikołajewski, D., & Kawala-Sterniuk, A. (2024). Digital twins generated by artificial intelligence in personalized healthcare. *Applied Sciences (Basel, Switzerland), 14*(20), 9404. DOI: 10.3390/app14209404

Makhdoom, I., Abolhasan, M., Abbas, H., & Ni, W. (2019). Blockchain's adoption in IoT: The challenges, and a way forward. *Journal of Network and Computer Applications, 125*, 251–279. DOI: 10.1016/j.jnca.2018.10.019

Moganti, J., Nookaratnam, P., Venkataramana, G., & Boddeda, B. (2025). Digital twin technology in graft vs host disease. *International Journal of Research in Pharmacy and Allied Science, 04*(03). Advance online publication. DOI: 10.71431/IJRPAS.2025.4311

Olatunde, R. V, Gyasiwaa, M. Y., Ayangeakaa, A. S., Usman, M. A., Olorundare, T. O., & Akpughe, O. V. (2025). Digital twin technology in precision medicine and public health: Transforming patient care and epidemiological forecasting. International Journal of Innovative Science and Research Technology, IJISRT25JUN719, 1044–1049. DOI: 10.38124/ijisrt/25jun719

Papachristou, K., Katsakiori, P. F., Papadimitroulas, P., Strigari, L., & Kagadis, G. C. (2024). Digital Twins' advancements and applications in healthcare, towards precision medicine. *Journal of Personalized Medicine*, *14*(11), 1101. DOI: 10.3390/jpm14111101 PMID: 39590593

Rahman, M. H., & Ansar, M. T. (2025). AI-powered QA in healthcare software: Leveraging predictive analytics and digital twins for safe, cost-effective, and agile medical systems. *Journal of Computer Science and Technology Studies*, *7*(9), 619–628. DOI: 10.32996/jcsts.2025.4.1.70

Rajput, A. R., Li, Q., Taleby Ahvanooey, M., & Masood, I. (2019). EACMS: Emergency access control management system for personal health record based on blockchain. *IEEE Access : Practical Innovations, Open Solutions*, *7*, 84304–84317. DOI: 10.1109/ACCESS.2019.2917976

Ravikumar, A. Olimbaevich, I. R., Mashkhura, S., & Musayeva, S. (2025). Transforming Healthcare with Large Language Models and AI agents. In Advances in Computational Intelligence and Robotics (pp. 51–82). IGI Global Scientific Publishing. DOI: 10.4018/979-8-3373-2008-3.ch003

Ravikumar, A. S., Saparbaevich, B. R., Kumar A., S., Jumaniyozova, M., & Toshova, S. (2025). AI-enhanced clinical decision-making through a collaborative approach. In Advances in Computational Intelligence and Robotics (pp. 249–280). IGI Global Scientific Publishing. DOI: 10.4018/979-8-3373-3311-3.ch010

Ravikumar, A. Sapayev, V., Atamuratova, Z., Kholboyev, N., & Sindhuja. (2025). The decentralized diagnostics revolution using federated Learning in medical imaging and beyond. In Advances in Computational Intelligence and Robotics (pp. 353–388). IGI Global Scientific Publishing. DOI: 10.4018/979-8-3373-3306-9.ch013

Ravikumar, R. S., Manujakshi, Aarthi, S., Urazbaeva, Y., & Tamilselvi, S. (2025). Navigating data privacy, security, and regulatory challenges in healthcare AI ensuring fairness, bias mitigation, interpretability, and trust. In Transformative Role of Transformer Models in Healthcare (pp. 25–54). IGI Global Scientific Publishing. DOI: 10.4018/979-8-3373-2038-0.ch002

Ravikumar, R. N., & Aarthi, S. (2025). AI-powered synergistic robotics and IoT ecosystems for predictive and preventive healthcare. In *Robotics and IoT Synergy in Next-Generation Healthcare* (pp. 1–32). IGI Global Scientific Publishing., DOI: 10.4018/979-8-3373-5447-7.ch001

Ravikumar, R. N., Aarthi, S., Kurbanova, S., Polvanov, S., Matchanova, B., & Sathya, K. (2025). Hybrid metaheuristic optimization for neural networks in biomedical imaging. In *Metaheuristic Algorithms and Optimizing Neural Networks for Biomedical Image Processing* (pp. 197–234). IGI Global Scientific Publishing., DOI: 10.4018/979-8-3373-0523-3.ch008

Šafran, V., Arioz, U., Sallauka, R., & Mlakar, I. (2025). A scalable and secured HL7 FHIR healthcare platform: Architecture, load testing, and preliminary findings. *International Journal of Education and Information Technologies*, *19*(13), 128–137. DOI: 10.46300/9109.2025.19.13

Saliha, C. B., & Ferhati, K. (2025). Real-world applications of digital twin technology in performance management: Lessons from global healthcare case studies. *International Journal of Innovative Technologies in Social Science*, *1*(45). Advance online publication. DOI: 10.31435/ijitss.1(45).2025.3197

Sasitharasarma, S., Alani, N. H. S., & Wisker, Z. L. (2025). Is the healthcare industry ready for Digital Twins? Examining the opportunities and challenges. *Future Internet*, *17*(9), 386. DOI: 10.3390/fi17090386

Sharma, A., Kaur, S., & Singh, M. (2024). A secure blockchain framework for the internet of medical things. *Transactions on Emerging Telecommunications Technologies*, *35*(1), e4917. Advance online publication. DOI: 10.1002/ett.4917

Singh, M., Fuenmayor, E., Hinchy, E., Qiao, Y., Murray, N., & Devine, D. (2021). Digital Twin: Origin to future. *Applied System Innovation*, *4*(2), 36. DOI: 10.3390/asi4020036

Sun, T., He, X., Song, X., Shu, L., & Li, Z. (2022). The digital twin in medicine: A key to the future of healthcare? *Frontiers in Medicine*, *9*, 907066. DOI: 10.3389/fmed.2022.907066 PMID: 35911407

Susilo, M. E., Li, C.-C., Gadkar, K., Hernandez, G., Huw, L.-Y., Jin, J. Y., Yin, S., Wei, M. C., Ramanujan, S., & Hosseini, I. (2023). Systems-based digital twins to help characterize clinical dose-response and propose predictive biomarkers in a Phase I study of bispecific antibody, mosunetuzumab, in NHL. *Clinical and Translational Science*, *16*(7), 1134–1148. DOI: 10.1111/cts.13501 PMID: 36908269

Taralunga, D. D., & Florea, B. C. (2021). A blockchain-enabled framework for mHealth systems. *Sensors (Basel)*, *21*(8), 2828. DOI: 10.3390/s21082828 PMID: 33923842

Thangaraj, P. M., Benson, S. H., Oikonomou, E. K., Asselbergs, F. W., & Khera, R. (2024). Cardiovascular care with digital twin technology in the era of generative artificial intelligence. *European Heart Journal*, *45*(45), 4808–4821. DOI: 10.1093/eurheartj/ehae619 PMID: 39322420

Turab, M., & Jamil, S. (2023). A comprehensive survey of digital twins in health-care in the era of metaverse. *BioMedInformatics*, *3*(3), 563–584. DOI: 10.3390/biomedinformatics3030039

Wang, D. H. (2020). IoT based Clinical Sensor Data Management and Transfer using Blockchain Technology. *Journal of ISMAC*, *2*(3), 154–159. DOI: 10.36548/jismac.2020.3.003

KEY TERMS AND DEFINITIONS

Artificial Intelligence (AI): Machine-based systems that analyze complex data to support diagnosis, treatment, and decision-making.

Blockchain: A decentralized ledger technology ensuring secure, transparent, and tamper-proof medical data management.

Clinical Decision Support System (CDSS): AI-assisted software that helps clinicians make data-driven and evidence-based medical decisions.

Cloud Computing: Remote storage and computation of healthcare data enabling large-scale analytics and model training.

Data Standardization: The process of formatting medical data consistently to enable compatibility across systems and devices.

Digital Twin (DT): A virtual replica of a physical patient, device, or hospital system that continuously updates with real-time data for monitoring and simulation.

Edge Computing: Processing of medical data near the source (e.g., hospital devices) to reduce delay and enhance response time.

Federated Learning: A decentralized AI training approach where models learn from distributed hospital data without transferring sensitive patient information.

Internet of Medical Things (IoMT): A network of connected medical devices and sensors that collect and share patient data for analysis and decision-making.

Interoperability: The ability of diverse healthcare systems and devices to exchange, understand, and use shared data seamlessly.

Machine Learning (ML): A subset of AI that learns from data patterns to improve prediction accuracy over time.

Predictive Diagnostics: The use of AI and data analytics to forecast diseases or complications before symptoms appear.

Predictive Maintenance: Use of digital twins to monitor medical equipment and predict failures before they occur.

Quantum Computing: Advanced computation method that uses quantum bits to accelerate complex healthcare simulations and data security.

Smart Hospital: A digitally connected healthcare environment that uses AI, IoMT, and digital twins for real-time, efficient, and patient-centered care.

Chapter 2
Secure and Intelligent Smart Hospitals:
A Blockchain-Enabled Digital Twin Architecture

Mutaz Abdel Wahed
http://orcid.org/0000-0002-4361-6185
Jadara University, Jordan

ABSTRACT

The rapid digitalization of healthcare has transformed hospitals into complex cyber–physical ecosystems integrating Internet of Medical Things (IoMT), artificial intelligence, and data-driven decision support systems. While these technologies enable intelligent and personalized healthcare services, they also introduce significant challenges related to data security, privacy, interoperability, and trust. This chapter proposes a blockchain-enabled digital twin architecture for secure and intelligent smart hospital ecosystems. Digital twins provide real-time virtual representations of patients, medical devices, and clinical workflows, enabling predictive analytics and operational optimization, while blockchain establishes a decentralized trust layer ensuring data integrity, provenance, and auditable governance. A six-layer reference architecture is presented, detailing cross-layer interactions between data acquisition, digital twin modeling, analytics, visualization, and blockchain-based consent and audit mechanisms.

1. INTRODUCTION AND BACKGROUND

The global healthcare sector is undergoing a profound digital transformation driven by advances in information and communication technologies, data analyt-

DOI: 10.4018/979-8-3373-8177-0.ch002

ics, and intelligent systems. Hospitals are no longer isolated clinical facilities but complex cyber–physical ecosystems that integrate medical devices, information systems, communication networks, and decision-support platforms. This evolution has given rise to the concept of *smart hospitals*, where real-time data, automation, and intelligence are leveraged to improve patient outcomes, operational efficiency, and system resilience (Arya et al., 2025).

Central to this transformation is the increasing adoption of the Internet of Medical Things (IoMT), which connects wearable sensors, implantable devices, diagnostic equipment, and hospital infrastructure into a unified digital environment. While IoMT-enabled systems offer unprecedented opportunities for continuous monitoring, personalized care, and predictive analytics, they also introduce significant challenges related to data security, privacy, interoperability, and trust. Sensitive patient data flows across heterogeneous platforms, often managed by multiple stakeholders, increasing the risk of unauthorized access, data tampering, and systemic failures (Dai et al., 2025).

In parallel, healthcare systems face growing pressure from demographic shifts, chronic disease prevalence, resource constraints, and global health crises. These challenges demand healthcare infrastructures that are not only intelligent but also secure, transparent, and resilient. Traditional centralized data management architecture struggles to meet these requirements, particularly in environments characterized by distributed data sources, dynamic system behavior, and stringent regulatory obligations (Wahed et al., 2025).

Within this context, Blockchain and Digital Twin technologies have emerged as two complementary paradigms with the potential to redefine how smart hospitals are designed and operated. Blockchain offers decentralized, tamper-resistant data management with built-in trust and transparency, while Digital Twins provide dynamic virtual representations of physical entities that enable simulation, prediction, and optimization (Kantaros et al., 2025). Individually, each technology addresses critical limitations of existing healthcare systems; collectively, they form a powerful foundation for next-generation smart hospital ecosystems.

This chapter explores how the integration of Blockchain and Digital Twin technologies can enable secure, intelligent, and trustworthy smart hospital infrastructures. By examining architectural models, operational mechanisms, and governance considerations, the chapter aims to provide a comprehensive understanding of how blockchain-enabled digital twins can transform healthcare delivery while addressing key technical, ethical, and regulatory concerns.

1.1 Theoretical Foundations

The proposed integration of blockchain and digital twins in smart hospitals is grounded in three complementary theoretical lenses: cyber–physical systems (CPS) theory, socio-technical systems theory, and decentralized trust architectures. First, CPS theory conceptualizes hospitals as tightly coupled environments in which physical processes (patients, devices, clinical procedures, and facility operations) are continuously sensed and controlled through computational systems. Digital twins operationalize CPS principles by maintaining a dynamic virtual representation of physical entities and workflows, enabling real-time monitoring, simulation, and predictive control. Second, socio-technical systems theory emphasizes that healthcare ecosystems are not purely technical infrastructures; rather, they involve complex interactions among clinicians, patients, administrators, and regulatory bodies. Consequently, any digital twin-driven intelligence must be aligned with human decision-making, accountability, and ethical governance. Third, decentralized trust architecture provides the conceptual basis for using blockchain as a trust anchor in multi-stakeholder environments. In smart hospitals, data is produced and consumed across organizational boundaries, and trust cannot be assumed solely through centralized institutional control. Blockchain contributes by enabling tamper-evident auditability, verifiable provenance, and policy enforcement through smart contracts. Together, these theoretical foundations justify the proposed architecture as a secure CPS-oriented and governance-aware approach to smart hospital intelligence.

1.2 Research Gap and Novel Contributions

Although prior studies have explored blockchain-based healthcare data sharing and digital twins for clinical and operational optimization, existing implementations often remain fragmented—either focusing on digital twin intelligence without end-to-end trust enforcement, or applying blockchain for auditability without continuous twin synchronization and actionable analytics. Moreover, many reported solutions are domain-specific pilots that lack a reusable reference architecture for secure, scalable, and regulation-aware deployment in hospital settings.

To address these gaps, this chapter makes the following novel contributions:

1. **A six-layer blockchain-enabled digital twin reference architecture** that explicitly models cross-layer interactions between sensing, twin synchronization, analytics, visualization, and decentralized governance.
2. **A dual-flow integration design** combining (i) a vertical data-to-intelligence pipeline and (ii) a horizontal blockchain trust anchoring mechanism to support provenance, non-repudiation, and compliance evidence generation.

3. **A consent-driven access and governance workflow** implemented through smart contracts to operationalize dynamic consent, traceability, and accountable interoperability without storing raw clinical data on-chain.
4. **Healthcare-oriented use cases with implementation considerations**, including latency constraints, stakeholder roles, and measurable impact indicators, enabling adoption beyond conceptual discussion.
5. **A validation-oriented perspective**, identifying limitations and proposing a phased evaluation strategy with operational KPIs to support real-world deployment readiness.

2. SMART HOSPITAL ECOSYSTEMS: CONCEPTS AND REQUIREMENTS

2.1 Defining Smart Hospitals

A smart hospital can be defined as a healthcare facility that leverages advanced digital technologies to enhance clinical care, optimize operations, and improve patient and staff experiences. Unlike traditional hospitals, which rely on siloed information systems and manual workflows, smart hospitals adopt integrated, data-driven approaches that enable real-time situational awareness and intelligent decision-making (Xue et al., 2025).

Key characteristics of smart hospital ecosystems include pervasive sensing through IoMT devices, interoperable health information systems, automated clinical workflows, and advanced analytics powered by artificial intelligence (AI) and machine learning (ML). These components work together to support applications such as remote patient monitoring, predictive diagnostics, asset tracking, and adaptive resource management (Hanna et al., 2025).

However, the increasing complexity of smart hospital ecosystems also amplifies systemic risks. As the number of connected devices and data sources grows, so does the attack surface for cyber threats. Furthermore, inconsistencies in data standards, proprietary platforms, and fragmented governance models hinder seamless interoperability and trust across systems.

2.2 Core Requirements of Smart Hospital Infrastructures

To function effectively and sustainably, smart hospital infrastructures must satisfy several critical requirements (Wahed et al., 2025):

Security and Privacy: Healthcare data is among the most sensitive categories of personal information. Smart hospitals must ensure confidentiality, integrity, and availability of patient data while complying with regulatory frameworks such as HIPAA and GDPR. This includes secure authentication, access control, and auditability across distributed systems.

Interoperability: Smart hospitals integrate diverse technologies, vendors, and data formats. Interoperability is essential to enable seamless data exchange between electronic health records (EHRs), IoMT devices, imaging systems, and analytics platforms.

Scalability and Resilience: Healthcare systems must handle high data volumes, real-time processing demands, and unpredictable workloads, particularly during emergencies. Scalable and resilient architecture is necessary to maintain continuity of care.

Transparency and Trust: Clinical decisions increasingly rely on automated systems and predictive models. Trust in data provenance, system behavior, and algorithmic outputs is essential for clinician adoption and patient acceptance.

Intelligence and Adaptability: Smart hospitals must move beyond reactive operations toward predictive and adaptive capabilities. This requires continuous monitoring, simulation, and optimization of both clinical and operational processes.

Traditional centralized architecture struggles to meet these requirements simultaneously. As a result, new paradigms are needed to support secure, intelligent, and interoperable smart hospital ecosystems.

While HIPAA and GDPR are among the most widely cited healthcare privacy frameworks, smart hospital deployments increasingly operate in multi-jurisdictional contexts. Therefore, global regulatory alignment should also consider China's Personal Information Protection Law (PIPL), which imposes strict requirements on sensitive personal information handling and cross-border transfers, as well as India's Digital Personal Data Protection Act (DPDPA), which emphasizes lawful processing, consent governance, and accountability. Incorporating such frameworks strengthens the global applicability of blockchain-enabled digital twin architectures and supports international interoperability without undermining national data sovereignty requirements.

3. DIGITAL TWIN TECHNOLOGY IN HEALTHCARE

3.1 Concept and Evolution of Digital Twins

The concept of the Digital Twin originated in manufacturing and aerospace, where virtual replicas of physical assets are used to monitor performance, predict failures, and optimize operations. A Digital Twin is not merely a static model but a dynamic, data-driven representation that evolves in real time alongside its physical counterpart (Chaparro-Cárdenas et al., 2025).

In healthcare, Digital Twins extend this concept to patients, medical devices, clinical workflows, and even entire hospital systems. By continuously synchronizing physical and virtual entities, digital twins enable advanced simulation, predictive analytics, and decision support across multiple levels of care.

The evolution of digital twin technology in healthcare has been driven by advances in sensing technologies, data integration platforms, AI algorithms, and computational infrastructure. These developments have made it possible to model complex physiological processes, equipment behavior, and system interactions with increasing accuracy.

3.2 Types of Digital Twins in Smart Hospitals

Digital Twins in healthcare can be categorized based on their scope and application (Awasthi et al., 2025):

Patient Digital Twins: Virtual representations of individual patients that integrate physiological data, medical history, and lifestyle information. These twins support personalized treatment planning, disease progression modeling, and outcome prediction.

Medical Device Digital Twins: Models of equipment such as MRI scanners, ventilators, or infusion pumps that enable predictive maintenance, performance optimization, and fault detection.

Process and Workflow Digital Twins: Representations of clinical pathways, patient flows, and administrative processes that support operational optimization and capacity planning.

Hospital System Digital Twins: Comprehensive models of entire hospital infrastructures, integrating physical assets, human resources, and digital systems to support strategic decision-making and resilience planning.

3.3 Benefits and Limitations of Digital Twins in Healthcare

Digital Twins offer numerous benefits for smart hospitals, including improved clinical outcomes, reduced operational costs, and enhanced system resilience. By enabling "what-if" simulations and predictive insights, they support proactive rather than reactive decision-making.

However, digital twins also introduce significant challenges. Their effectiveness depends on the availability of accurate, timely, and trustworthy data. Data quality issues, model uncertainty, and lack of transparency can undermine trust in digital twin outputs. Moreover, the continuous data exchange required for real-time synchronization raises concerns about data security, privacy, and accountability.

These limitations highlight the need for robust data governance and trust mechanisms that can ensure the integrity and reliability of digital twin systems in healthcare environments.

While Digital Twins provide the dynamic intelligence layer for smart hospitals, ensuring the trustworthiness of the data they consume requires equally robust security foundations. This brings us to blockchain technology, which offers complementary capabilities in decentralized trust and data integrity assurance.

4. BLOCKCHAIN FOUNDATIONS FOR HEALTHCARE SYSTEMS

4.1 Overview of Blockchain Technology

Blockchain is a distributed ledger technology (DLT) that enables secure, transparent, and tamper-resistant recording of transactions across a decentralized network of participants (Pokharel et al., 2025). Unlike traditional centralized databases, blockchain systems rely on consensus mechanisms to validate and append new records, ensuring that no single entity has unilateral control over the data. Each transaction is cryptographically linked to previous records, forming an immutable chain that provides strong guarantees of data integrity and traceability (Barbaria et al., 2025).

Key characteristics of blockchain include decentralization, immutability, transparency, and fault tolerance. These properties have positioned blockchain as a promising solution for environments where trust must be established among multiple stakeholders who may not fully trust one another. In healthcare, where data is shared among hospitals, laboratories, insurers, regulators, and patients, blockchain offers a novel approach to managing trust and accountability in complex ecosystems.

Blockchain platforms can be broadly classified into public, private, and permissioned blockchains. Public blockchains allow open participation and transparency but often suffer from scalability and privacy limitations. Private blockchains are controlled by a single organization, offering higher performance but reduced decentralization. Permissioned blockchains, which restrict participation to authorized entities, are particularly well suited for healthcare environments, as they balance decentralization, performance, and regulatory compliance.

4.2 Blockchain Applications in Healthcare

Blockchain technology has been explored across a wide range of healthcare applications, primarily focusing on data security, interoperability, and trust. One of the most prominent use cases is electronic health record (EHR) management, where blockchain serves as a secure index or access-control layer that governs data sharing without storing sensitive medical data directly on-chain. This approach enhances interoperability while preserving patient privacy and compliance with data protection regulations (Wahed et al., 2025).

Another key application is identity and access management. Blockchain-based digital identities enable secure authentication of patients, healthcare professionals, and medical devices. By decentralizing identity management, healthcare systems can reduce reliance on vulnerable centralized identity providers and improve resilience against identity theft and unauthorized access.

Blockchain has also been applied to medical supply chain management, ensuring traceability and authenticity of pharmaceuticals and medical devices. By recording supply chain events on an immutable ledger, healthcare organizations can combat counterfeit drugs, monitor recalls, and improve inventory transparency.

Additionally, smart contracts are self-executing programs deployed on blockchain platforms enable automated enforcement of policies and agreements. In healthcare, smart contracts can support automated consent management, insurance claims processing, compliance checks, and data access control, reducing administrative overhead and minimizing human error.

4.3 Security, Privacy, and Governance Implications

Despite its potential, blockchain adoption in healthcare raises important security, privacy, and governance considerations. While blockchain provides strong integrity guarantees, it does not inherently ensure data confidentiality (Arigbabu et al., 2024). Sensitive healthcare data must be encrypted and managed carefully to prevent unauthorized disclosure. Moreover, the immutability of blockchain records can conflict with regulatory requirements such as the "right to be forgotten" under the General Data Protection Regulation (GDPR) (Wahed & Wahed, 2025).

Governance is another critical challenge. Blockchain networks require clear rules regarding participation, consensus, data ownership, and dispute resolution. In healthcare ecosystems involving multiple stakeholders, defining governance structures that balance decentralization with accountability is essential for sustainable adoption (George, 2025).

These considerations underscore the importance of designing blockchain solutions that are tailored to healthcare-specific requirements and integrated with complementary technologies that provide intelligence and adaptability, such as Digital Twins.

Having established the individual capabilities of Digital Twins and blockchain, we now examine why their integration creates synergistic value greater than either technology alone. The convergence addresses fundamental gaps in current smart hospital architectures (Roumeliotis et al., 2024).

5. MOTIVATION FOR INTEGRATING BLOCKCHAIN AND DIGITAL TWINS

5.1 Complementary Strengths and Limitations

While Blockchain and Digital Twin technologies each offer significant benefits for smart hospitals, they also exhibit inherent limitations when deployed independently. Digital Twins excel at modeling complex systems, enabling simulation, prediction, and optimization. However, their reliance on continuous data streams exposes them to risks related to data tampering, unauthorized access, and lack of accountability. Without trusted data provenance, the accuracy and reliability of digital twin outputs can be compromised (Suleiman et al., 2025).

Conversely, blockchain provides a robust trust infrastructure for data management, ensuring integrity, traceability, and controlled access. However, blockchain lacks the analytical intelligence and real-time modeling capabilities needed to optimize healthcare operations and clinical decision-making. Blockchain systems are fundamentally transactional rather than predictive (Wahed & Wahed, 2025).

Integrating these technologies allows each to compensate for the other's limitations. Blockchain can serve as the trust layer that guarantees the authenticity and integrity of data feeding digital twins, while digital twins act as the intelligence layer that transforms trusted data into actionable insights. Together, they enable secure, intelligent, and transparent smart hospital ecosystems.

5.2 Trusted Data Pipelines for Digital Twins

A critical requirement for effective digital twins is the availability of high-quality, trustworthy data. In smart hospitals, data originates from heterogeneous sources, including IoMT devices, clinical information systems, and administrative platforms. Ensuring the integrity and provenance of this data is essential for reliable modeling and prediction (Lomotey et al., 2024).

Blockchain-enabled data pipelines can address this challenge by recording data transactions, metadata, and access events on a distributed ledger. Each data update can be cryptographically signed and timestamped, providing a verifiable audit trail that ensures accountability. This approach enhances trust in digital twin models by enabling clinicians and administrators to trace insights back to their data sources (Wahed, 2024).

Furthermore, blockchain-based access control mechanisms can enforce fine-grained permissions, ensuring that only authorized entities can contribute data to or retrieve insights from digital twins. This is particularly important in healthcare environments where data sensitivity and regulatory compliance are paramount.

5.3 Auditable Simulations and Decision Support

Digital twins are increasingly used to support clinical and operational decision-making through simulations and predictive analytics. Examples include evaluating treatment options, forecasting patient demand, and optimizing resource allocation. However, the use of algorithmic decision-support tools raises concerns about transparency, accountability, and trust—especially when decisions have significant clinical or ethical implications (Zhao et al., 2025).

By integrating blockchain, digital twin simulations and decisions can become auditable and verifiable. Blockchain records can store hashes of simulation models, parameters, and outputs, enabling independent verification without exposing sensitive data. This supports transparency and accountability, facilitating regulatory oversight and ethical governance.

In addition, smart contracts can automate decision-support workflows by triggering predefined actions based on digital twin insights. For example, a smart contract could automatically schedule equipment maintenance when a digital twin predicts imminent failure, while recording the decision logic and execution on the blockchain.

5.4 Enabling Automated Governance and Compliance

Healthcare systems operate under complex regulatory frameworks that govern data protection, clinical safety, and operational accountability. Ensuring compliance across dynamic, data-driven environments is a significant challenge for smart hospitals (Wahed, 2025).

The integration of blockchain and digital twins enables automated governance by embedding compliance rules directly into system architectures. Smart contracts can enforce regulatory policies, consent agreements, and organizational rules in real time, reducing reliance on manual oversight. Digital twins, in turn, provide continuous monitoring and simulation capabilities that support proactive risk management and compliance assessment (Mazlan et al., 2025).

This synergy supports a shift from reactive compliance to continuous assurance, where governance mechanisms are integrated into everyday operations rather than applied retrospectively (Wahed et al., 2025).

To operationalize the theoretical integration of blockchain and Digital Twins, we propose a layered reference architecture. This framework translates complementary capabilities into a practical ecosystem design for secure, intelligent smart hospitals.

6. PROPOSED ARCHITECTURE FOR BLOCKCHAIN-ENABLED DIGITAL TWIN ECOSYSTEMS IN SMART HOSPITALS

This section introduces an enhanced reference architecture that integrates blockchain technology with Digital Twins (DTs) to support secure, intelligent, and interoperable smart hospital operations. To enhance interpretability and reproducibility, Figures 1–3 are intentionally designed as conceptual reference diagrams that translate the proposed framework into implementable workflows. Each figure is explicitly linked to the surrounding discussion to clarify (i) the layered structure of the architecture, (ii) cross-layer data and trust flows, and (iii) governance and compliance enforcement mechanisms. This visual integration enables both technical and non-technical readers (e.g., healthcare administrators and compliance officers) to validate the architectural logic without requiring supplementary materials. Figure 1 presents the proposed blockchain-enabled digital twin smart hospital architecture as a six-layer workflow that integrates cyber–physical data acquisition, real-time modeling, and decentralized trust anchoring. The figure clarifies how data originating from IoMT devices and clinical information systems is first integrity-protected through hashing at ingestion, then synchronized into patient, asset, and process digital twins. Governance is enforced through blockchain smart contracts that regulate consent, access permissions, and policy execution. The analytics layer consumes verified twin states to produce predictive insights, while visualization interfaces provide clinicians, administrators, and patients with interpretable outputs and traceable provenance indicators. Importantly, the blockchain ledger does not store raw health data; instead, it anchors trust by recording hashes, metadata, model versions, and consent transactions, enabling tamper-evident auditing across the entire ecosystem.

Figure 1. Proposed Multi-Layer Framework Workflow

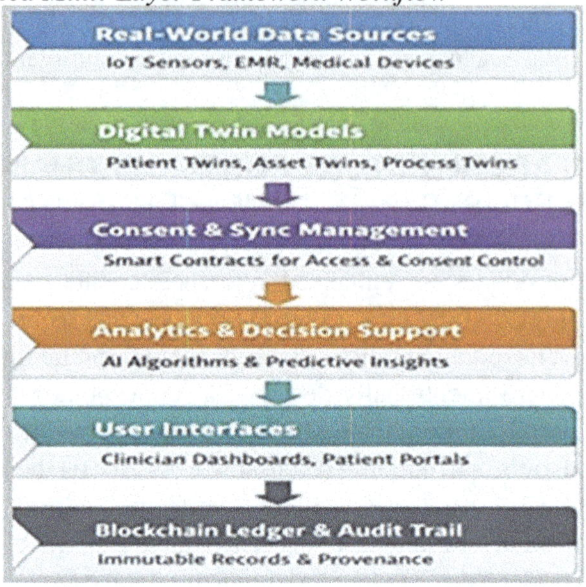

As illustrated in Figure 1, the architecture is designed around two complementary flows: (i) a vertical data-to-intelligence pipeline from sensing to analytics, and (ii) a horizontal trust anchoring mechanism provided by the blockchain. In the vertical flow, continuous physiological and operational signals are captured, standardized, and streamed to their corresponding digital twins to maintain real-time state alignment. In the horizontal flow, every critical event (e.g., data ingestion, model update, consent change, or access request) generates a blockchain transaction that provides immutable traceability and non-repudiation. This dual-flow design ensures that digital twins remain both intelligent (through real-time synchronization and analytics) and trustworthy (through verifiable provenance and decentralized governance).

6.1 Real-World Data Sources: Clinical Systems and IoT-Driven Environments

Smart hospitals are inherently data-intensive environments, characterized by continuous interaction between clinical information systems and cyber-physical assets. The data acquisition layer includes patient-worn biomedical sensors (e.g., ECG, glucose monitors, smart wearables), smart beds, infusion pumps, MRI and CT scanners, environmental monitoring devices (e.g., humidity and operating-room temperature sensors), Electronic Medical Records (EMR/EHR), and Laboratory Information Systems (LIS) (Can et al., 2024).

To strengthen integrity and provenance assurance, ingested data is cryptographically hashed at the point of collection. Rather than storing raw clinical data on the blockchain, only the hash (a tamper-evident digital fingerprint) is committed to the distributed ledger. This enables later verification that the stored off-chain data has not been altered, while maintaining privacy, scalability, and regulatory compliance. In this way, blockchain functions as a verifiable trust layer that ensures authenticity, traceability, and non-repudiation of clinical and operational data streams without imposing latency or storage overhead on hospital systems.

6.2 Digital Twin Models of Patients, Assets, and Clinical Processes

The digital twin layer represents the core intelligence and simulation environment of the smart hospital ecosystem. Three primary classes of twins are modeled:

- **Patient Digital Twins**, which dynamically integrate real-time physiological signals with historical EMR records to support personalized monitoring, deterioration risk assessment, and treatment simulation.
- **Asset Digital Twins**, representing critical medical devices (e.g., ventilators, MRI units) to track operational performance, usage fatigue, maintenance cycles, and failure probability.
- **Process Digital Twins**, modeling complex workflows such as surgical theater scheduling, emergency department triage pathways, or sepsis response protocols.

To support accountability and clinical validation, key model parameters, update states, and version histories are recorded on the blockchain. This creates an auditable evidence trail demonstrating which model version informed a particular decision, who modified the model, and when changes occurred. Such provenance tracking is particularly important in medicolegal contexts, safety-critical environments, and AI-assisted decision pipelines.

6.3 Synchronization, Consent Management, and Governance Layer

The synchronization and consent governance layer represents one of the most critical and complex components of the architecture. Data exchanged between physical systems and their corresponding digital twins must adhere to patient-defined consent policies, institutional governance rules, and regulatory mandates (Ogut, 2025).

A permissioned blockchain network hosts smart contracts that function as automated policy enforcement mechanisms. These contracts encode patient-specific consent preferences (e.g., "cardiology data may be accessed by treating clinicians and research units, but not by non-clinical departments") and regulate how, when, and by whom data may be accessed or processed.

Every access request, authorization event, and data-sharing transaction is immutably logged on-chain, creating a comprehensive audit trail for HIPAA, GDPR, and institutional compliance. This mechanism enables:

- transparent consent administration
- fine-grained access control
- automated compliance verification
- forensic accountability in breach events

Thus, blockchain shifts governance from static documentation to programmable, traceable, and enforceable consent ecosystems.

While Figure 1 introduces the overall layered framework, the practical enforcement of privacy and patient sovereignty requires a detailed access-control workflow. Figure 2 therefore illustrates the secure consent-driven data access sequence in which clinician dashboards interact with digital twins through blockchain-based governance. The figure highlights that access decisions are not based on institutional discretion alone; rather, consent policies are encoded as executable smart contracts. Each access request is validated against patient-defined permissions, and the resulting authorization outcome is immutably recorded to enable continuous compliance verification and forensic accountability.

Figure 2. Secure Data Flow and Consent Management Workflow

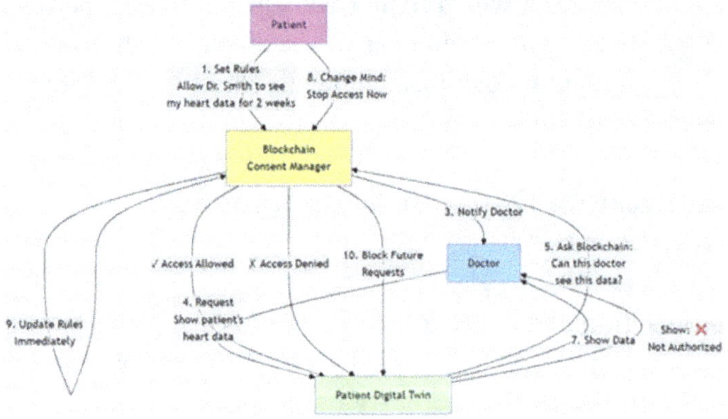

Specifically, Figure 2 depicts a stepwise interaction where (1) a clinician initiates a request through the interface layer, (2) the request invokes the consent smart contract within the governance layer, (3) the smart contract evaluates the request using cryptographically verifiable policy states anchored on-chain, and (4) if approved, the system issues a tokenized authorization key for time-bound access. The digital twin then retrieves the permitted data from secure off-chain repositories, while (5) the blockchain ledger logs the transaction as an immutable evidence record. This design enables dynamic consent (grant/revoke), minimizes privacy leakage by avoiding on-chain raw data storage, and strengthens trust through verifiable audit trails.

6.4 Analytics, Prediction, and Clinical Decision-Support Intelligence

The analytics layer integrates AI- and ML-based engines that operate on digital twin environments to support (Sarani Rad et al., 2024):

- early warning and deterioration prediction
- diagnostic assistance
- personalized therapy optimization
- operational demand and capacity forecasting

Blockchain enhances trust and reliability at this layer through model provenance recording, where metadata regarding training datasets, validation procedures, certification status, and deployment versions are written to the ledger. This ensures that clinicians and regulators can verify that models have not been tampered with and that decisions are generated from validated versions.

Additionally, federated learning processes across multiple hospitals may be coordinated using blockchain smart contracts. This approach allows distributed model training while preserving data locality and privacy, ensuring that sensitive medical records do not leave their institutional repositories. Contributions to joint models can be securely tracked and credited — supporting collaborative innovation without compromising confidentiality.

6.5 Visualization and Interaction Interfaces

User-focused visualization tools provide actionable insights to clinicians, patients, administrators, and governance authorities. Three interface domains are emphasized:

- **Clinical Dashboards**, presenting real-time patient digital twin states, anomaly alerts, and treatment simulation scenarios.

- **Patient Portals**, enabling individuals to view selected aspects of their digital twin, manage consent settings, and review who accessed their records.
- **Operational Command Views**, supporting administrators with equipment health status, operating room utilization analytics, and workflow efficiency indicators.

The interface layer retrieves only consent-authorized and integrity-verified data, while also enabling transparency by displaying blockchain-based access histories and chain-of-custody indicators for sensitive clinical events.

6.6 Blockchain Ledger and Immutable Audit Infrastructure

At the foundation of the architecture lies a permissioned blockchain network (e.g., Hyperledger Fabric) operated by hospitals, research partners, and regulatory stakeholders. The ledger stores:

- cryptographic hashes of clinical and sensor datasets
- digital twin state checkpoints
- consent and policy enforcement transactions
- AI model provenance metadata
- system-wide access and audit records

Meanwhile, high-volume raw data remains in secure off-chain repositories, such as hospital databases and HIPAA-compliant cloud environments. Blockchain therefore functions not as a data warehouse, but as a secure integrity index and access-control backbone, enabling trustworthy linkage, verification, and accountability across distributed smart hospital infrastructures

7. SMART HOSPITAL USE CASES AND CASE SCENARIOS

To ground the theoretical framework in practical reality, we present three representative case scenarios that demonstrate the transformative potential of blockchain-enabled digital twins across different dimensions of smart hospital operations:

7.1 Patient-Centric Digital Twins for Personalized Care

One of the most impactful applications of blockchain-enabled digital twins is personalized patient care. Patient-centric digital twins create dynamic virtual representations of individual patients by integrating real-time physiological data, clinical history, genomic information, and lifestyle factors. These models enable clinicians to simulate disease progression, evaluate treatment options, and personalize care plans (Kuponiyi & Akomolafe, 2024).

Blockchain plays a critical role in ensuring the trustworthiness of patient digital twins. All data contributions from wearable devices to laboratory systems are cryptographically validated and logged onto the blockchain. This guarantees data integrity and provides an auditable history of how patient data is used in simulations and decision-making.

For example, in chronic disease management, a patient digital twin can continuously monitor health indicators and predict potential complications. Smart contracts can trigger alerts or interventions when predefined thresholds are exceeded, while ensuring that patient consent and privacy preferences are respected. This approach enhances patient safety, improves outcomes, and reduces hospital readmissions.

Implementation Considerations:

- **Latency requirement:** Real-time alerts (e.g., ICU monitoring) should target sub-second to a few seconds response time; therefore, edge processing is recommended for critical signals.
- **Data volume:** Continuous physiological sensing (PPG, ECG, BP, SpO_2) generates high-frequency streams that require buffering and feature extraction prior to twin synchronization.
- **Stakeholder roles:** Hospital IT and clinical engineering units maintain the twin infrastructure; clinicians consume insights; patients retain consent control via governance contracts.

7.2 Predictive Maintenance of Medical Equipment

Medical equipment failures can have serious consequences for patient safety and hospital operations. Digital twins of medical devices such as MRI scanners, ventilators, or infusion pumps enable predictive maintenance by modeling equipment behavior and identifying early signs of malfunction (Sriram et al., 2025).

By integrating blockchain, maintenance records, sensor data, and service logs are securely recorded and shared among manufacturers, hospitals, and service providers. This ensures transparency and accountability across the equipment lifecycle. Smart contracts can automate maintenance scheduling and warranty management based on digital twin predictions, reducing downtime and maintenance costs.

This case illustrates how blockchain-enabled digital twins can enhance operational resilience and safety in smart hospitals.

Implementation Considerations:

- **Reliability constraint:** Maintenance models must tolerate missing sensor packets and calibration drift; robust preprocessing and anomaly filtering are required.
- **Operational KPIs:** Typical targets include reducing unplanned downtime by 10–20% and improving equipment utilization rates through early fault detection.
- **Node responsibility:** Equipment vendors or biomedical engineering departments may operate consortium nodes for maintenance evidence logging.

7.3 Secure Data Sharing and Interoperability

Interoperability remains a persistent challenge in healthcare, as data is often fragmented across incompatible systems. Blockchain-enabled digital twins provide a framework for secure, standardized data sharing among stakeholders while preserving patient privacy.

In this scenario, blockchain acts as a decentralized coordination layer that manages access rights and data provenance, while digital twins aggregate and contextualize data for analysis. Standardized data models and APIs facilitate interoperability between IoMT platforms, hospital information systems, and external healthcare providers.

Implementation Considerations:

- **Interoperability profile:** Data exchange should align with HL7 FHIR resources and standardized ontologies to avoid semantic mismatch.
- **Access governance:** Cross-hospital access must be purpose-limited and time-bounded to reduce privacy risk and consent fatigue.
- **Audit objective:** Blockchain logs can reduce audit time from day to minute by providing tamper-evident provenance trails.

This approach supports continuity of care, enables collaborative research, and enhances public health surveillance without compromising data security or ownership. The representative applications described above are synthesized and compared in Table 1, which outlines key smart hospital use cases of blockchain-enabled digital twins across clinical, operational, and interoperability domains. This table summarizes the digital twin functions, corresponding blockchain roles, and expected benefits for each use case, providing a concise reference for practitioners and researchers.

Table 1. Key Smart Hospital Use Cases of Blockchain-Enabled Digital Twins

Use Case	Digital Twin Function	Blockchain Role	Expected Benefits
Personalized patient care	Patient modeling and simulation	Data integrity, consent management	Improved outcomes, personalized treatment
Equipment maintenance	Device behavior modeling	Auditability, smart contracts	Reduced downtime, enhanced safety
Data interoperability	System-level digital twins	Access control, traceability	Secure data sharing, compliance
Resource optimization	Operational simulations	Trusted data pipelines	Efficiency, cost reduction

8. SECURITY, PRIVACY, AND REGULATORY CONSIDERATIONS

8.1 Data Privacy and Confidentiality

Healthcare data is among the most sensitive categories of personal information, making privacy protection a paramount concern in smart hospital systems. While blockchain provides strong integrity and transparency guarantees, it must be carefully designed to avoid unintended data exposure.

This chapter emphasizes the use of off-chain storage for sensitive data, with blockchain storing only cryptographic hashes and metadata. Encryption techniques, such as attribute-based encryption and secure multi-party computation, can further protect data confidentiality. Permissioned blockchain networks enable controlled access, ensuring that only authorized entities can participate.

8.2 GDPR "Right to Erasure" vs. Blockchain Immutability: A Practical Pattern

A key tension in blockchain-enabled healthcare systems is the conflict between blockchain immutability and GDPR requirements such as the "right to erasure." To resolve this conflict in a technically feasible manner, this chapter adopts a **pointer-based ledger pattern** in which sensitive clinical content is stored off-chain in encrypted repositories, while the blockchain stores only (i) cryptographic hashes, (ii) metadata, and (iii) access and consent transactions. When erasure is required, the off-chain encrypted payload can be deleted or rendered inaccessible by destroying encryption keys (crypto-shredding), while the on-chain record remains as a non-sensitive proof of event occurrence. In addition, **proxy re-encryption** can be used to support controlled revocation and re-delegation of access rights without exposing raw data. For advanced regulatory alignment, **redactable blockchain techniques** (e.g., chameleon hash–based editing) can be considered in permissioned hospital consortia to support legally authorized redaction while preserving audit integrity. This approach preserves compliance feasibility without undermining provenance, auditability, or institutional accountability.

8.3 Regulatory Compliance and Ethical Governance

Compliance with regulations such as HIPAA and GDPR requires careful consideration of data ownership, consent, and the right to erasure. Blockchain immutability can conflict with these requirements, necessitating hybrid approaches that allow data modification or deletion off chain while preserving auditability.

Ethical governance is equally important, particularly when digital twins and AI-driven analytics influence clinical decisions. Transparency, explainability, and accountability must be prioritized to maintain trust among patients and clinicians. Blockchain-based audit trails support ethical oversight by enabling traceability of data usage and decision logic.

9. CHALLENGES, LIMITATIONS, AND RESEARCH GAPS

While blockchain-enabled digital twins offer significant potential, their implementation faces multidimensional challenges that must be carefully addressed. Table 2 provides a structured analysis of benefits and considerations across technical, organizational, ethical, and governance domains. These considerations inform both the research gaps discussed in this section and practical implementation strategies.

Table 2. Benefits and Challenges of Blockchain–Digital Twin Integration

Category	Benefits	Challenges & Considerations
Technical	**End-to-End Verifiability:** Creates an immutable chain of custody from sensor to decision. **Enhanced Security:** Combines DT's anomaly detection with blockchain's tamper-proof logging. **True Interoperability:** Enables autonomous machine-to-machine communication with baked-in trust.	**Performance & Throughput:** Blockchain consensus can introduce latency unsuitable for real-time, life-critical alerts. **Data Storage:** On-chain storage of all DT data is impractical; requires robust hybrid models (off-chain storage with on-chain hashes). **System Complexity:** Integrating two complex technologies exponentially increases architectural and debugging complexity.
Organizational	**Operational Transparency:** Unprecedented visibility into workflows, supply chains, and resource utilization. **Automated Compliance:** Smart contracts can auto-enforce regulations (GDPR, HIPAA) in data sharing. **New Business Models:** Enables data marketplaces for anonymized research, outcome-based contracts, and fractional asset ownership.	**High Initial Cost & Expertise:** Significant investment in new infrastructure and scarce talent (blockchain architects, DT modelers). **Cultural Shift:** Requires move from centralized control to a decentralized, shared-governance mindset. **Legacy Integration:** Difficult and costly integration with existing hospital information systems (HIS, EHR).
Ethical & Legal	**Enhanced Patient Sovereignty:** Puts patients in control of their digital twin and data footprint. **Improved Accountability:** Non-repudiable audit trail clarifies responsibility for adverse events. **Ethical AI:** Provides a framework to audit training data and decisions made by AI within the DT.	**Liability Attribution:** If a smart contract executes an erroneous automated action. **Immutable Mistakes:** The "right to be forgotten" (GDPR) conflicts with blockchain's immutability. Data deletion is impossible; solutions require advanced cryptography. **Algorithmic Bias:** Bias in DT simulation models or training data, once anchored on-chain, could become perpetuated and harder to challenge.
Governance & Regulatory	**Standardized Provenance:** Creates a universal framework for data and device provenance that regulators can directly audit. **Streamlined Reporting:** Automated, verifiable reporting to health authorities.	**Lack of Standards:** No universally accepted standards for DT data models or blockchain implementations in healthcare. **Regulatory Uncertainty:** Most health regulators have no clear framework for approving decentralized, algorithmically governed systems. **Cross-Border Data Flow:** While blockchain is borderless, health data sovereignty laws create complex technical and legal hurdles.

9.1 Scalability and Performance

Scalability remains a significant challenge for blockchain-enabled digital twin systems, especially in large hospitals with thousands of IoMT devices. High transaction volumes and real-time data requirements can strain blockchain networks.

Solutions such as layer-2 scaling, off-chain processing, and edge computing are critical to addressing these limitations.

9.2 Interoperability and Standardization

The lack of standardized data models and protocols hinders interoperability across healthcare systems. While efforts such as HL7 FHIR provide a foundation, further alignment with blockchain and digital twin frameworks is needed. Research into standardized architectures and ontologies remains an open area.

9.3 Organizational and Cultural Barriers

Beyond technical challenges, organizational and cultural factors can impede adoption. Healthcare institutions may lack the expertise or resources needed to implement complex digital infrastructures. Change management, training, and stakeholder engagement are essential for successful deployment.

10. POLICY, STANDARDIZATION, AND GOVERNANCE FRAMEWORKS

10.1 Governance Challenges in Smart Hospital Ecosystems

As smart hospitals evolve into highly interconnected cyber–physical environments, governance becomes a central concern. Governance in this context refers not only to regulatory compliance but also to the organizational, ethical, and technical mechanisms that ensure responsible, transparent, and accountable use of digital technologies. The integration of blockchain and digital twins introduces new governance complexities due to their decentralized nature, automation capabilities, and reliance on continuous data flows.

Traditional healthcare governance models are often hierarchical and institution-centric, relying on centralized control and manual oversight. In contrast, blockchain-enabled digital twin ecosystems operate in distributed environments involving multiple stakeholders, including hospitals, device manufacturers, cloud service providers, patients, regulators, and researchers. This multiplicity of actors necessitates new governance frameworks that can manage shared responsibility, data ownership, and decision authority.

One key governance challenge lies in defining accountability when automated systems influence clinical or operational decisions. For example, if a digital twin simulation informs a treatment plan or triggers a maintenance action through a smart contract, determining liability in the event of adverse outcomes becomes complex. This chapter argues that governance frameworks must explicitly address accountability allocation across technical systems, organizations, and human actors.

To validate feasibility in real hospital environments, evaluation should follow a phased strategy. Phase 1 can use simulation and synthetic workloads to benchmark throughput, latency, and audit logging overhead. Phase 2 can pilot non-critical workflows (e.g., equipment maintenance logging or cross-department audit trails). Phase 3 can extend to clinical decision support with strict safety constraints. Recommended KPIs include (i) reduction in audit preparation time, (ii) improvement in provenance verification accuracy, (iii) reduction in unplanned equipment downtime, (iv) alert latency under high-load conditions, and (v) clinician acceptance measures such as perceived trust and usability.

10.2 Role of Blockchain in Governance Automation

Blockchain technology offers unique capabilities for embedding governance directly into digital infrastructures. Smart contracts enable the codification and automatic enforcement of rules related to data access, consent, compliance, and service-level agreements. By embedding governance logic into blockchain protocols, smart hospitals can move from retrospective compliance audits to proactive and continuous governance. Beyond technical architecture and secure data flows, operational success depends on governance mechanisms that translate institutional policies into enforceable digital rules.

Figure 3 provides a governance and compliance framework showing how hospital policies, regulatory requirements, and ethical constraints can be operationalized through smart contracts. The framework emphasizes continuous assurance rather than retrospective auditing: compliance checks occur at the time of access and decision execution, and each enforcement event is immutably logged for later verification by internal auditors or regulators.

Figure 3. Governance and Compliance Framework

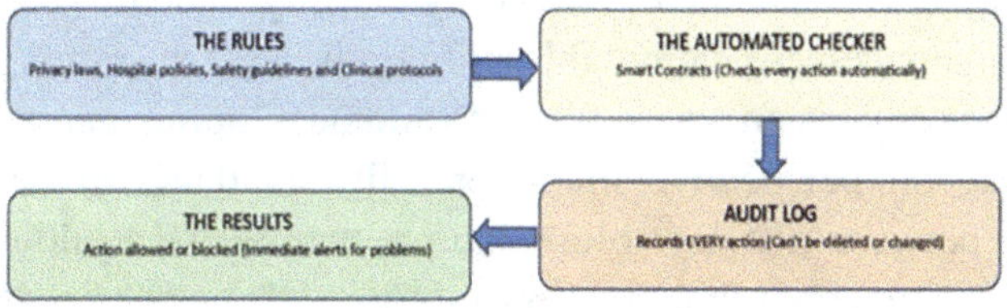

As shown in Figure 3, governance operates as a closed-loop control system. Policies and regulatory requirements are encoded into smart contracts that validate actions such as data access, digital twin updates, and automated clinical or operational triggers. If an action violates policy constraints (e.g., missing consent, expired authorization, unauthorized stakeholder role), the system blocks execution and records the failed attempt as a compliance event. Conversely, approved actions generate a verifiable audit trail, enabling transparent accountability and supporting legal defensibility. This model strengthens institutional trust by ensuring that governance is not merely documented but technically enforced within daily smart hospital workflows.

For instance, consent management can be automated through smart contracts that dynamically enforce patient preferences regarding data sharing. When a digital twin requests access to patient data for simulation or analysis, the blockchain can verify consent conditions before granting access. This reduces administrative burden while enhancing transparency and trust.

Moreover, blockchain-based governance supports auditability and traceability. All transactions, policy executions, and access events are recorded in an immutable ledger, enabling regulators and internal auditors to verify compliance without relying solely on institutional reports. This capability is particularly valuable in cross-organizational collaborations, such as regional health information exchanges or research consortia.

10.3 Standardization Efforts and Interoperability Frameworks

Standardization is critical to the successful integration of blockchain and digital twins in healthcare. Without common standards, interoperability between devices, systems, and organizations remains limited, undermining the potential benefits of smart hospital ecosystems.

In healthcare data exchange, standards such as HL7 FHIR (Fast Healthcare Interoperability Resources) provide a foundation for structured and interoperable data representation. However, these standards were not originally designed with blockchain or digital twins in mind. Extending existing standards to support decentralized identity management, immutable audit trails, and real-time synchronization with digital twins remains an active research and development area.

From a blockchain perspective, interoperability standards are needed to enable communication between different blockchain networks and healthcare platforms. Initiatives focusing on cross-chain interoperability and standardized smart contract templates can facilitate broader adoption while avoiding vendor lock-in.

Digital twin standardization is still at an early stage, particularly in healthcare. Efforts to define reference models, ontologies, and lifecycle management practices are essential for ensuring consistency and scalability. This chapter emphasizes the need for coordinated standardization across healthcare informatics, blockchain systems, and digital twin platforms to enable seamless integration.

Standardization is essential for scaling blockchain-enabled digital twins beyond isolated pilots. A practical roadmap should involve (i) aligning digital twin definitions and lifecycle models with emerging initiatives such as IEEE P2806, (ii) adopting healthcare interoperability standards such as HL7 FHIR for data exchange, and (iii) implementing decentralized identity mechanisms through W3C Decentralized Identifiers (DIDs) to support verifiable stakeholder authentication and role-based authorization. In addition, interoperability profiles should specify a minimal handshake model between the digital twin layer and blockchain governance layer, including required metadata fields (twin identifier, timestamp, model version, consent state, and provenance hash). Such alignment supports cross-vendor integration, reduces deployment friction, and enables regulator-friendly auditability.

11. ETHICAL, LEGAL, AND SOCIAL IMPLICATIONS

11.1 Ethical Considerations in Blockchain-Enabled Digital Twins

The deployment of blockchain-enabled digital twins in healthcare raises profound ethical questions related to autonomy, fairness, transparency, and trust. Digital twins increasingly influence clinical decisions, resource allocation, and risk assessment, making it essential to ensure that these systems align with ethical principles.

One ethical concern is the potential for algorithmic bias in digital twin models. If training data reflects historical inequities or incomplete representations of patient populations, digital twins may perpetuate or amplify disparities in healthcare delivery. Ethical governance requires continuous monitoring, validation, and adjustment of models to ensure fairness and inclusivity.

Transparency is another critical ethical requirement. Clinicians and patients must be able to understand how digital twin recommendations are generated. Blockchain can support transparency by providing verifiable records of data sources, model updates, and decision logic. However, transparency must be balanced with privacy and intellectual property considerations.

11.2 Legal and Regulatory Implications

From a legal perspective, the integration of blockchain and digital twins challenges existing regulatory frameworks. Healthcare regulations such as HIPAA and

GDPR impose strict requirements on data protection, consent, and individual rights. Blockchain's immutability, while valuable for auditability, may conflict with rights such as data rectification or erasure.

To address this tension, hybrid architecture that separates immutable audit records from mutable data storage are essential. Legal frameworks must evolve to recognize these architectures and provide clear guidance on compliance responsibilities. Additionally, jurisdictional differences in data protection laws complicate cross-border data sharing in global healthcare networks.

Liability and accountability are also central legal concerns. As digital twins and smart contracts automate decisions, determining responsibility for errors or harm becomes complex. This chapter suggests that legal frameworks should explicitly define shared liability models that reflect the distributed nature of smart hospital ecosystems.

11.3 Social Acceptance and Trust

Beyond legal and ethical considerations, social acceptance plays a decisive role in the success of smart hospital technologies. Patients and healthcare professionals must trust that blockchain-enabled digital twins serve their interests and protect their rights.

Building trust requires transparency, education, and participatory governance. Patients should be informed about how their data is used and have meaningful control over consent. Healthcare professionals must be trained to interpret and critically evaluate digital twin outputs rather than relying on them unquestioningly.

By embedding trust mechanisms into both technical design and organizational practices, smart hospitals can foster social acceptance and long-term sustainability.

Beyond algorithmic bias, continuous digital twin monitoring introduces additional ethical risks that require explicit safeguards. Persistent sensing and simulation may create psychological pressure on patients, particularly in chronic care scenarios, where individuals may feel constantly observed. Furthermore, questions arise regarding digital twin ownership (i.e., whether the twin belongs to the patient, hospital, or platform provider) and whether patients can meaningfully control downstream use of simulated outputs. A further concern is consent fatigue, where repeated requests for authorization can overwhelm patients and reduce informed decision-making quality. Finally, the risk of digital determinism must be considered: clinicians and administrators may over-rely on twin predictions and treat model outputs as definitive rather than probabilistic decision support. Ethical deployment therefore requires human-in-the-loop governance, transparency about uncertainty, and patient-centered consent mechanisms that remain understandable and manageable over time.

12. FUTURE TRENDS AND RESEARCH DIRECTIONS

12.1 AI-Driven and Autonomous Digital Twins

The future of digital twins in healthcare lies in increased autonomy and intelligence. AI-driven digital twins will be capable of continuous learning, adaptive modeling, and real-time decision support. When combined with blockchain, these systems can ensure that autonomous behaviors remain auditable, accountable, and aligned with governance rules.

Research into explainable AI, federated learning, and human-in-the-loop systems will be critical for balancing autonomy with oversight. Blockchain can support these approaches by enabling secure collaboration and model validation across institutions.

12.2 Edge Computing and Scalable Architectures

Scalability challenges are likely to drive the adoption of edge computing and hierarchical architectures. Processing data closer to the source reduces latency and bandwidth requirements, enabling real-time digital twin updates. Blockchain systems will need to evolve to support edge-based deployments through lightweight consensus mechanisms and localized trust models.

12.3 Toward Quantum-Safe and Resilient Healthcare Systems

As quantum computing advances, cryptographic resilience becomes an emerging concern. Research into quantum-resistant cryptographic algorithms and their integration into blockchain infrastructures will be essential for long-term security. Smart hospitals must proactively address these challenges to ensure future-proof digital infrastructures.

13. SYNTHESIS AND DISCUSSION

This chapter has demonstrated that the integration of blockchain and digital twins represents a transformative approach to building secure, intelligent, and resilient smart hospital ecosystems. By combining blockchain's trust and governance capabilities with the analytical power of digital twins, healthcare systems can address long-standing challenges related to data integrity, interoperability, and decision transparency.

The transformative impact of this integration becomes particularly evident when comparing architectural paradigms, as detailed in Table 2. This comparative analysis highlights fundamental shifts across nine critical dimensions of hospital operations.

However, realizing this vision requires more than technological innovation. Effective governance frameworks, ethical oversight, standardization efforts, and stakeholder engagement are equally essential. The chapter underscores the importance of interdisciplinary collaboration among technologists, healthcare professionals, policymakers, and researchers.

13.1 Comparative Analysis

Table 3 provides a comparative view between conventional smart hospital architectures and the proposed blockchain–digital twin integrated model. Importantly, "conventional" does not imply that all existing hospitals are fully centralized; many institutions already adopt hybrid cloud, federated analytics, or partially distributed interoperability solutions. However, such deployments often lack end-to-end verifiable provenance and programmable governance. The comparison therefore highlights how blockchain-enabled digital twins enhance trust, accountability, and compliance across multi-stakeholder ecosystems.

Table 3. Traditional Smart Hospitals vs. Blockchain-Enabled Digital Twin Hospitals

Aspect	Traditional Smart Hospital	Blockchain-Enabled Digital Twin Hospital
Core Architecture	Centralized or federated IT systems. Data stored in siloed databases.	Decentralized ecosystem. Physical entities have synchronized Digital Twins, with trust anchored on a distributed ledger.
Data Security & Integrity	Relies on perimeter security (firewalls, access controls). Data can be altered or deleted centrally. Logs are mutable.	**Cryptographic integrity:** Data provenance is ensured via hashing. Critical events are immutable. Tamper-evident by design.
Interoperability	Achieved through HL7/FHIR APIs and middleware. Requires trusted intermediaries and constant reconciliation.	**Trustless interoperability:** Smart contracts enable automated, verifiable data exchange between DTs without a central broker.
Audit & Governance	Periodic, sample-based audits. Logs are centralized and potentially unreliable for forensics.	**Real-time, pervasive audit:** Every interaction with a DT (access, consent, command) is immutably logged, enabling continuous compliance.

continued on following page

Table 3. Continued

Aspect	Traditional Smart Hospital	Blockchain-Enabled Digital Twin Hospital
Patient Agency & Consent	Static, often broad consent forms managed by the institution. It is difficult for patients to track or revoke.	**Dynamic consent:** Patients use cryptographic wallets to grant/revoke granular, time-bound access to their DT in real-time.
Trust Model	**Institutional trust:** Trust is placed in the hospital as a single entity.	**Distributed trust (Trustless):** Trust is shifted to cryptographic proofs and consensus mechanisms among network participants.
Scalability	Scales vertically (bigger servers) or via cloud. Data sharing with external partners creates complex integration projects.	Scales horizontally via a distributed network. New entities (insurer, research lab) join as permissioned nodes, simplifying ecosystem growth.
Decision Intelligence	Analytics and AI operate on potentially stale or siloed data, raising questions about input data quality.	AI/ML models operate on a **verified, real-time data stream** from DTs, with model versions and training data hashed for auditability.
Failure Resilience	Central points of failure (central server, identity provider). Downtime can cripple operations.	**Inherent resilience:** Distributed ledger and DT architecture reduce single points of failure. DTs can continue simulation/analysis even if some data streams are interrupted.

14. REPRESENTATIVE CASE STUDIES AND PRACTICAL APPLICATIONS

14.1 Blockchain-Enabled Digital Twin for Smart Hospital Operations

One representative application of blockchain-enabled digital twins can be observed in smart hospital operational management. In this scenario, a digital twin models hospital infrastructure components such as medical equipment, energy systems, patient flow, and staff allocation. Real-time data from IoT sensors continuously updates the twin, allowing administrators to simulate operational scenarios and optimize resource utilization.

Blockchain plays a critical role by ensuring the integrity and provenance of the data feeding the digital twin. Sensor data is hashed and registered on the blockchain, enabling tamper detection and verifiable audit trails. Smart contracts automate maintenance workflows by triggering alerts or service requests when digital twin simulations predict equipment failure. This integration reduces downtime, improves patient safety, and enhances accountability across departments.

14.2 Secure Patient-Centric Digital Twin for Clinical Decision Support

A second case study focuses on patient-centric digital twins used for personalized care. In this model, a digital twin represents a virtual profile of a patient, integrating physiological data, medical history, imaging results, and treatment responses. Clinicians can simulate treatment options and predict outcomes using the digital twin before applying interventions in the physical world.

Blockchain ensures secure data sharing among stakeholders while preserving patient autonomy. Through decentralized identity and consent mechanisms, patients retain control over who can access their digital twin data and for what purpose. Each access request and modification is recorded on the blockchain, enabling transparent oversight. This approach enhances trust while enabling advanced analytics and personalized medicine.

14.3 Regional Healthcare Networks and Interoperable Digital Twins

At a broader scale, blockchain-enabled digital twins support interoperability across regional or national healthcare systems. Digital twins can model healthcare networks, including hospitals, laboratories, emergency services, and supply chains. Policymakers can use these twins to simulate crisis scenarios such as pandemics, natural disasters, or supply shortages.

Blockchain facilitates secure cross-institutional data exchange and coordination. By providing a shared and trusted infrastructure, blockchain reduces fragmentation and enables collaborative decision-making. These capabilities are particularly relevant for public health planning and emergency response, where timely and reliable information is critical.

15. CONCLUSION

In conclusion, blockchain-enabled digital twins represent far more than a technological innovation, they signify a strategic paradigm shift toward secure, resilient, and trustworthy digital healthcare ecosystems. By enabling trustworthy data exchange, auditable simulations, and automated governance, this convergence addresses persistent challenges in data integrity, interoperability, and patient-centric care. However, realizing this potential requires coordinated efforts across technological development, policy design, and organizational transformation. Future success will depend not only on technical excellence but also on ethical governance, stakeholder engagement, and sustained public trust. As healthcare systems worldwide continue to digitalize, the thoughtful integration of blockchain and digital twins will play an increasingly central role in shaping next-generation smart hospitals that are secure, transparent, and adaptive.

Future work should include longitudinal studies, pilot implementations, and quantitative evaluations to validate the proposed models in real-world settings. In closing, the chapter calls for coordinated action among researchers, healthcare leaders, and policymakers. Hospital IT leaders should begin with controlled pilots of blockchain-enabled digital twins in non-critical workflows to build organizational readiness and validate governance mechanisms. Researchers should prioritize lightweight consensus, explainable twin analytics, and regulation-aware privacy engineering to address adoption barriers. Policymakers and regulators are encouraged to establish sandbox environments that enable experimentation with decentralized governance models while maintaining patient safety. Such collaborative efforts are essential to transition secure digital twin ecosystems from conceptual architectures to measurable impact in next-generation smart hospitals.

REFERENCES

Arigbabu, A. T., Olaniyi, O. O., Adigwe, C. S., Adebiyi, O. O., & Ajayi, S. A. (2024). Data governance in AI-enabled healthcare systems: A case of the project nightingale. *Asian Journal of Research in Computer Science*, *17*(5), 85–107. DOI: 10.9734/ajrcos/2024/v17i5441

Arya, S., Aggarwal, S., & Ansar, S. A. (2025). Transforming healthcare with blockchain and digital twins: innovations in IoMT for smart hospitals. In *Blockchain and Digital Twin for Smart Hospitals* (pp. 497–510). Elsevier. DOI: 10.1016/B978-0-443-34226-4.00025-3

Awasthi, M., Raghuvanshi, C. S., Dudhagara, C., & Awasthi, A. (2025). Exploring virtual smart healthcare trends using digital twins. In *Digital twins for smart cities and villages* (pp. 377–406). Elsevier. DOI: 10.1016/B978-0-443-28884-5.00017-8

Barbaria, S., Jemai, A., Ceylan, H. İ., Muntean, R. I., Dergaa, I., & Boussi Rahmouni, H. (2025, October). Advancing compliance with HIPAA and GDPR in healthcare: A blockchain-based strategy for secure data exchange in clinical research involving private health information. [). MDPI.]. *Health Care*, *13*(20), 2594. PMID: 41154272

Can, O., Dag, T., & Kantarcioglu, M. (2024). A blockchain based hybrid architecture for auditable consent management. *IEEE Access : Practical Innovations, Open Solutions*, *12*, 100419–100445. DOI: 10.1109/ACCESS.2024.3431292

Chaparro-Cárdenas, S. L., Ramirez-Bautista, J. A., Terven, J., Córdova-Esparza, D. M., Romero-Gonzalez, J. A., Ramírez-Pedraza, A., & Chavez-Urbiola, E. A. (2025, July). A technological review of digital twins and artificial intelligence for personalized and predictive healthcare. [). MDPI.]. *Health Care*, *13*(14), 1763. PMID: 40724790

. Dai, H. J., Mir, T. H., Chen, C. T., Chen, C. C., Yang, H. P., Lee, C. H., ... & Jonnagaddala, J. (2025). Leveraging large language models for the deidentification and temporal normalization of sensitive health information in electronic health records. *npj digital medicine*, *8*(1), 517.

George, B. (2025). Blockchain-Based Land Tenure Systems: A Conceptual Model for Using Decentralized Technologies in Managing Land Rights and Ownership Disputes. *Land Management and Utilization*, *1*(2), 32–48. DOI: 10.54963/lmu.v1i2.1527

Hanna, M. G., Pantanowitz, L., Dash, R., Harrison, J. H., Deebajah, M., Pantanowitz, J., & Rashidi, H. H. (2025). Future of artificial intelligence (AI)-machine learning (ML) trends in pathology and medicine. *Modern Pathology*, *38*(4), 100705. DOI: 10.1016/j.modpat.2025.100705 PMID: 39761872

Kantaros, A., Ganetsos, T., Pallis, E., & Papoutsidakis, M. (2025). From Mathematical Modeling and Simulation to Digital Twins: Bridging Theory and Digital Realities in Industry and Emerging Technologies. *Applied Sciences (Basel, Switzerland)*, *15*(16), 9213. DOI: 10.3390/app15169213

. Kuponiyi, A., & Akomolafe, O. O. (2024). Utilizing AI for Predictive Maintenance of Medical Equipment in Rural Clinics. *International Journal of Advanced Multidisciplinary Research and Studies*.

Lomotey, R. K., Kumi, S., Ray, M., & Deters, R. (2024, June). Synthetic data digital twins and data trusts control for privacy in health data sharing. In *Proceedings of the 2024 ACM Workshop on Secure and Trustworthy Cyber-Physical Systems* (pp. 1-10). DOI: 10.1145/3643650.3658605

Mazlan, E. M., Sarman, A. M., Kamaruddin, S. S., & Bakar, R. A. (2025). Digital Twin for Dynamic Construction Site Monitoring and Control. *Journal of Technology Management and Business*, *12*(2), 1–13.

Ogut, E. (2025). Artificial intelligence in clinical medicine: Challenges across diagnostic imaging, clinical decision support, surgery, pathology, and drug discovery. *Clinics and Practice*, *15*(9), 169. DOI: 10.3390/clinpract15090169 PMID: 41002784

Pokharel, B. P., Kshetri, N., Sharma, S. R., & Paudel, S. (2025). blockHealthSecure: Integrating Blockchain and Cybersecurity in Post-Pandemic Healthcare Systems. *Information (Basel)*, *16*(2), 133. DOI: 10.3390/info16020133

Roumeliotis, C., Dasygenis, M., Lazaridis, V., & Dossis, M. (2024). Blockchain and digital twins in smart industry 4.0: The use case of supply chain-a review of integration techniques and applications. *Designs*, *8*(6), 105. DOI: 10.3390/designs8060105

Sarani Rad, F., Hendawi, R., Yang, X., & Li, J. (2024). Personalized diabetes management with digital twins: A patient-centric knowledge graph approach. *Journal of Personalized Medicine*, *14*(4), 359. DOI: 10.3390/jpm14040359 PMID: 38672986

Sriram, V., Conard, A. M., Rosenberg, I., Kim, D., Saponas, T. S., & Hall, A. K. (2025). Addressing biomedical data challenges and opportunities to inform a large-scale data lifecycle for enhanced data sharing, interoperability, analysis, and collaboration across stakeholders. *Scientific Reports*, *15*(1), 6291. DOI: 10.1038/s41598-025-90453-x PMID: 39984563

Suleiman, R., Maradapu Vera Venkata Sai, A., Yu, W., & Wang, C. (2025). Blockchain for Security in Digital Twins. *Future Internet*, *17*(9), 385. DOI: 10.3390/fi17090385

Wahed, M. A. (2024, November). Real-Time Intrusion Detection and Traffic Analysis Using AI Techniques in IoT Infrastructure. In *2024 1st International Conference on Emerging Technologies for Dependable Internet of Things (ICETI)* (pp. 1-6). IEEE. DOI: 10.1109/ICETI63946.2024.10777213

. Wahed, M. A. (2025). ICAIMT_Real-Time Federated Learning for Autonomous Defense Robots: Enhancing Distributed Threat Detection and Response. *Journal of Information & Knowledge Management*, 2550073.

Wahed, M. A., Alzoubi, A. E., Wahed, S. A., & Kursheva, J. (2025, April). AI-Driven Approach to Predict High-Risk Newborns to Reduce NICU Admission Overcrowding. In *2025 1st International Conference on Computational Intelligence Approaches and Applications (ICCIAA)* (pp. 1-6). IEEE. DOI: 10.1109/ICCIAA65327.2025.11013654

Wahed, M. A., Halasa, A., & Alzboon, M. S. (2025, August). Enhancing Real-Time Detection of Distributed Denial of Service (DDoS) Attacks on IoT Infrastructure. In *2025 5th International Conference on Emerging Smart Technologies and Applications (eSmarTA)* (pp. 1-6). IEEE.

Wahed, M. A., & Wahed, S. A. (2025). Autonomous Defense Systems for Surgical Robots Ensuring Cybersecurity in Robotic-Assisted Surgery. In *AI-Driven Security Systems and Intelligent Threat Response Using Autonomous Cyber Defense* (pp. 407–438). IGI Global Scientific Publishing. DOI: 10.4018/979-8-3373-0954-5.ch014

Wahed, M. A., Wahed, S. A., & Alzoubi, A. E. (2025). AI-Driven Cybersecurity for Telemedicine: Enhancing Protection Through Autonomous Defense Systems. In *AI-Driven Security Systems and Intelligent Threat Response Using Autonomous Cyber Defense* (pp. 375-406). IGI Global Scientific Publishing.

Wahed, S. A., & Wahed, M. A. (2025). AI-Driven Digital Well-being: Developing Machine Learning Model to Predict and Mitigate Internet Addiction. *LatIA*, *3*(3), 73. DOI: 10.62486/latia202573

Wahed, S. A. W. A., Shdefat, R. S., & Wahed, M. A. (2025). A Machine Learning Model for Diagnosis and Differentiation of Schizophrenia, Bipolar Disorder and Borderline Personality Disorder. *LatIA*, *3*, 133–133. DOI: 10.62486/latia2025133

Xue, J., Li, Z., & Zhang, S. (2025). Multi-resource constrained elective surgical scheduling with Nash equilibrium toward smart hospitals. *Scientific Reports*, *15*(1), 3946. DOI: 10.1038/s41598-025-87867-y PMID: 39890977

Zhao, T., Song, C., Yu, J., Xing, L., Xu, F., Li, W., & Wang, Z. (2025). Leveraging Immersive Digital Twins and AI-Driven Decision Support Systems for Sustainable Water Reserves Management: A Conceptual Framework. *Sustainability (Basel)*, *17*(8), 3754. DOI: 10.3390/su17083754

Chapter 3
Architecting Smart Hospitals:
Integrating Blockchain Security With Digital Twin Intelligence

Vikash Kumar Maurya
http://orcid.org/0009-0006-3860-5090
Independent Researcher, India

Sumit Kumar
Galgotias University, India

Avanish Kumar Varma
Galgotias University, India

Shrikant Tiwari
http://orcid.org/0000-0001-6947-2362
Galgotias University, India

ABSTRACT

The speedy digital change of healthcare has led to the quick adoption of hospital facilities with smart infrastructures that are able to deliver services which are efficient, secure, and patient-centric. This chapter deals with how blockchain technology and digital twin intelligence work together as one integrated unit to constitute hospital ecosystems that are resilient, transparent, and interoperable. Digital twins, or virtual replicas of physical assets, clinical workflows, and patient pathways, provide the capacity for real-time monitoring, predictive analytics, and optimised resource management. Nevertheless, their performance is largely dependent on the integrity,

DOI: 10.4018/979-8-3373-8177-0.ch003

privacy, and security of the data they use. In order to overcome these obstacles, blockchain offers a decentralized and tamper-resistant arrangement that is able to ensure secure data sharing, traceability, and trust management among stakeholders.

1. INTRODUCTION TO SMART HOSPITAL ARCHITECTURES

Smart hospital architectures signal a fundamental change of traditional healthcare models, in essence, they are integrated, digital, and intelligent systems aimed at improving patient care, hospital efficiency, and clinical decision-making.(Catarinucci et al., 2015) Smart hospitals powered by technologies such as IoT, AI, cloud computing, digital twins, and blockchain provide continuous monitoring, predictive insights, and automated workflows. Besides, they emphasize giving personalized care, enhancing the use of resources, and providing secure and easily accessible data exchange. This chapter is about the baseline of the smart hospital metamorphosis and it features the technological, organizational, and strategic factors that turn this change around, thus preparing the ground for advanced healthcare .

1.1 Introduction to Digital Transformation in Healthcare

Digital transformation in healthcare is the use of cutting-edge technology to revamp clinical services, patient management, and hospital operational processes. The transformation is about discarding paper-based systems in favor of digital tools, thus allowing data-driven decision-making, care quality improvement, and patient engagement enhancement. This is how the digital revolution in healthcare delivery is explained in this section. The changes brought about by digital transformation in healthcare are not only helping the sector to adapt to the current times but are also enabling the provision of personalized treatment and the setting up of smart hospitals .

1.2 Traditional vs. Smart Hospital Models

Traditional hospitals mainly rely on manual processes, have very limited data integration, and follow reactive care approaches. Most of the time, patient records are kept in silos, which slows down decision-making and lowers the hospital's output. On the other hand, smart hospitals use interconnected systems, real-time monitoring, automated workflows, and data analytics to provide proactive and personalized care. The hospital network becomes a healthy ecosystem through the integration of IoT devices, AI models, cloud platforms, and digital twins. Here we compare the differences in the infrastructural condition, level of technology adoption, patient experience, and operational efficiency that exist between traditional and smart hospital .

1.3 Role of IoT, AI, Cloud, Edge Computing

IoMT technologies enable real-time data acquisition within hospital environments, supplying trusted inputs to blockchain-secured digital twin models that support predictive analytics and operational intelligence. (Tyagi et al., 2024) AI goes through huge datasets to help clinical decision-making, diagnostics, and predictive analytics. Cloud computing offers storage and computing capabilities that can be expanded as per need and thus, allows remote access to medical records and applications. By dealing with data close to the source, edge computing lessens the delay, thus, speeding up the responses for the healthcare functions that are of utmost need. (Ficili *et al.*, 2025)

Figure 1. Edge AI vs. Cloud AI in Smart Hospital Data Processing

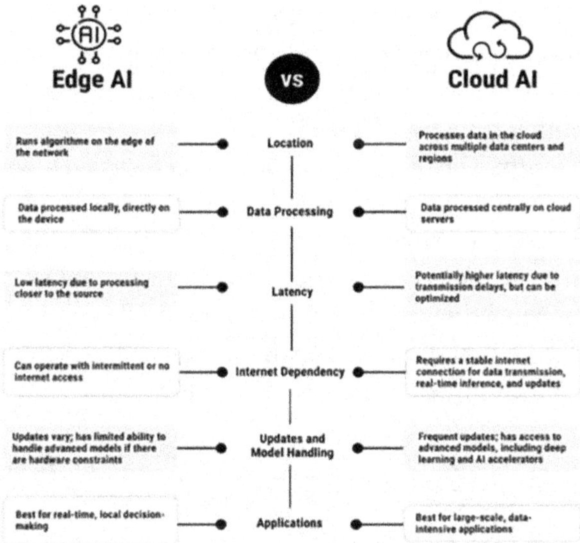

1.4 Benefits of Intelligent Hospital Systems

Smart hospital technologies lead to better patient results, smoother operations, and increased safety in the clinical area. (Pradeep et al., 2024)These units allow continuous observation, prompt identification of health concerns, and customized therapies based on AI-derived information. The use of robots relieves the administration of non-medical tasks that hamper the work and reduces the expenses of the hospital. Digitally-integrated units facilitate efficient utilization of resources, accurate scheduling, and quickening of the process of responding to emergencies. Intelligent hospitals, moreover, impart to the patients the benefits of a top notch experience through effortless communication, lessened waiting periods, and improved transparency. This part describes the far-reaching benefits of smart infrastructure for the healthcare.

1.5 Key Challenges and Opportunities

Even though they are full of promise, intelligent medical facilities have issues like expensive setup costs, difficult integration, security threats, and employees not wanting to accept the technological change in their work. Communicability between data of different systems is still the biggest challenge. On the other hand, enhanced patient outcomes, predictive medicine, efficient resource usage, and robust data protection with the support of blockchain and digital twin technologies are among the possibilities. The adoption of smart hospitals is becoming more and more facilitated by the positive climate created due to the acceptance of digital healthcare initiatives by governments and organizations. This part is about their problems and the great opportunities to be transformed into a.

While traditional smart healthcare models mainly focus on IoMT connectivity or AI, powered analytics, this chapter presents a blockchain, based digital twin-centric viewpoint for the design of smart hospital systems. Here, blockchain and digital twins serve as the architectural backbone, providing a reliable framework for data exchange, real-time synchronization, and predictive intelligence. Meanwhile, IoMT, AI, cloud, and edge computing technologies are considered as the enabler layers that help in data collection, processing, and analytics.

2. FUNDAMENTALS OF BLOCKCHAIN TECHNOLOGY IN HEALTHCARE

Blockchain is a perfect match for a decentralized and tamper-resistant system that is necessary for handling extremely sensitive healthcare data. It gives the healthcare industry the qualities of transparency, permanence, and safe communication between the different stakeholders. Blockchain technology in healthcare is a boon as it helps in patient identity management, easy sharing of medical records, drug traceability, and auditing of clinical data. Smart contracts are there to do the work automatically, while consensus mechanisms are the ones that take care of the correctness of the data. The given part is a brief overview of blockchain concepts and an explanation of how these features foster trust and security in digital healthcare.

2.1 Introduction to Blockchain Technology

Blockchainis a decentralized digital ledger that tracks transactions across many nodes in a network. Every transaction is kept in a block, which is linked cryptographically to the previous blocks, thus creating an unchangeable chain. By allowing peer-to-peer validation via consensus algorithms, blockchain eliminates the need for central authorities. It was only a short time ago that the blockchain was purely associated with the creation of cryptocurrencies, but now it has become a trendy topic in various industries such as the healthcare industry where the management of secure and traceable data is regarded as an absolute must. The section aims at equipping one with fundamental knowledge of blockchain's core concepts and its ultimate .

2.2 Architecture of Distributed Ledgers

A distributed ledger is a shared database that is replicated across several nodes and thus keeps the records synchronized and consistent. Blockchain is one type of distributed ledger technology (DLT), where the data is divided into blocks that are secured using cryptographic methods. It has elements such as nodes, peer-to-peer networks, consensus layers, and storage layers in its structure. Each node has its own copy of the ledger, which, therefore, elevates the system's fault tolerance and transparency. Changes are made only if they are agreed upon by the whole group thus, stopping the alterations from being done by the unauthorized parties. Distributed ledgers are designed for traceability, security, and auditability—features that are indispensable to healthcare data .

2.3 Consensus Mechanisms (PoW, PoS, PBFT, etc.)

Consensus methods are the means by which distributed nodes come to an agreement on which transactions are valid. In a Proof of Work (PoW) system, computational power is used to solve puzzles, thus securing the network but at a very high energy cost. A Proof of Stake (PoS) mechanism picks validators on the basis of the number of tokens they own, and thus, the energy consumption is considerably lowered. Practical Byzantine Fault Tolerance (PBFT) provides quick and reliable consensus capabilities to permissioned networks, such as those in the healthcare sector. These very mechanisms are the ones which uphold the integrity of the ledger, stop double spending, and ward off any kind of malicious attacks. Determining the right consensus model for a system is essentially a matter of its scalability, security requirements, and the nature of its operating.

In smart hospital environments, it is more appropriate for permissioned blockchain networks to be used rather than permissionless systems considering the stricter latency, privacy, and regulatory requirements. Consensus methods like Practical Byzantine Fault Tolerance (PBFT) allow for quick transaction finality and limited involvement of only trusted hospital stakeholders. Additionally, smart contracts help in automatically managing consents, controlling access to digital twins, and enforcing compliance, thus ensuring that only authorized clinicians, devices, and systems have the capability to interact with sensitive hospital data.

2.4 Smart Contracts and Automation

Smartcontracts refer to self-executing code saved in the blockchain that automatically carries out stipulated agreements and performs operations without human intervention when set criteria are fulfilled. They do away with intermediaries, lessen the time taken for operations, and make trust possible among the participants. Smart contracts in the healthcare industry can be used to automate insurance claims, consent management, data access permissions, and supply chain processes. Their openness and permanence serve as a means of accountability. Nevertheless, it is very important to provide for accuracy and security of such agreements so as not to get results which were not intended. The section here is about how healthcare workers can use smart contracts as a tool to help their work be done faster and more securely .

2.5 Security Properties of Blockchain

Table 1. Blockchainis a tech that comes with a punch of security properties, among them are:

Security Property	Description (Short)	Benefit in Healthcare
Immutability	Data cannot be altered once recorded	Ensures tamper-proof medical records
Decentralization	No single point of control or failure	Enhances system reliability and trust
Transparency	All transactions are verifiable	Enables auditability and accountability
Cryptographic Security	Uses hashing and digital signatures	Protects data integrity and authenticity
Consensus Mechanisms	Network agrees on valid transactions	Prevents fraud and unauthorized changes
Traceability	Full historical record of data events	Supports secure tracking of data and devices

2.6 Blockchain Suitability for Healthcare

Healthcareis an industry that <em>needs</em> (or: depends on) highly secure, transparent, and interoperable data environments—exactly the areas in which blockchain performs best. Among other things, it makes medical records that cannot be altered, the confirmed data sharing, the patient-centric access control, and the increased supply chain trust possible. By integrating the different data sources, which are usually heavily fragmented, and at the same time making sure that privacy regulations are observed, blockchain facilitates interoperability. Because of its decentralized structure, it is less vulnerable to cyber-attacks and failures. Furthermore, blockchain enhances the performance of digital twin systems by making sure that the data is accurate and reliable. This part deals with the reasons why blockchain is the only technology that can solve the problems of data integrity and security in .

2.7 Limitations and Considerations

Whileblockchain brings many advantages, it is not without several limitations such as scalability problems, increased storage requirements, and latency issues, notably in big healthcare organizations. Conforming to regulations may become a challenge because of the unchangeable nature of the records and data privacy issues. Compatibility with the current IT infrastructure is a matter of substantial integration work. The power usage is quite high for certain consensus mechanisms although there are some alternative mechanisms. Besides that, if a smart contract is not written properly, it may become a security risk. This goes to show that this section is about the necessity of a thorough assessment before the implementation of blockchain in healthcare .

3. DIGITAL TWIN INTELLIGENCE: CONCEPTS AND APPLICATIONS IN HOSPITALS

Digital twin intelligence refers to the practice of making virtual representations of hospital systems, equipment, processes, and even patients to let healthcare providers track in real-time, forecast through data analytics, and make decisions. Such digital models get fresh data from sensors, IoT devices, and clinical systems all the time, thus they can figure out the future situations and make the operations best. Digital twins in hospitals are instruments to raise the quality of patient care, to expedite the work processes, and to refine the management of hospital structures by offering insightful information that can be acted upon. This section is about the introduction of digital twins as well as the sign of their being a tool that changes the present healthcare world through better precision, productivity, and .

3.1 Understanding Digital Twins

A digital twin refers to a constantly changing virtual model of a physical object, a process, or a system, which reflects the real-time behavior through the continuous data input. It mixes IoT sensors, analytics, and simulation tools to monitor the performance, locate the deviations, and predict the results. In healthcare, digital twins represent patient physiology, medical devices, hospital workflows, or the whole network of healthcare facilities. They assist clinicians and administrators in condition monitoring, treatment impact evaluation, and operations optimization. Digital twins are the means to connect the physical and digital worlds, thus providing accurate decision support, automation, and predictive maintenance capabilities in .

3.2 Types of Digital Twins

Digital twins in the health sector are available at different levels. Process twins capture the movement of the clinical staff through such processes as patient admissions or surgery scheduling. Device twins stand for medical equipment." enable "real-time monitoring and predictive maintenance. Patient twins generate unique models of a patient's biology for diagnosis, treatment planning, and risk prediction. System twins portray the whole hospital scenarios such as energy consumption, staff movement, and resource allocation. Every one of them improves hospital operations in terms of visibility, efficiency, and personalization. In effect, they make up a complete intelligent healthcare .

3.3 Data Acquisition and Flow Models

Digital twins require ongoing data collection through IoT sensors, medical devices, electronic health records, imaging tools, and hospital management systems. Information travels through interlinked levels, beginning with data capture and moving on to preprocessing, storage, analytics, and real-time visualization. Such a flow guarantees precise alignment between the physical and digital systems. In most cases, edge computing takes care of the data locally so that the response is faster, whereas cloud platforms are used for storage and analytics of a large volume of data. (Veeramachaneni, 2025)

3.4 Analytics and Simulation Capabilities

Analyticsand simulation form the core of digital twin intelligence. ML and AI models consume real-time as well as historical data to output predictions, anomaly detection, and decision optimization. Simulation or virtual reality tools enable to recreate different clinical or operational scenarios, thus giving the staff the opportunity to see the results of their changes and confirm before executing them. Predictive analytics can be used to anticipate patient deterioration, equipment failure, or workflow bottlenecks. These features allow for greater accuracy, safety, and.

3.5 Applications in Patient Care and Hospital Operations

Digital twins are an ingenious idea, which goes a long way in the medical field. They are used to show the changes in the vital signs, the development of a disease, the responses to treatment, and preoperative planning in patient care. Besides that, they facilitate personalized medicine, monitor patients remotely, control the ICU, and determine the probability of an event .

Figure 2. Virtual Assistants & Remote Monitoring

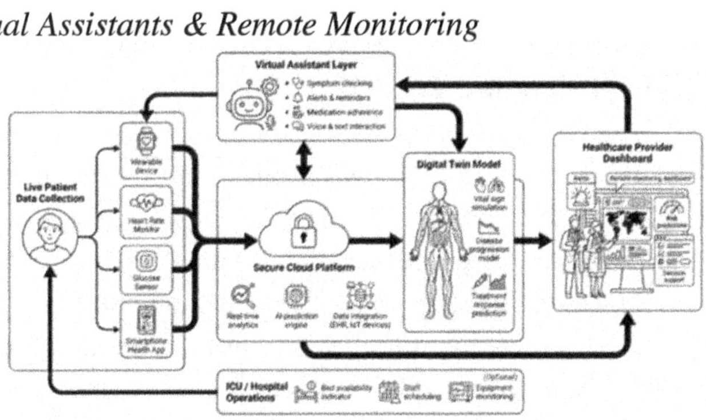

Moreover, hospital digital twins facilitate bed allocation, staff scheduling, and monitoring of the hospital environment, among other hospital management tasks made efficient by the use of digital twins. Further, they increase the effectiveness of the hospital's maintenance program and lessen the idle time of the most critical hospital machinery. By combining clinical and operational data, digital twins become a single source that supports better coordination, efficiency, and patient s.

In operational hospital environments, digital twins keep on receiving real-time IoMT (Internet of Medical Things) data to check on patient vitals, equipment status, and environmental conditions. These data streams are checked via blockchain, secured pipelines before they are used to update digital twin states, thus ensuring reliable simulations and predictions. Operational digital twins of this kind make it possible for healthcare professionals to spot patient deterioration early, carry out predictive maintenance of critical medical equipment, and optimize hospital workflows.

3.6 Benefits and Adoption Challenges

The use of digital twins leads to better decision-making, safety of patients can be raised, maintenance can be made predictive, operational costs can be lowered and healthcare can be made more personalized. (Vallée, 2023) Thus, these devices are means for hospitals to perform diagnosis faster and to manage resources more efficiently in addition to providing them with real-time visibility. On the other hand, there still exist the difficulties of adoption represented by such factors as the complex integration of data, the high costs of implementation, the problem of interoperability, the risk of cyber-attacks, and the necessity of having skilled personnel. Care for the accuracy of the data and conforming to regulations is another requirement. Regardless of the barriers, digital twins are a powerful option for hospitals to achieve efficiency, strength, and innovation in health care .

4. INTEGRATING BLOCKCHAIN WITH DIGITAL TWINS: A UNIFIED FRAMEWORK

Integrating blockchain with digital twins builds an environmentally friendly ecosystem that is secure, transparent and tamper-resistant, for healthcare data as well as for managing operational processes. Patient data on blockchain is encrypted and secure guaranteeing data integrity, traceability and decentralized access control, whereas digital twins offer real-time monitoring, simulation, and predictive analytics. By achieving these, the hospital is empowered with more trust, reliability and efficiency stemming from the use of IoT in smart hospital environments. It is indeed such a combined architecture that makes the sharing of data safe, the flows of work easy, and the communication between the consorts un-interrupted. The union, in turn, facilitates accurate updates of digital twins, helps in the security of sensitive data and deepens clinical as well as operational decision-making which is the core of futuristic intelligent healthcare .

4.0 Unified Reference Architecture Blockchain, Enabled Digital Twin Smart Hospitals

It is incredibly necessary to have a unified reference architecture to explain in detail how blockchain and digital twin intelligence could provide smart hospital infrastructures together. Figure 3 shows a multi, layered architecture where data pipelines secured by blockchain and digital twin intelligence gradually become the fundamental operational backbone in a hospital ecosystem.

The architecture defines five layers that are both physically and logically interconnected. The Physical Layer captures real-time data through IoMT devices, medical equipment, wearables, and hospital infrastructure sensors. The Edge and Data Processing Layer carries out local preprocessing, latency reduction, and initial analytics to help time, critical clinical operations. Blockchain Middleware Layer offers data security validation, decentralized identity management, immutable audit trails, and automated access control through smart contracts. The Digital Twin Intelligence Layer holds patient, device, workflow, and hospital infrastructure virtual models in real-time, thus providing simulation, prediction, and optimization. Lastly, the Application Layer features clinical dashboards, hospital management systems, and decision, support tools for use by healthcare professionals and administrators.

On this architecture, data from the hospital in real-time are always in sync with the digital twins, and cryptographic hashes along with metadata of digital twin updates are put on the blockchain to guarantee data integrity, provenance, and trust. Such a combined model facilitates not only runs securely and transparently but also intelligently. As illustrated in Figure 3, blockchain and digital twin intelligence form the core architectural backbone enabling secure data exchange and real-time hospital intelligence.

Figure 3. Proposed layered architecture for blockchain-enabled digital twin smart hospitals.

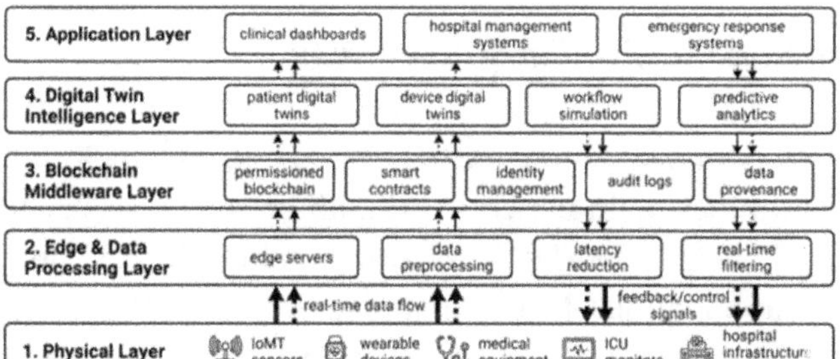

At the edge layer of this architecture, real, time IoMT data are initially processed and then the blockchain middleware validates these data. After checking, only cryptographic hashes of incrementally updated data are saved on the blockchain, before digital twin states are synchronized, thus guaranteeing the integrity, traceability, and trusted decision, making.

4.1 Need for Integration

Digital twins cannot function without precise, up-to-the-minute data, but their performance still hinges on the data being secure, trustworthy, and verifiable. To meet these requirements, blockchain offers immutable data storage, decentralized confirmation, and stakeholder communication that is visible to all. The merger makes sure that digital twins get verified data and generate trustworthy simulations. Moreover, it elevates patient confidentiality, stops data alteration, and sets up secure access control. With the increasing interconnection of healthcare systems, the use of blockchain along with digital twins is a must if the aim is to keep trust, guarantee data correctness, and facilitate collaborative decision-making in the network of intelligent .

4.2 Architectural Layers

Afederated blockchain–digital twin framework pervades several strata: the data procurement stratum which is the realm of sensors and devices that fetch real-time data; the integration stratum that takes the data and sends it to digital twin models; the blockchain stratum that carries out secure storage, consensus validation, and transaction logging; and the application stratum where clinical systems, analytics tools, and dashboards get to work with the digital twin. Smart contracts are there to automate workflows while APIs are there to allow communication across the layers. Such a layered structure guarantees that the hospital systems are interoperable, secure, and operating in sync and thus is the backbone of intelligent hospital .

4.3 Data Interoperability Requirements

Interoperability is a must if there are to be no barriers in the joining-up of digital twin platforms and blockchain networks. Health organizations need to adopt data standards like HL7, FHIR, and DICOM to maintain uniform communication between devices and applications. Proper mapping, semantic alignment, and ontology frameworks help different systems to get and share data correctly. With blockchain in the picture, the problems of interoperability are solved by the provision of a single, trustworthy data exchange layer. Nevertheless, issues of real-time data synchronization, high throughput, and support for legacy systems are still there. By fulfilling these interoperation standards, it is possible to have the most accurate twin models and the efficient collaboration of systems.

4.4 Synchronization Between Physical and Virtual Systems

Synchronization is what keeps the digital twins as close to the reality of the hospital systems, devices, and patients as possible. Continuous data streaming from IoT sensors is what allows real-time updates, while blockchain records every update to guarantee authenticity and immutability. Smart contracts cause automated twin changes if certain conditions happen. Edge computing helps synchronization get faster by handling data nearer to the source. This smooth coordination between the physical and the virtual worlds is what makes predictive analytics, operational optimization, and proactive clinical interventions possible. Without synchronized twins, the whole system would not be trustworthy and decision-making would not be . (Wang et al., 2023)

4.5 Blockchain-Based Secure Communication

By guaranteeing data integrity, authentication, and access control, blockchain essentially makes communication between digitally twinned components more secure. Consensus validates the encrypted transactions thus there is no room for unauthorized manipulation. To make sure that only authorized users or systems get access to sensitive information smart contracts automate permission management. As blockchains are decentralized, there are no single points of failure hence hospital networks become more resilient because of this. This is a secure communication system that shields patient data, the interaction of medical devices, and the hospital's operational processes which is what makes it possible for digital twins to be trustworthy, transparent, and accountable when collaborating with other hospital .

4.6 Reference Framework/Model Diagram

A reference framework for blockchain-enabled digital twins generally consists of five layers: the physical layer (sensors, devices, hospital infrastructure), the data processing layer (edge and cloud analytics), the digital twin layer (models and simulations), the blockchain layer (ledger, consensus, smart contracts), and the application layer (clinical dashboards, management systems). Data moves upward from the physical systems, gets verified by the blockchain, and is then utilized by digital twin models to make predictions and optimize processes. Though depicted here in a linear fashion, this layered architecture is actually a conceptual diagram that helps in the planning of the implementation. It makes possible secure data exchange, real-time synchronization, and seamless integration of intelligence across hospital (Khan & Abaoud, 2023).

5. SECURE DATA MANAGEMENT FOR SMART HOSPITALS

Careful handling of stored data is a must in smart health care institutions considering that patient data of a very sensitive nature keeps on being generated by IoT devices, clinical systems, and digital twin platforms. To keep data confidential, accurate, and available, strong privacy measures, data encryption, user account management, and conforming to regulations are needed. Blockchain secures data by providing tamper-proof records and distributed access control. This section talks about the whole data lifecycle, the major protection methods, and the sophisticated auditing techniques. The integration of state-of-the-art cybersecurity instruments with blockchain and smart systems enables healthcare organizations to create a secure, stable, and reliable digital healthcare environment of the (Wenhua et al., 2023).

5.1 Data Lifecycle in Smart Hospitals

The data lifecycle in smart hospitals spans the stages of collecting, storing, processing, analyzing, sharing, and archiving medical information. Data comes from sensors, medical devices, patient records, imaging systems, and operational platforms. Effective lifecycle management guarantees that the data is accurate, available, and secure at every stage. Immediate data use is essential for digital twins, clinical decision support, and automated workflows. Safe lifecycle management safeguards against breaches, unauthorized access, and data corruption. Hospitals need to put in place stringent governance policies, standardized protocols, and secure infrastructure to ensure that data remains accurate and trustworthy throughout its entire life .

5.2 Privacy Preservation Techniques

Privacy protection methods keep patients' confidential information safe and secure and ensure that unauthorized data exposure does not happen. The commonly used methods are anonymization, pseudonymization, data masking, and differential privacy that protect the identifiable parts of the data while allowing the data to be analyzed. Access control policies limit who can see sensitive information to only those authorized. Homomorphic encryption and secure multi-party computation are two ways that allow calculations to be done on encrypted data without decryption. These methods are indispensable for digital twin models, remote monitoring systems, and inter-hospital data sharing. Proper privacy protection helps in maintaining patient trust and is a must for healthcare regulations (Shahid et al., 2022).

5.3 Identity and Access Management

Identity and Access Management (IAM) is the technology that limits the interaction of authorized users, devices, and applications with healthcare data and systems. An IAM framework typically has various authentication methods such as biometrics, multi-factor authentication (MFA), digital certificates, and role-based access control (RBAC). In smart hospitals, the scope of IAM goes to the IoT devices, cloud platforms, and digital twin parts as well. Blockchain makes IAM more secure by providing the means for decentralized identity (DID) systems through which individuals are the only ones who decide the permissions for their data. Implementing the right IAM measures will reduce the risk of insider threats, eliminate unauthorized access, and make the organization's cybersecurity discipline .

5.4 Encryption and Key Management

Encryption is the primary means of ensuring data confidentiality, wherein sensitive data are converted into formats that are non-readable by utilizing cryptographic algorithms. As an example, medical centers implement a symmetric method of encryption when they need to quickly process data while using an asymmetric method when they want to communicate securely. Good key management covers all aspects such as the creation, distribution, changing, and safe storage of keys used in cryptography. If key management is done poorly, it can turn a situation where the strongest cryptographic algorithms are at risk of being broken into just to be secure. Blockchain technology can be utilized as a platform for the decentralized key management as well as for ensuring the security of the exchanged keys (Wang et al., 2018).

5.5 Compliance Standards (HIPAA, GDPR, etc.)

Intelligent hospitals are required to follow healthcare privacy and security regulations such as HIPAA in the US, GDPR in Europe, and other national data protection laws. These norms lay down very detailed regulations in respect of data handling, patient consent, access control, breach reporting, and cross-border data transfers. Being compliant with the requirements is the management of patient information in an ethical and legal way while also lowering the risks for the organization. Hospitals should be putting in place technical protections, conducting regular audits, risk assessments, and keeping records so as to be able to prove their conformity. There are also new requirements that serve as a source of support for the implementation of secure and interoperable healthcare operations for digital health and IoT .

5.6 Blockchain for Secure Data Auditing

Blockchain offers a clear and secure-from-tampering record of all interactions with healthcare data. In fact, every operation - e.g., data access, updates, or transfers - is permanently logged, thus, allowing total traceability. Smart contracts implement auditing regulations automatically and notify administrators when there is a suspicious activity. Auditing through blockchain increases the healthcare providers' accountability, makes compliance reporting easier, and stops any unauthorized changes. Additionally, it guarantees data origin which is very important for digital twins that need correct historical records. Trust in hospital data systems gets increased as blockchain decentralizes audit control, thus, lessening the risk of single points of (Yaqoob et al., 2022).

6. BLOCKCHAIN-ENABLED DIGITAL TWIN APPLICATIONS IN CLINICAL SETTINGS

One of the ways how digital twins powered by a blockchain can revolutionize healthcare is by their ability to combine real-time data modeling with a secure and tamper-proof data management system. Digital twins replicate patient scenarios, help in early diagnosis, make treatment decisions more efficient, and increase the accuracy of the monitoring process. On the other hand, blockchain technology guarantees data authenticity, privacy, and sharing with the clinical stakeholders in a secure way. In short, this union makes it possible to have very reliable digital twins which, in turn, lead to patient safety and care coordination improvements (Mihai et al., 2022).

6.1 Virtual Patient Modeling

Virtual patient modeling employs digital twins to develop real-time, data-driven simulations of a person's body, development of a disease, and the effects of the treatment. Such models fuse medical records, sensor data, the results of scans, and genomic data to create precise digital replicas. Medical practitioners utilize virtual models to trial treatments, foresee dangers, and tailor treatments, thus, there is no harm to the real patient (Choppara & Lokesh, 2025).

6.2 Predictive Diagnostics and AI Integration

AI-powered digital twins can carry out predictive diagnostics by evaluating streaming patient data to locate the earliest signs of illness or weakening. Machine learning techniques recognize deviations, predict health crises, and facilitate the making of decisions based on data. (Rastogi et al., 2025) Blockchain is there to keep the diagnostic data accurate and unalterable, thus providing reliable sources to AI models. Such a combination results in fewer diagnostic errors, the patient's condition being better tracked, and the preventive healthcare being facilitated. Predictive insights give clinicians the opportunity to intervene at an early stage, thus, patient outcomes get better, and hospital readmissions become fewer. Thus, AI, digital twins, and blockchain together constitute a potent triad for diagnostics that are ready.

6.3 Intensive Care Monitoring and Emergency Response

Digital twins in intensive care units keep track of patient vitals, device performance, and environmental conditions in real-time to be able to detect any critical changes immediately. They help quick decision-making by modeling body responses and forecasting next complications. Digital twins are also used to the best effect in resource management, staff coordination, and treatment strategies when there is an emergency situation.

6.4 Surgical Planning and Digital Twin-Assisted Operations

Digital twins help to plan surgeries more effectively through detailed anatomical simulations and predictions of patient-specific surgical results. Doctors are able to see how operations would work, assess the dangers, and even try different approaches without actually doing the experiments. In addition, twins provide up-to-the-minute support during the operation by delivering the latest physiological data.

Blockchain is the technology that makes sure imaging data, surgical plans, and intraoperative updates are kept safe and can be traced. (Tyagi et al., 2025)The unchangeable records that are created are meant to improve the accountability and collaboration of the surgical teams. Operations with the help of a digital twin are less likely to have the risk of complications, the accuracy will be higher, and the recovery after the surgery will be better. The combination of this technology is a big step forward in surgical safety and clinical making.

6.5 Personalized Treatment Pathways

By simulating the characteristics of an individual patient, a digital twin can figure out how soon a patient reacts to a treatment and can even suggest the best possible treatment plan. They include everything from medical history and lifestyle data to genomic information and also real-time monitoring metrics in order to be highly specific with interventions. Blockchain adds to the personalization feature by giving the most secure way of access control and also patient-consent management for very sensitive data. Healthcare professionals get enough accurate data with which they are able to adjust dosages of medicines, create programs for rehabilitation, and even outline care plans for a patient's longer stay at the hospital. Such personalized pathways make therapy more effective, less likely to cause side effects, and more patient satisfaction, which is in line with precision medicine initiatives in the present healthcare .

6.6 Benefits and Technical Challenges

Healthcare AI-textbook: Digital twins enabled by blockchain technology have a number of advantages like increased data trust, precise forecasts, customized treatment, better monitoring, and fewer clinical risks. (Tyagi et al., 2025)They facilitate the use of automation, interoperability, and the coordination of care between different units. But there are still obstacles in the way, for example, difficulties in data integration, limitations in scalability, problems with latency, a high computational load, and a requirement for highly-skilled technical personnel. Apart from these, ensuring conformity to healthcare regulations and keeping the synchronization in real-time also bring up some problems. However, the combination has a huge potential to be a game-changer in terms of clinical quality, safety, and efficiency in smart.

6.7 End-to-end Blockchain, Enabled Digital Twin Use, Case in a Smart Hospital ICU

Within a smart hospital intensive care unit (ICU), IoMT sensors are constantly recording the vital signs of patients, ventilator functioning, and the surrounding environment. To lessen the latency, these data are initially handled at the edge and then sent through a blockchain middleware layer, where data integrity and access permissions are maintained with the help of smart contracts. After verification, data changes are merged with patient, specific digital twins that allow real-time simulations of the physiological responses as well as risk prediction.

Physicians can get to the digital twin discoveries via secure dashboards that send them alerts regarding the worsening of the patient's condition, suggest treatments that are optimized, and also inform about the status of the equipment. Clinical records that cannot be altered, blockchain, based audit trails ensure accountability, compliance with regulations, and the whole clinical process. This complete chain of operations shows how blockchain, secured digital twins bring about improvements in safety of the patient, functioning of the hospital, and decision-making in the case of hospital emergencies.

7. OPERATIONAL DIGITAL TWINS FOR HOSPITAL INFRASTRUCTURE MANAGEMENT

Operational digital twins enable hospital infrastructure management through the creation of up-to-date virtual copies of the hospital buildings, utilities, equipment, and operational workflows. Such models facilitate regular checking, predictive maintenance, and even the optimization of the performance of the hospital facilities. Operational digital twins, by the use of IoT sensor data, analytics, and automation extend the hospital management to the best possible use of the resources, energy-saving, and the making of equipment trustworthy. They furnish administrators with the means to enhance sustainability, lower costs, and raise operational resilience through the implementation of these insights. Digital twins are also instrumental in the facilitation of emergency planning and the security of the hospital infrastructure. This chapter is devoted to how they can be used to create intelligent, data-driven hospital environments that can function in an efficient and reliable r.

7.1 Digital Twins for Hospital Buildings and Utilities

Hospitalbuilding digital twins are essentially detailed representations of the structural aspects, utility systems, environment, and operations of the facilities. Based on this, these models are updated with live data obtained from the sensors which are installed in the walls, equipment, lighting systems, and utility networks. They are being utilized by administrators for the purpose of keeping a check on the use of space, quality of air, water flow, and energy consumption. Digital twins, by means of simulation of such situations as normal working conditions, enable the determination of inefficiencies in the system, the prediction of failures and the facilitation of the planning of renovations. They are also a great help in the process of ensuring compliance with various safety, hygiene, and infrastructure standards. As a result of being aware of what is going on at any given moment, hospital buildings turn into more flexible, clever, and capable of making less harm to the environment, thus patient comfort and operational reliability are .

7.2 Energy Management and Sustainability

Through observing consumption patterns, forecasting peak loads, and imitating energysaving strategies, digital twins significantly enhance energy management. They pull in data from power grids, HVAC are, lighting, and medical devices to be energy-efficient at the best level possible. Hospitals can try out clean growth measures—like renewables and energy-saving mode–usage—before they actually commit to them in the real world. Anomalies in energy use are detected in real time by the alert system, thus giving the user a chance to stop energy wastage and prevent equipment overwork. This is how these technologies become a considerable portion of the solution for the climate crisis, help earn green building certifications, and save the operating budget. Digital twins are a great tool for hospitals that want to make a successful shift toward intelligent, environmentallyfriendly buildings that also respect the global sustainability .

7.3 HVAC, Power, and Infrastructure Monitoring

With the help of digital twins, the exact performance of HVAC systems, power networks, and other essential infrastructure can be closely followed. They follow changes in the hospital environment in terms of temperature, humidity, air quality, pressure, and power distribution in different hospital zones. Any deviation from the norm is quickly identified by the real-time models, which also predict system failures and make recommendations for changes to be at the ideal environmental level. This is very important for operating rooms, ICUs, and storage areas that need stringent environmental control. Digital twins also rehearse power cuts and other emergency situations to help staff be ready for them. As a result of offering healthcare institutions a thorough look into the behavior of their infrastructure, they become safer, more reliable, and their operational flow is not interrupted.

7.4 Equipment Tracking and Predictive Maintenance

Through giving up-to-the-minute locations, usage levels, and performance data of medical devices and machinery, digital twins are a great tool for equipment tracking. Predictive maintenance algorithms, on the other hand, look at changes in the vibration, temperature, and operation of a machine to be able to predict when a failure is going to happen before it actually does. In this way, the downtime of ventilators, imaging machines, infusion pumps, and in general, any kind of critical devices is avoided. Blockchain makes it possible for maintenance activities as well as device history to be securely logged. The combination is very powerful in terms of reliability, it also makes the equipment lifespan longer and repair costs lower. The hospitals are thus enabled to improve their asset management, have fewer disruptions and the essential medical tools may be used more .

7.5 Workflow Automation and Process Optimization

Digital twins replicate and refine hospital workflows of the patient admission, surgery scheduling, discharge processes, and emergency response coordination, etc. They figure out bottlenecks and inefficiencies by analyzing staff movements, resource usage, and task dependencies. Automated workflows—powered by AI and smart contracts—are getting rid of the most common tasks and thus, they are giving a raise to the level of operational synchronization. On-the-fly process optimization is delivering hospitals the means to improve patient flow, cut down on waiting times, and raise staff productivity.

7.6 Cost Reduction and Efficiency Gains

Operational digital twins are a key factor in cost reduction through the processes of lessening energy waste, decreasing equipment failures, and improving resource utilization. Predictive maintenance is a tool that lessens repair costs and prolongs asset life. Workflow optimization is a tool that lessens the occurrence of delays, makes the throughput higher, and lessens the administrative overhead. Better tracking ensures that staff, space, and equipment are used in the most efficient way. Moreover, digital twins can be an important element of a data-driven financial planning system by forecasting operational demands. These efficiency improvements have a major impact on cost savings while hospital performance is being enhanced at the same time. Consequently, digital twins become indispensable instruments in the achievement of sustainable, high-quality healthcare .

8. INTEROPERABILITY CHALLENGES AND SOLUTIONS IN SMART HOSPITAL ECOSYSTEMS

Interoperability is a must for smart hospitals, as it allows for smooth communication among different medical systems, devices, platforms, and digital twin environments. Nevertheless, healthcare ecosystems are riddled with fragmented data sources, incompatible formats, and isolated legacy systems. These problems make it difficult to provide coordinated care, make decisions in real time, and carry out operations efficiently. To be interoperable, hospitals need standardized protocols, secure data-sharing frameworks, and strong integration layers. Blockchain provides a decentralized and trustable platform for the different systems to be united. This chapter identifies the main interoperability issues and gives the technological solutions that lead to efficient, connected, and data-driven hospital .

8.1 Importance of Interoperability

Interoperability is the core functionality that allows healthcare systems, hardware, and software to share information in a proper, safe, and user-friendly manner. By doing away with different data storage methods, it facilitates the delivery of care that is well-coordinated and more efficient through the integration of clinical records, diagnostic machines, IoT (Internet of Things) sensors, and enterprise management platforms. Proper interoperability results in better decision-making, fewer mistakes, and increased operational efficiency across different hospital units.

8.2 Standards (FHIR, HL7, DICOM)

Interoperability in healthcare is dependent on fixed standards like FHIR that make the data sharing easy by using modern web technologies; HL7, which regulates clinical messaging and communication; and DICOM, which is the standard for medical imaging formats. These standards allow different vendor systems to understand, exchange, and process the data in the same way. FHIR is responsible for API-based interoperability, whereas HL7 is used for communication with a certain structure.

8.3 Data Exchange Models

Data exchange models outline the movement of data from one healthcare system to another. Typical models are peer-to-peer exchange, centralized repositories, and federated architectures. Peer-to-peer structures enable direct communication; however, they might not be able to handle a large number of users. Centralized structures provide effortless access, but they also entail security vulnerabilities and the risk of complete system failure from a single point. Federated structures give the option to keep the data at the source while permitting the regulated access to different systems—thus, they are perfect for extensive hospital networks.

8.4 Integration With Legacy Systems

Infrastructures of old hospital systems like old EHR platforms and single-use diagnostic tools that have different data formats and limited connectivity are the main reasons for interoperability issues. To integrate these systems, it is necessary to use middleware solutions, APIs, interface engines, and data translation techniques. Digital twins and intelligent systems require that the data be timely and accurate, hence the need for compatibility with the old system. A blockchain may be instrumental in closing the integration gaps by providing a single layer for the exchange of data in a secure manner. This part is about the strategies for upgrading the heritage structures without the hospital's working hours being affected and thus making the transition to the fully connected digital health ecosystems.

8.5 Cross-Platform Interoperability Solutions

Cross-platform interoperability refers to the ability of different healthcare software, devices, and systems to exchange information and collaborate effectively. The solutions consist of API gateways, middleware integration platforms, semantic ontologies, cloud-based interoperability hubs, and microservices architectures. These instruments are there to convert, synchronize, and verify data in different environments. Digital twins, in particular, are very dependent on standardized data flows that are made possible by such solutions. Sophisticated models even use AI-driven mapping to ensure that they are consistent and that the manual integration work is minimized. Proper cross-platform interoperability has a great impact on the hospital network by increasing the efficiency, clinical accuracy, and system scalability, and at the same time, it lowers the fragmentation that is present in hospital.

8.6 Blockchain as an Interoperability Enabler

Blockchain improves interoperation through a decentralized, transparent, and tamper-resistant platform for data exchange. To prevent the transfer of whole datasets, blockchain keeps references, hashes, or access permissions, thus allowing security and verification between communication systems. Automating data-sharing rules through smart contracts and enforcing standardized workflows are the ways in which these smart contracts operate. By guaranteeing uninterrupted data integrity and traceability, blockchain unites the old systems, IoT devices, and modern platforms for a seamless transition. Due to its distributed character, there is no need for a centralized integration hub. Here, we see blockchain as a trusted layer of interoperability which, by facilitating collaboration, joins different smart hospital .

9. CYBERSECURITY THREATS AND RISK MITIGATION STRATEGIES

Becauseof their dependence on interconnected systems, IoT devices, digital twins, and cloud platforms, smart hospitals are increasingly exposed to cybersecurity risks. (Jimenez et al., 2019) Cyberattacks have the potential to not only disrupt the hospital's operations but also to endanger patient safety and, even further, to expose sensitive data. Ransomware, device tampering, and network intrusions are some of the ways through which the attackers can target the most vulnerable parts of hospital infrastructures. On the other hand, risk mitigation at the highest level requires well-established security policies, continuous monitoring of the system, and cutting-edge technologies such as blockchain for data integrity and secure communication.

9.1 Cybersecurity Landscape in Smart Hospitals

Smart hospitals are part of a very complicated cybersecurity environment that is influenced by their digital integration, remote connectivity, and heavy data usage. While clinical and operational systems are getting digitized, attackers look for vulnerabilities in networks, medical devices, and cloud setups to exploit them. In general, hospitals become victims of ransomware attacks, data breaches, and system shutdowns, which not only jeopardize patient safety but also hospital continuity. Indeed, the expansion of telemedicine and remote monitoring has further increased the number of exposure points. Therefore, hospitals need to implement cybersecurity frameworks that are adaptive, multi-layered and capable of safeguarding data, devices, and users in any part of the ecosystem. Knowing the changing landscape is the first step towards creating smart healthcare systems that are resilient.

9.2 Threat Models and Attack Surfaces

Threat models are a great tool for understanding who the potential adversaries are, how they can attack, and what vulnerabilities exist in hospital systems. The hospital systems that can be attacked include networks, IoT devices, medical equipment, EHR systems, and digital twin platforms. The most frequent attacks are malware infections, phishing, DDoS attacks, man-in-the-middle intrusions, and unauthorized data access. Insider threats, therefore, empower the risk through the misuse of privilege. With the development of smart hospitals, the interconnected architecture of the hospitals makes them more vulnerable to both external and internal threats. By using efficient modeling, hospitals can decide which defenses to put up, where to install security controls, and be able to foresee the new risks. This part is about the main attack surfaces that have an influence on cybersecurity .

9.3 Vulnerabilities in IoT and Digital Twins

TheInternet of Things (IoT) equipment in intelligent medical facilities are ill-equipped to have a robust security system, hence they are susceptible to hacking, spoofing, and unauthorized control. The devices with weak authentication, firmware that is still unpatched, and communication channels that are not secure make the environment riskier. Digital twins require that they get data uninterrupted from IoT devices, so if the data are compromised, the simulations will be distorted, and this may result in wrong clinical decisions. Malicious parties may alter the data of medical devices, cause desynchronization, or even take advantage of digital twin platforms. On the bright side, these security loopholes can be mitigated by employing encryption, proper management of device identities, and securing data pipelines so as not to jeopardize the hospital functions and cause loss of trust in the digital twin technology .

9.4 Blockchain for Threat Detection and Response

Blockchain enhances cybersecurity by offering unchangeable audit trails, decentralization for validation, and data storage that is highly resistant to any kind of tampering. Transparent transaction logs along with automated smart contract alerts enable the detection of suspicious activities at a very fast pace. Identity management implemented through the blockchain guarantees authentication that is safe and thus, the unauthorized access is minimized. Consensus achieved in a distributed manner forbids any kind of manipulation in the case of medical records or digital twin data.

9.5 Real-Time Risk Mitigation Strategies

Continuous monitoring, automated threat detection, and a quick incident response are some of the ways through which real-time risk mitigation is achieved. The AI-driven analytics figure out the anomalies in network traffic, device behavior as well as digital twin data. Zero-trust frameworks thus, guarantee that users and devices are authenticated at every interaction. Encryption, segmentation, and secure communication protocols thus, ensure that the most critical are safe. Regular patching and vulnerability scanning are also part of the measures taken to reduce system risks. Blockchain is Real-time Mitigation's best friend as it ensures data integrity and gives out transparent logs. By employing these measures in smart hospitals, the risks of downtime, data breaches, and operational continuity are kept at .

9.6 Best Practices for Secure Deployment

Elaborate safety measures in the form of cybersecurity policies must be the first line of defense in any smart hospital system. Other ways to keep the system safe is to do an audit of the security risks regularly and control the access to different parts of the system rigorously. Health institutions ought to implement encryptions standards, secure coding practices and continuous monitoring systems to ensure security. By using network segmentation, it becomes very hard for the cybercriminal to spread their attacks laterally as the most important devices are isolated from the network. Training of the hospital personnel is very important as it helps reduce human mistakes and also increases employees' alertness to cyber threats. One of the ways blockchain can be of help is by facilitating secure data workflows, device authentication and compliance auditing automation. It is very crucial to provide security-by-design principles as foundations for digital twins, IoT systems and cloud platforms if we want to have a healthcare environment that is both resilient and.

10. CASE STUDIES OF BLOCKCHAIN AND DIGITAL TWIN INTEGRATION IN HEALTHCARE

Thischapter features case studies from the real world that illustrate the impact of blockchain and digital twin technologies on healthcare systems. (Yaqoob et al., 2020)Such implementations incite the evolution of patient monitoring, clinical decision-making, medical device management, and hospital operations to new levels. Worldwide initiatives are paving the way for enhanced data security, transparency, and predictive capabilities. Experimental projects unveil the potential of these technologies in the elevation of care coordination and the streamlining of operational efficiency. The chapter, through the examination of achievements, obstacles, and experiences, offers a glance at on-the-ground tactical rollout and a horizon of possibilities for the extensive infusion of these .

10.1 Global Use Cases

Worldwide, healthcare organizations are turning to blockchain and digital twins to enhance data privacy, patient care, and operational efficiency. There are examples such Europe-based patient monitoring systems through digital twins, USmedical supply chains secured by blockchain, and hospital management tools using AI in Asia. Certain nations have implemented blockchain-based national networks for health records sharing securely. These usage scenarios reveal how combined technologies facilitate clinical precision, accelerate administrative tasks, and lessen healthcare systemrisks. Moreover, they reflect the extent and different functionalities of blockchain-powered digital twin healthcare can be in various .

10.2 Pilot Projects and Prototypes

Pilot projects investigate whether blockchain could be combined with digital twins to create highly targeted healthcare applications. Some of the prototype systems are smart ICU monitoring, blockchain-verified digital patient twins, AI-driven predictive care models, and real-time surgical simulation platforms. These pilot programs have shown to deliver better diagnostic accuracy, increased security, and the effectiveness of resource use. They have also identified issues like integration complexity, latency, and regulatory barriers. The results help a great deal in the preparation of the next step, which is hospital-wide implementation of these .

10.3 Digital Twins in Clinical Operations

By modeling patient conditions, workflows, and treatment pathways, digital twins help clinical operations achieve their goals. In these instances, hospitals have reportedly used twins to make the most of surgery schedules, ICU beds, emergency responses, and chronic disease management. Blockchain helps to make the patient data flow secure, thus ensuring that the synchronization is done accurately, and also improving the auditability. Such changes lead to fewer medical errors, better coordination, and shorter waiting times for treatment. The power of digital twins to transform clinical decision-making through the provision of predictive insights and real-time operational visibility is emphasized in the local . (Ahmadi-Assalemi et al., 2020)

10.4 Blockchain-Based Healthcare Networks

Healthcare networks powered by blockchains allow for secure and easily interoperable sharing of data among hospitals, clinics, laboratories, and insurers. Examples of such systems are health record networks at the national level, platforms for managing consent in a decentralized way, and repositories for imaging files that are powered by blockchain technology.When combined with digital twins, the data becomes even more accurate and reliable. Hospitals that have such systems in place say that they have achieved better care continuity, increased patient engagement, and have administrative processes that are more efficient. These networks are an example of how blockchain can serve as a fundamental infrastructure for interconnected and secure healthcare .

10.5 Success Factors and Key Insights

Successful deployments have in common key factors: support from strong leadership, clear objectives, strong data governance, interoperability standards, and technically skilled teams. Engaging stakeholders early, testing through pilots, and gradual rollout help to lessen the risks. Blockchain provides a means for safe and clear data sharing, while digital twins improve forecasting accuracy. Case studies point to factors such as the ability of the architecture to scale, continuous training, and going deeper with the integration of existing hospital systems to be of great importance. One of the biggest revelations is that blockchain and digital twins, when used together with AI, IoT, and cloud technologies, bring about the greatest effect. The most effective change management is the key to sustaining success in the long (Errida & Lotfi, 2021).

10.6 Limitations and Future Potential

While the results may seem promising, actual implementations in the real world are limited by factors such as expensive deployment costs, difficulties in interoperability, obstacles imposed by regulations, and the requirement of having highly skilled technical personnel.The adoption will be faster because of the emerging standards and the government support. When the technologies become mature, there will be less human intervention needed in the integrated blockchain-digital twin systems, which will allow for more personalized and secure healthcare models to be developed .

11. ETHICAL, LEGAL, AND REGULATORY CONSIDERATIONS

Innovativehospitals using blockchain and digital twins are facing complicated ethical, legal, and regulatory issues (Bruynseels et al., 2018). Laws need to change to allow for the safe, responsible, and compliant use of these advanced digital tools. From an ethical point of view, it is very important to preserve patient trust, avoid discrimination, and guarantee that the data are used in a transparent manner. This chapter deals with the main issues and provides principles as a guide for the ethical use of these technologies in healthcare so that the tech could be a tool to support patient rights and societal

11.1 Ethical Issues in Smart Hospitals

Smart hospitals encounter ethical problems in different scenarios, including issues related to patient privacy, informed consent, data misuse, transparency of automated decisions, and unequal access to digital technologies.The use of health data for secondary research without proper consent may result in ethical conflicts in healthcare. Hospitals should not only innovate but also make sure patient rights are safeguarded. They implement ethical principles, communicate openly, and have strict data governance measures in place, which together help them to be responsible while using digital healthcare systems that are also effective and of high.

11.2 Data Ownership and Consent

Data ownership in smart hospitals can be described as a complicated issue since patients are the ones generating the data while healthcare providers are the ones that have the power to store and use it.Blockchain technology is capable of enabling decentralized consent management whereby patients are allowed to give as well as take back their permissions in a secure manner. By giving patients control over their data, healthcare providers will be able to win patients' trust, be in line with the law and at the same time, support the implementation of ethical digital healthcare .

11.3 Bias, Fairness, and Transparency

Artificial intelligence-powered digital twins might get biases from their training data, which in turn might lead to unjust or incorrect clinical forecasts. To make sure that the system is fair, it is necessary to have diverse datasets, methods for detecting bias, and a model that is developed in a transparent way. It is very important for the doctors to know how the digital systems arrive at the recommendations that they give, hence the need for transparency.

11.4 Legal Frameworks for Emerging Technologies

Table 2. Key healthcare laws and regulatory frameworks governing data protection, cybersecurity, AI, and digital health

Framework / Law	Region	Focus Area
HIPAA	USA	Health data privacy & security
GDPR	EU	Data protection, consent, user rights
NIST Framework	USA	Cybersecurity standards & risk management
EU AI Act	EU	Regulation of AI systems, transparency, safety
MDR / FDA Regulations	EU / USA	Medical device certification & safety
Telemedicine Guidelines	Global/National	Remote care, licensing, digital consultations
Blockchain Governance Drafts	Global	Smart contracts, data integrity, decentralized identity

11.5 Ethical Use of Virtual Patient Models

Ethical concerns are raised by virtual patient models regarding their accuracy, consent, and their use in a responsible manner. As these models represent human physiology and how the treatment will affect the patient, it follows that misleading predictions may affect the actual clinical decisions. To be sure of the ethical use of these devices, it is the requirement of such use to be thoroughly tested, supervised by the clinician, and communicated transparently with regard to the limitations of the model. Patients need to agree that their data can be used to make their digital twins. Ethical standards set virtual models as assistants to clinical judgment rather than substitutes, thus ensuring patient safety and trust while allowing the implementation of personalized (Mennella et al., 2024).

11.6 Accountability and Governance

Accountabilityin intelligent healthcare facilities entails well-defined roles and responsibilities for handling data, automated systems, and the digital twin activities. The management structures should guarantee openness, the possibility of an audit, and adherence to moral and legal norms. Incorporating blockchain technology into the system of accountability makes it more robust due to unchangeable records, however, healthcare institutions need to specify who holds the responsibility in case AI or digital twins are used for decision-making. In addition, governance includes evaluating the performance of the system, handling the risks, and providing fair access to digital technologies. Effective supervision is a guarantee that high-level systems will function safely, courteously, and in accordance with the values of .

11.7 Ethical Governance Framework for Blockchain, Digital Twin Hospitals

The authors propose in this chapter an ethical governance framework that merges blockchain, based accountability with clinician supervision of digital twin decisions. Transparent audit trails, consent mechanisms controlled by patients, and explainable digital twin models are the key operators that allow for ensuring fairness, trust, and regulatory compliance in the implementation of smart hospitals.

12. FUTURE RESEARCH DIRECTIONS AND EMERGING TRENDS

Futuristically, the trends revolving around smart hospitals will primarily entail a much profound harmonious functioning of AI, blockchain, IoT, and digital twins to actualize self-governing, clever, and safe healthcare systems. Studies are progressing in predictive modeling, decentralized AI, quantum-safe security, and fully interoperable digital ecosystems.

12.1 Intelligent Automation with AI-Driven Digital Twins

Digital twins powered by AI represent a radical change that redefines the hospital of tomorrow with intelligent automation. Twins leverage real-time data and artificial intelligence to enable them to predict patient risks, manage the work flow, and even adjust system parameters remotely without any human intervention on their own. The implementation of smart automation in healthcare decision support has been a major factor in relieving the heavy manual work and making the overall management more .

12.2 Federated Learning and Decentralized AI Systems

Federated learning enables AI models to be trained at various hospitals without the need to share sensitive patient data and thus, privacy is preserved. The outcome of this decentralized AI method is that collaborative intelligence is enabled, the model becomes more precise, and data silos are prevented. Moreover, if used together with blockchain, federated learning allows for secure model updates, easily verifiable contributions, and a tamper-proof audit trail. (V. Ziegler et al.,)

12.3 Advancements in IoT-Blockchain Integration

The integration of IoT with blockchain technology enhances the security, interoperability, and trust of interconnected medical devices. Upcoming inventions will mainly revolve around energy-efficient consensus mechanisms, on-device blockchain processing, and scalable IoT identity management. These developments will enable on-demand verification, encrypted data transmissions, and tamper-proof device.

12.4 Quantum-Safe Blockchain for Healthcare

With the rise of Quantum computing, traditional cryptographic techniques might become ineffective. So, to tackle such a problem, quantum-safe blockchains employ post-quantum crytographic algorithms to not only make the healthcare data safe but also to keep them away from a quantum attack. These types of cryptographic techniques like lattice-based cryptography, hash-based signatures, and quantum key distribution will be the security measures for medical records and digital twin communication. The paper mainly focuses on the scalability, performance, and integration of hospital systems. Quantum-safe blockchain as a smart hospital security solution can be considered as the next wave of cyber attack immune technology which can ensure digital healthcare resilience in the future digital healthcare landscape. (H. Khodaiemehr et al., 2023)

12.5 Vision for Next-Generation Smart Hospital Ecosystems

The future technologies of hospitals will be represented by such institutions will be ecosystems that are fully interconnected, autonomous, and patient-centered, powered by AI, digital twins, and blockchain. Hospitals will be transformed into intelligent networks capable of making decisions in real-time, having predictive functionalities, and being equipped with self-optimizing systems.

Table 3. Vision for Next-Generation Smart Hospital Ecosystems

Category	Future Vision (Short)	Key Features (Short)	Benefits (Short)
Clinical Care	AI-driven personalized care	Digital twins, predictive diagnostics	Higher accuracy, faster diagnosis
Hospital Operations	Automated, self-optimizing workflows	Robotics, smart scheduling	Efficiency, reduced delays
Patient Experience	Seamless digital care	Virtual consults, smart rooms	Comfort, real-time monitoring
Data Ecosystem	Decentralized health networks	Blockchain, federated learning	Secure data sharing, privacy
Infrastructure	Autonomous smart buildings	Smart HVAC, analytics	Lower costs, predictive maintenance
Cybersecurity	Quantum-safe systems	PQC, blockchain auditing	Strong protection, fewer breaches
Emergency Response	AI-enhanced crisis management	Simulations, IoT sensors	Faster response, fewer errors
Research	Global research integration	AI collaboration, biobanks	Faster innovation, ethical research

12.6 Summary

The chapter explains that smart hospital infrastructures will be most effective when the two technologies, blockchain and digital twin intelligence, are integrated as a single, cohesive architectural paradigm. The former establishes a framework of reliable data governance, security, and transparency. The latter supplies the hospital environment with real-time intelligence, prediction, and optimization in clinical and operational arenas. The combination of these technologies will lead to well-equipped capable, efficient, and patient, focused hospital ecosystems that offer advanced healthcare services.

REFERENCES

Ahmadi-Assalemi, G., Al-Khateeb, H., Maple, C., Epiphaniou, G., Alhaboby, Z. A., Alkaabi, S., & Alhaboby, D. (2020). Digital twins for precision healthcare. In *Cyber defence in the age of AI, smart societies and augmented humanity* (pp. 133–158). Springer., DOI: 10.1007/978-3-030-35746-7_8

Bruynseels, K., Santoni de Sio, F., & Van den Hoven, J. (2018). Digital twins in health care: Ethical implications of an emerging engineering paradigm. *Frontiers in Genetics*, *9*, 31. DOI: 10.3389/fgene.2018.00031

Catarinucci, L., De Donno, D., Mainetti, L., Palano, L., Patrono, L., Stefanizzi, M. L., & Tarricone, L. (2015). An IoT-aware architecture for smart healthcare systems. *IEEE Internet of Things Journal*, *2*(6), 515–526. DOI: 10.1109/JIOT.2015.2417684

Choppara, P., & Lokesh, B. (2025). Efficient task scheduling and load balancing in fog computing for crucial healthcare through deep reinforcement learning. *IEEE Access : Practical Innovations, Open Solutions*, *13*, 26542–26563. DOI: 10.1109/ACCESS.2025.3539336

Errida, A., & Lotfi, B. (2021). The determinants of organizational change management success: Literature review and case study. *International Journal of Engineering Business Management*, *13*, 18479790211016273. DOI: 10.1177/18479790211016273

Ficili, I., Giacobbe, M., Tricomi, G., & Puliafito, A. (2025). From sensors to data intelligence: Leveraging IoT, cloud, and edge computing with AI. *Sensors (Basel)*, *25*(6), 1763. DOI: 10.3390/s25061763

Jimenez, J. I., Jahankhani, H., & Kendzierskyj, S. (2019). Health care in the cyberspace: Medical cyber-physical system and digital twin challenges. In *Digital twin technologies and smart cities* (pp. 79–92). Springer., DOI: 10.1007/978-3-030-18732-3_7

Khan, M. F., & Abaoud, M. (2023). Blockchain-integrated security for real-time patient monitoring in the Internet of Medical Things using federated learning. *IEEE Access : Practical Innovations, Open Solutions*, *11*, 117826–117850. DOI: 10.1109/ACCESS.2023.3326155

Khodaiemehr, H., Bagheri, K., & Feng, C. (2023). Navigating the quantum computing threat landscape for blockchains: A comprehensive survey. Authorea Preprints. DOI: Not available (preprint)

Mennella, C., Maniscalco, U., De Pietro, G., & Esposito, M. (2024). Ethical and regulatory challenges of AI technologies in healthcare: A narrative review. *Heliyon, 10*(4), e26297. Advance online publication. DOI: 10.1016/j.heliyon.2024.e26297

Mihai, S., Yaqoob, M., Hung, D. V., Davis, W., Towakel, P., Raza, M., & Nguyen, H. X. (2022). Digital twins: A survey on enabling technologies, challenges, trends and future prospects. *IEEE Communications Surveys and Tutorials*, *24*(4), 2255–2291. DOI: 10.1109/COMST.2022.3208773

Pradeep, M., Kumari, S., Tyagi, A. K., & Tiwari, S. (2024). Smart hospital in smart cities. In Tyagi, A. K. (Ed.), *Digital twin and blockchain for smart cities*. John Wiley & Sons., DOI: 10.1002/9781394303564.ch24

Rastogi, D., Johri, P., Donelli, M., Agarwal, T., Tiwari, S., & Singh, P. (2025). XAI-BT-EdgeNet: Explainable edge-aware deep learning with squeeze-and-excitation for brain tumor detection and prediction. *Frontiers in Artificial Intelligence*, *8*, 1676524. DOI: 10.3389/frai.2025.1676524

Shahid, J., Ahmad, R., Kiani, A. K., Ahmad, T., Saeed, S., & Almuhaideb, A. M. (2022). Data protection and privacy of the Internet of Healthcare Things (IoHTs). *Applied Sciences (Basel, Switzerland)*, *12*(4), 1927. DOI: 10.3390/app12041927

Tyagi, A., Kumari, S., & Tiwari, S. (2024). Internet of Things for smart healthcare: A survey. In Sharma, A. K., Chanderwal, N., Tyagi, S., & Upadhyay, P. (Eds.), *Future of AI in medical imaging*. IGI Global., DOI: 10.4018/979-8-3693-2359-5.ch002

Tyagi, A. K., Balogun, B. F., & Tiwari, S. (2025). Digital twin for blockchain-enabled intelligent transportation systems in smart cities. In Tyagi, A. K., & Tiwari, S. (Eds.), *Human-centric integration of 6G-enabled technologies for modern society*. Academic Press., DOI: 10.1016/B978-0-443-27434-3.00006-4

Tyagi, A. K., Tripathi, K., Tiwari, S., & Kaushik, S. (2025). An efficient technique for privacy preservation, trusted and secure patient-centric services in smart healthcare. In *Proceedings of the 6th International Conference on Recent Trends in Communication & Intelligent Systems (ICRTCIS 2025)* (pp. 31–47).DOI: https://doi.org/DOI: 10.1049/icp.2025.2731

Vallée, A. (2023). Digital twin for healthcare systems. *Frontiers in Digital Health*, *5*, 1253050. DOI: 10.3389/fdgth.2023.1253050

Veeramachaneni, V. (2025). Edge computing: Architecture, applications, and future challenges in a decentralized era. *Recent Trends in Computer Graphics and Multimedia Technology*, *7*(1), 8–23. DOI: 10.5281/zenodo.14166793

Wang, S., Zhang, Y., & Zhang, Y. (2018). A blockchain-based framework for data sharing with fine-grained access control in decentralized storage systems. *IEEE Access : Practical Innovations, Open Solutions*, *6*, 38437–38450. DOI: 10.1109/ACCESS.2018.2851611

Wang, Y., Su, Z., Guo, S., Dai, M., Luan, T. H., & Liu, Y. (2023). A survey on digital twins: Architecture, enabling technologies, security and privacy, and future prospects. *IEEE Internet of Things Journal*, *10*(17), 14965–14987. DOI: 10.1109/JIOT.2023.3263909

Wenhua, Z., Qamar, F., Abdali, T. A. N., Hassan, R., Jafri, S. T. A., & Nguyen, Q. N. (2023). Blockchain technology: Security issues, healthcare applications, challenges and future trends. *Electronics (Basel)*, *12*(3), 546. DOI: 10.3390/electronics12030546

Yaqoob, I., Salah, K., Jayaraman, R., & Al-Hammadi, Y. (2022). Blockchain for healthcare data management: Opportunities, challenges, and future recommendations. *Neural Computing & Applications*, *34*(14), 11475–11490. DOI: 10.1007/s00521-020-05519-w

Yaqoob, I., Salah, K., Uddin, M., Jayaraman, R., Omar, M., & Imran, M. (2020). Blockchain for digital twins: Recent advances and future research challenges. *IEEE Network*, *34*(5), 290–298. DOI: 10.1109/MNET.001.1900661

Ziegler, V., Schneider, P., Viswanathan, H., Montag, M., Kanugovi, S., & Rezaki, A. (2021). Security and trust in the 6G era. *IEEE Access : Practical Innovations, Open Solutions*, *9*, 142314–142327. DOI: 10.1109/ACCESS.2021.3120143

Chapter 4
Integration of Blockchain and Digital Twins in Healthcare:
Trust, Transparency, and Immutability in Smart Hospital Data Ecosystems

Boopathi Raja G.
http://orcid.org/0000-0003-3345-4503
Velalar College of Engineering and Technology, India

ABSTRACT

The rise of blockchain technology had a significant impact on healthcare by creating a new paradigm for storing, sharing, and protecting sensitive healthcare information through a distributed platform in a secure and transparent manner. The purpose of blockchain is eliminating single points of failure and providing auditable transactions on all stages of the transaction process. It also enhances trust between patients, providers and regulators. This chapter will showcase the ability of blockchain to provide interoperability across the fragmented system used by most hospitals, to support predictive analytics when combined with digital twins and to protect against cyber attacks through the use of cryptography are a few of the many uses blockchain technology provides to smart hospital systems. Finally, this chapter will provide a framework to position blockchain technology as a foundational enabler for secure, resilient, patient-centric smart hospitals by providing the basis for future integration with digital twins and AI-driven healthcare systems.

DOI: 10.4018/979-8-3373-8177-0.ch004

1. INTRODUCTION

The healthcare industry has entered a massive digital transformation. It is caused by the influx of new technologies, including artificial intelligence (AI), Internet of Medical Things (IoMT), blockchain, and digital twins. This is not only a technological but structural change that will transform the storage, sharing, and trust of medical data among various stakeholders. The essential of this paradigm shift is the blockchain technology that provides the solution with certain features of trust, transparency, and immutability. These are invaluable in managing medical data within the framework of a smart hospital (Abbas, Qureshi, Khan, Chandio, & Ali, 2022; Arbabi et al., 2022; Saeed et al., 2022). The healthcare systems have long been facing the problems of fragmented data silos, interoperability issues, and patient privacy vulnerabilities. The need for reliable, secure, and transparent data management systems has grown due to the growing demand of IoT-connected monitoring devices, telemedicine, and electronic health records (EHRs) (Alam et al., 2023; Sharma, Kaur, & Singh, 2021). Blockchain as a decentralized framework based on cryptography offers expected response to these issues because it assures that medical records are immutable, audit-traceable, and can only be accessed by authorized individuals (Taherdoost, 2023; Yaqoob, Salah, Jayaraman, & Al-Hammadi, 2022).

Patients have to provide their most private information to the healthcare professional, and doctors must have trust in the accuracy of the data they employ for diagnosis and treatment. By removing single points of failure and enabling distributed consensus mechanisms to validate transactions among several nodes, blockchain further enhances this confidence (Ali, Norman, & Azzuhri, 2023). In contrast to conventional centralized databases, blockchain also means that the information that has been logged cannot be modified without agreement, thus minimizing the risks of fraud or manipulation (Attaran, 2022). The research has shown that blockchain can enhance the relationships among patients and providers by providing a transparent audit trail of what data has been accessed and used (Hasselgren, Hanssen Rensaa, Kralevska, Gligoroski, & Faxvaag, 2021; Velmovitsky, Bublitz, Fadrique, & Morita, 2021). The transparency is especially important when it comes to the following situations: clinical trials, where the data integrity has a direct effect on patient safety and scientific validity (Emma & Adams, 2025; Leiva & Castro, 2025).

The distributed ledger of blockchain offers unchanging documentation of all operations, encompassing regulators and auditors to make certain that the standards like HIPAA and GDPR are met without involving any intermediary (Singh, Sharma, Mehrotra, Bhatt, & Kaurav, 2022; Villarreal, García-Alonso, Moguel, & Alegría, 2023). This will play a crucial role in intelligent hospital solutions, in which numerous systems, including IoT sensors and AI-based diagnostic applications, have to communicate with each other with a high level of accountability. Transparency also enables interoperability which has been one of the persistent issues in healthcare. Blockchain-powered systems enable dissimilar systems to share information safely to guarantee that patient data is reliable through the providers and institutions (Hussain, Rahman, Abdulsaheb, Al-Khawaja, & Khalaf, 2023; Tahir et al., 2024). For example, emergency care can be an instance where interoperability made with the blockchain can help when a quick access to correct patient history is important. In addition, the supply chain management transparency (i.e., pharmaceuticals monitoring between the manufacturer and the patient) minimizes the risks of using the counterfeit drugs and improves patient safety (Akram et al., 2024; Kavinraja & Mithula, 2025).

The most distinguishing feature of blockchain is immutability. Medical records are also reliable in the long term because when information is added to the blockchain, it can be accessed and modified only in certain situations (Ngabo et al., 2021; Zaabar, Cheikhrouhou, Jamil, Ammi, & Abid, 2021). The stated feature is especially useful in the healthcare sector where precise longitudinal data is a key to the successful treatment, research, and policy-making. Records that cannot be changed help in avoiding malpractice, fraud and other unintentional mistakes (Chen et al., 2024). Immutability in clinical trials ensures that the information about patients and trial outcomes are not altered which prevents scientific integrity and promotes trust between the participants (Emma & Adams, 2025). Similarly, predictive analytics and digital twin simulation can be facilitated with sensor data immutable logs in the IoMT application to allow hospitals to model patient outcomes and optimize resource allocation (Ghadi et al., 2024; Ramani, Mary, Raja, & Shunmugam, 2024).

Intelligent medical systems benefited from the interaction between blockchain and digital twins. In order to replicate hospital procedures, patient health states, and treatment outcomes, digital twins—real-world models of physical infrastructure—have to be fed with precise and reliable information in real-time. Blockchain ensures that the data supporting these simulations is authentic, transparent, and unchangeable (V. Ali et al., 2023; Nguyen et al., 2025). For example, a blockchain-based digital twin of a hospital may replicate patient flow, resource usage, and emergency response scenarios with assurance on the accuracy of underlying data.

In addition to digital twins, blockchain is becoming more connected with AI, IoT, and metaverse to improve care delivery. The analytics driven by AI use the blockchain as a source of reliable datasets, whereas the IoT devices use blockchain to provide secure communication and data storage (Alam et al., 2023; Khan et al., 2023). Explainable AI and blockchain can be used to collaborate with the metaverse and provide patients with immersive healthcare experiences without jeopardizing patient data security and trust (S. Ali et al., 2023). Zero-knowledge proofs and smart contracts are examples of other ethical frameworks that extend the use of blockchain in transparent data governance (Ezz, Alaerjan, & Mostafa, 2025). Although blockchain use in healthcare is encouraging, there are significant obstacles to overcome. Scalability is another issue since healthcare systems generate massive amounts of data that may be too much for blockchain to handle at this time (Dong, Abbas, Li, & Kamruzzaman, 2023; Wenhua et al., 2023). Widespread adoption is also hampered by issues with energy consumption, latency, and storage needs. Furthermore, a substantial investment and organizational change will be necessary for the integration of blockchain technology with the current systems (Atadoga et al., 2024).

Privacy is another significant issue. Even though blockchain technology has the advantage of immutability, one can question how to keep medical data without compromising its secrecy. Some of the techniques being developed for achieving a balance between immutability and privacy include off-chain storage, encryption, and permissioned blockchains (Masood, Daud, Wang, Banjar, & Alharbey, 2024; Thantharate & Thantharate, 2023). The implementation of blockchain in healthcare governance is further complicated by the ethical problems of informed consent and equitable access (Ezz et al., 2025). Digital twins based on blockchain-secured smart hospitals will be increasingly used to optimise hospital operations, anticipate patient outcomes, as well as improve crisis resilience. The interoperability frameworks will be enhanced to facilitate a smooth sharing of data between institutions, and technologies that do not violate privacy will be developed to deal with the ethical issues (Nguyen et al., 2025; Taherdoost, 2025).

The expanding significance of technology in the healthcare industry is demonstrated by recent advancements in decentralized clinical trials, blockchain-enabled federated learning, and IoT-based medication tracking systems (Kavinraja & Mithula, 2025; Ramani et al., 2024). Advancement in blockchain and its integration with AI, IoT, and metaverse technologies will revolutionize healthcare delivery and establish trust, transparency, and immutability as the guiding principles of smart hospital infrastructures as well as technological aspects (Ahmed, 2025; Leiva & Castro, 2025). Future healthcare systems will be secure, interoperable, and patient-centered because of the ongoing research and advancements that guarantee blockchain's relevance is being simplified despite the current challenges. Blockchain can support the establishment of strong, dependable, and transparent healthcare systems by keeping consideration of both technological and ethical factors (Abbas et al., 2022; Arbabi et al., 2022; Saeed et al., 2022; Yaqoob et al., 2022).

2. BLOCKCHAIN FUNDAMENTALS IN HEALTHCARE

2.1 Understanding Blockchain in the Healthcare Context

A blockchain is a distributed ledger technology that allows recording of transactions in a safe, transparent, and unalterable way in numerous nodes. In contrast to conventional central databases, blockchain results in the absence of single points of failure and the integrity of the data. This is considered by consensus mechanism (Dong et al., 2023). This architecture is specifically useful in a healthcare environment since medical data is extremely sensitive. It is often shared as well as regulated among institutions (Abbas et al., 2022; Arbabi et al., 2022).

Cyberattack susceptibility and non-interoperable data silos are two additional challenges faced by healthcare systems. The blockchain solution can assist in overcoming these difficulties by providing a decentralized system that enables secure and transparent handling of patient information, clinical trial data, and supply chain of pharmaceutical businesses(Saeed et al., 2022; Yaqoob et al., 2022). Because of its encryption, data cannot be altered without consent after it has been saved, protecting against fraud and unauthorized changes (Attaran, 2022).

Figure 1. Blockchain as a foundational framework for smart healthcare ecosystem

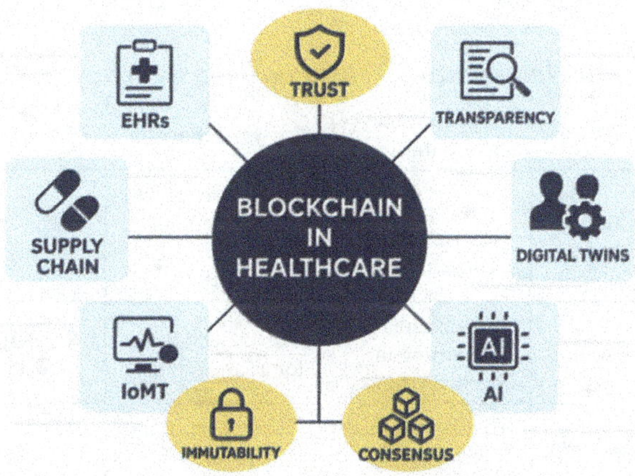

Figure 1 depicts that blockchain supports the modernization of healthcare systems. The key characteristics of blockchain are decentralisation, consensus mechanism, transparency, and immutability by embedding into all aspects of healthcare. For example, these are implemented through Electronic Health Records (EHRs), clinical trials, and pharmaceutical supply chain management and cyber security in smart hospitals. The outer layer illustrates how blockchain integrates with new and emerging technologies such as IoT, AI, Digital Twins, and the Metaverse. These technologies enable secure and real-time monitoring of patients using predictive analytics and immersive experience of clinical care. This illustrates the importance of blockchain in creating patient-centric, interoperable and ethically managed healthcare systems (Abbas et al., 2022; Emma & Adams, 2025; Nguyen et al., 2025).

2.2 Trust as a Foundational Principle

The foundation of healthcare delivery is trust. It includes patient faith in the clinicians, provider confidence in the useful data, and the institution's accountability. Because blockchain integrates accountability and transparency into the data management system, it raises the degree of confidence. These concerns will be reduced since patients will have control over who receives their records, when, and why (Hasselgren et al., 2021; Velmovitsky et al., 2021). This auditability improves patient-provider relationships and fosters confidence in digital health infrastructures. The blockchain system ensures that no alteration is done on trial data hence preserving scientific integrity and establishing trust among the participants and regulators (Emma & Adams, 2025; Leiva & Castro, 2025). Also, blockchain is decentralized, which removes the dependence on third parties, which limits the possibility of corruption and manipulation (V. Ali et al., 2023).

Table 1. Blockchain in Healthcare – Trust and Transparency

Reference	Focus Area	Transparency Contribution	Trust Mechanism	Limitations	Key Application
(Hasselgren et al., 2021)	Virtual healthcare	Transparent virtual consultations	Proof-of-concept blockchain for patient-provider trust	Early-stage prototype	Telemedicine
(Velmovitsky et al., 2021)	Public health	Transparent reporting in health systems	Distributed ledger for accountability	Scalability issues	Public health monitoring
(Emma & Adams, 2025)	Clinical trials	Transparent trial data sharing	Immutable trial records	Regulatory adoption	Clinical research
(Leiva & Castro, 2025)	Clinical trials + AI	Transparent trial oversight	Blockchain + AI governance	Integration complexity	Data governance
(V. Ali et al., 2023)	Blockchain characteristics	Transparency via consensus	Trust through decentralization	Conceptual framework	General healthcare

Table 1 demonstrates the function of blockchain in healthcare. It is to provide increased transparency and build trust in multiple areas such as telemedicine, public health, clinical trials, etc. Transparency can be provided by utilizing characteristics of blockchain technology for example, immutable records, distributed ledgers, consensus mechanisms, while trust can be established by using characteristics of blockchain technology such as decentralisation, accountability, and governance models.

2.3 Transparency in Medical Data Management

The distributed registry of blockchain offers irreversible logs of every interaction and allows governmental bodies to ensure that the regulation is followed, including HIPAA and GDPR (Singh et al., 2022; Villarreal et al., 2023). This visibility is especially essential in intelligent hospital systems, where various systems, such as sensors in the IoT, AI-driven diagnostic applications, and so forth, need to communicate with each other seamlessly and hold them accountable.

Transparency is another way to create interoperability. Because different systems may communicate data utilizing secure blockchain-based frameworks, the distributed system can be utilized to establish consistency across providers and institutions (Hussain et al., 2023; Tahir et al., 2024). For example, blockchain-enabled interoperability can be applied in emergency care scenarios where prompt access to accurate patient histories is essential. Transparency enhances patient safety and reduces the possibility of fake medications in pharmaceutical supply chains (Akram et al., 2024; Kavinraja & Mithula, 2025).

2.4 Immutability and Data Integrity

Immutability is the key feature of blockchain technology. The validity of medical records throughout time is ensured by their inability to make any modifications after data collection (Ngabo et al., 2021; Zaabar et al., 2021). This quality is crucial in the healthcare industry, where accurate longitudinal data is essential for appropriate treatment, research, and policy development. Unchangeable records lower risks by ensuring that fraud, malpractice, and inadvertent errors are minimized (Chen et al., 2024). In order to preserve scientific integrity, immutability also ensures that no patient information or trial outcomes will be changed in clinical trials (Emma & Adams, 2025). Hospitals may model patient outcomes and improve resource allocation in IoMT applications by using digital twins with immutable sensor data logs and predictive analytics (Ghadi et al., 2024; Ramani et al., 2024).

Table 2. Blockchain for Immutability and Data Integrity

Reference	Data Integrity Approach	Healthcare Use Case	Immutability Mechanism	Challenges	Security Strength
(Taherdoost, 2023)	Medical data sharing	Patient record exchange	Cryptographic hashing	Adoption barriers	Strong immutability
(Masood et al., 2024)	Patient privacy	Patient data security	Immutable audit logs	Storage scalability	High
(Hovorushchenko, Moskalenko, & Osyadlyi, 2023)	Data management methods	Medical data lifecycle	Block linking	Complexity of deployment	Reliable
(Singh et al., 2022)	Efficient data management	Hospital data systems	Tamper-proof records	Regulatory compliance	Moderate
(Tahir et al., 2024)	Records management framework	Interoperable EHR	Permissioned blockchain	Integration with legacy systems	Strong

Table 2 illustrates how blockchain will ensure immutability and integrity of data in healthcare by using a combination of mechanisms; including cryptographic hashing, audit logs, linking blocks into chains, tamper-proof records, and permissioned frameworks. Each of these mechanisms will enhance trust in the exchange of patient data, privacy protection, and hospital system management by providing security against tampering and unauthorized modifications of records. However, various adoption barriers and technical, institutional, and regulatory challenges must be overcome to achieve seamless implementation of blockchain applications. In summary, blockchain technologies can provide robust security and reliability.

In figure 2, the use of blockchain technology is represented to provide a decentralized, secure backbone for the exchange of medical records among various stakeholders such as patients, physicians, laboratory workers, pharmacists, data analysts, and health insurance providers. Each of these stakeholders is able to use the blockchain for their own unique and important roles: patients use the blockchain to obtain medical recommendations and give permission to view their data; physicians use the blockchain to make clinical decisions based on an unaltered history of patient records; laboratory workers provide authenticated test results to physicians and patients; pharmacists provide verified prescriptions through the blockchain; data analysts utilize the blockchain's available audit trails to identify trends, and health insurance providers utilize smart contract technology for administering policies. The trust, transparency, and security that are inherent in blockchain solutions will be applied to medical records in order to prevent fraud, ensure accountability, and promote ethical governance among all stakeholders involved in the medical record industry. This stakeholder-centric framework is consistent in regard to the development of interoperable systems, consent management systems, and the secure integration of AI, IoT, and Digital Twins into an overall cohesive environment (V. Ali et al., 2023; Ezz et al., 2025; Velmovitsky et al., 2021).

Figure 2. Stakeholder-centric Blockchain integration in Smart Healthcare Systems

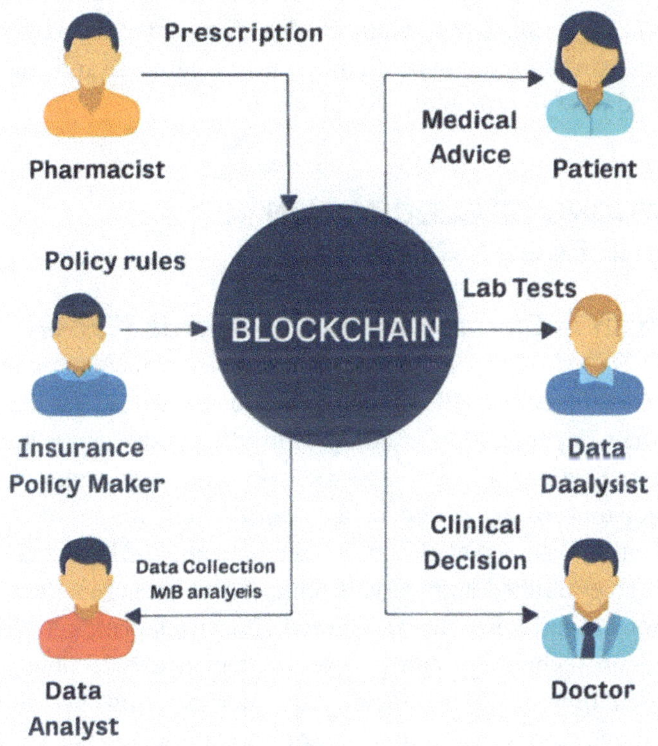

2.5 Integration with IoT, AI, and Digital Twins

The incorporation of blockchain to IoT, AI, and digital twins is one of the frontiers of smart hospital systems. The IoT gadgets provide a steady flow of patient data, which is to be defended against interference and hacking. Blockchain is also a decentralized model of storing and verifying such data, which is reliable and trustworthy (Alam et al., 2023; Khan et al., 2023). Digital twins, the virtual projections of physical systems, need the correct and reliable information to model hospital processes and patient outcomes. Blockchain verifies and immutably stores the data that powers these simulations (V. Ali et al., 2023; Nguyen et al., 2025). For example, a blockchain-protected digital twin in hospital may replicate patient flow, resource distribution, and critical situations with the assurance that the underlying data is of the highest caliber.

Blockchain has reliable datasets in AI-driven analytics as well. Blockchain improves the credibility of AI models applied in the field of diagnostics and treatment planning by eliminating the risks of errors in training data and protecting it from manipulation (Jadav et al., 2023). Combined with explainable AI and blockchain, the metaverse can provide patients with immersive healthcare and guarantee patient data security and trust (S. Ali et al., 2023).

3. APPLICATIONS OF BLOCKCHAIN IN HEALTHCARE ECOSYSTEMS

3.1 Blockchain in Electronic Health Records (EHRs)

Electronic Health Records (EHRs) are the foundation of contemporary healthcare systems, but their dependability is compromised by issues with interoperability, privacy, and data fragmentation. The blockchain offers a decentralized EHR management solution that ensures patient data is confidential, immutable, and accessible to authorized entities (Ngabo et al., 2021; Zaabar et al., 2021). Because blockchain does not require centralized authority, it reduces the danger of data breaches and illegal alterations by utilizing the distributed consensus principle (Masood et al., 2024). Blockchain technology can be used to enhance EHR interoperability. A blockchain-based approach to healthcare data interoperability which makes it easier for data to move across institutions and protects patient privacy (Hussain et al., 2023). In similar fashion, Tahir et al. (2024) have developed a blockchain-based approach for managing medical records that can enhance interoperability, security, and privacy(Tahir et al., 2024).

Figure 3 shows flowchart begins at Patient/Doctor interaction and ends with the storage of the medical data as EHRs. Once created, EHRs undergo a process of defining customized access control and storing them within a centralized repository. Next, using blockchain technology, the medical data via an EHR will be secured (immutability, auditability, and privacy) with scalable cloud based storage of EHRs so that the healthcare provider can access the medical data through permissioned channels. Overall, the flowchart and life cycle processes show how blockchain technology is becoming the transformative enabler of secure, interoperable, and patient centric EHR systems (Masood et al., 2024; Ngabo et al., 2021).

Figure 3. Electronic Health Records (EHRs) in a blockchain-based Healthcare System.

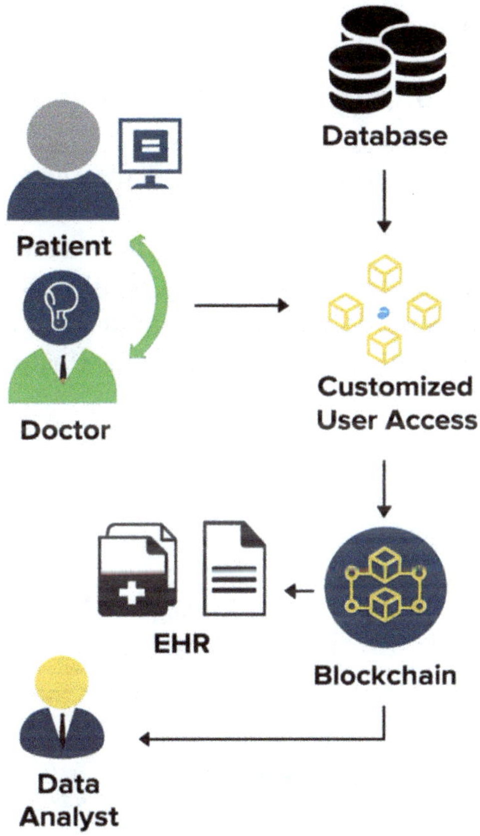

3.2 Clinical Trials and Research Data Integrity

Clinical trials play a vital role in the further development of medical knowledge, but they are also characterized by issues with the integrity of data, its transparency, and the confidence of patients. Blockchain can make sure that data of a trial is unrestricted thus eliminating manipulation and instilling confidence among participants and regulators (Emma & Adams, 2025). Unalterably recorded records ensure that once the results of a trial are documented, no one is able to modify them and ensure scientific integrity and ethical practices (Leiva & Castro, 2025). Transparency of clinical trials can also be improved by blockchain which offers auditable data collection, data analysis and reporting records. This openness limits the risks of selective disclosure and enhances regulation (Velmovitsky et al., 2021). Moreover, the smart contracts enabled by blockchain can be used to automate the consent management process, in which patients are in control of their data but are involved in trials (Ezz et al., 2025). These apps demonstrate how blockchain can transform clinical research by integrating trust and transparency in all phases of the procedure.

3.3 Pharmaceutical Supply Chain Management

Counterfeit drugs are a great risk to the health of the patients and the population. Blockchain is a transparent and unchangeable system that handles pharmaceutical distribution through the producer to the patient and could minimize the chances of fraud and guarantee authenticity (Akram et al., 2024). Blockchain allows stakeholders to confirm the provenance of drugs and monitor the allegations in real time by registering every activity in the supply chain on a distributed registry (Kavinraja & Mithula, 2025).

Figure 4. Pharmaceutical Supply Chain Management

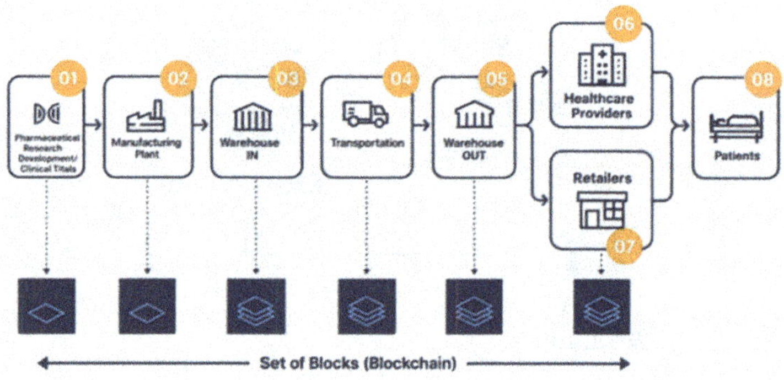

The blockchain-related solutions to supply chain management also increase regulatory compliance, as they offer auditory records of drug distribution. The compliance with the safety standards can be checked, and violations can be detected using these records, which strengthen the accountability throughout the supply chain (Singh et al., 2022). Furthermore, integration with IoT-powered containers can be used to monitor the state of drug storage in real-time so that pharmaceuticals could be transported and stored in the most favorable conditions (Alam et al., 2023). Collectively, these apps illustrate how blockchain could be used in the future to protect the pharmaceutical supply chains and ensure patient well-being.

Figure 4 demonstrates how blockchain technology improves visibility, tracking ability, and security throughout each phase of the healthcare supply chain - from Pharmaceutical R&D to Patient Delivery - in an easy-to-understand manner. The eight stages in the healthcare supply chain correspond to blocks within the blockchain, therefore providing an immutable record of important data points related to each phase (Clinical Trials, Manufacturing, Warehousing, Transportation, and Retail) as well as enabling a secure connection between these points. Because all stages are linked via the blockchain, a clear, tampering-proof view of the product's life cycle will be available, thereby preventing the possibility of counterfeit products entering the healthcare supply chain, supporting compliance with regulatory agencies, and creating trust between Healthcare Providers and Patients.

3.4 Internet of Medical Things (IoMT) and Remote Monitoring

IoMT includes wearable devices, sensors, and remote monitoring systems which produce constant patient data streams. Although the IoMT positively impacts healthcare delivery because it allows real-time monitoring, it provokes the issue of data safety and privacy. Blockchain can be used to solve these issues through its decentralized design of IoMT data storage and verification (Ghadi et al., 2024; Khan et al., 2023).

Figure 5. Blockchain-based Remote Healthcare Monitoring System using IoMT

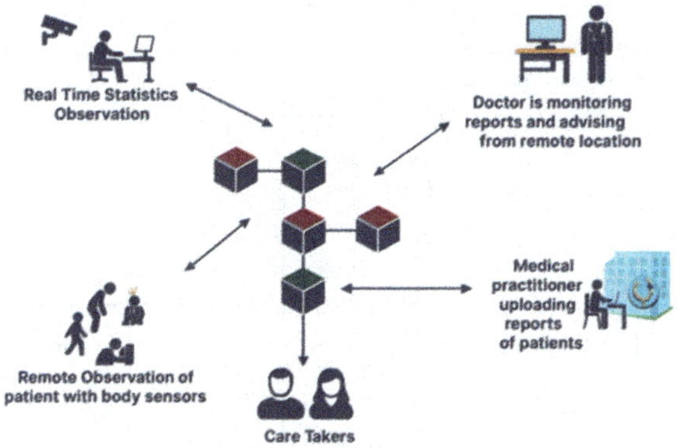

Unchangeable blockchain documents make sensor data immutable, which facilitates predictive analytics and digital twin simulations (Ramani et al., 2024). As an example, the model of patient outcomes and optimization of hospital resources that can be made with the help of blockchain-secured IoMT data. Alam et al. (2023) stated that blockchain-IoT represents the key to effective and safe monitoring of health records, and it can help to increase trust and transparency in remote healthcare systems(Alam et al., 2023).

Figure 5 shows blockchain-based remote healthcare monitoring system using IoMT. It enables continual access to patient records through a centralized data network and allows for the sharing of information between all parties involved in a patient's care. Body sensors monitor the health condition of patients and send live metrics directly to a central system. Physicians post diagnostic reports into the central system that can be viewed by a remote physician who will typically analyse the data from the report and offer suggestions or recommendations for follow-up care. Caregivers will receive continual updates and/or instructions to follow in providing appropriate care, and analysts will monitor the live reports for all patients to facilitate intervention if required. The interconnectivity of the various systems provides for improved efficiency, extended periods of proactive care, and ongoing monitoring of patients without the need to have the patient present at the office for continuous monitoring.

Table 3. Blockchain Integration with Smart Hospital Infrastructures

Reference	Blockchain Contribution	IoT Role	Integration Focus	Smart Hospital Application	Limitations
(Alam et al., 2023)	Secure health record streams	IoT sensors for monitoring	IoT integration	Real-time patient monitoring	Energy consumption
(Ghadi et al., 2024)	Blockchain-secured IoMT	Internet of Medical Things	IoMT security	Device-to-cloud security	Latency issues
(Ramani et al., 2024)	Blockchain for secure FL	IoMT data aggregation	Federated learning	AI-driven hospital analytics	Computational overhead
(Khan et al., 2023)	Blockchain for data security	IIoT devices	Industrial IoT	Smart hospital infrastructure	Network complexity
(Raja, 2021, 2024; Raja, Vigneashwaran, Rohan, Praveen, & Vijay, 2025)	Blockchain for adaptive systems	IoT-enabled systems	Industry 4.0 + IoT	Smart hospital + sanitation monitoring	Implementation cost

Table 3 shows the blockchain integration with smart hospital infrastructures. The combination of IoT and IoMT systems integrated with the hospital smart infrastructure and blockchain enhances security, integrity of data, and interoperability. Blockchain provides support for secure streaming of health information (electronic health records). It provides a secure link between IoMT medical devices and the cloud with federated learning to develop AI-based analytics and adaptive systems to support Industry 4.0 applications. Blockchain also allows for real-time monitoring, advanced analytics, and the ability to manage sanitation. However, like all technology, blockchain solutions present several barriers including high energy consumption, latency, computational overhead, increased network complexity and higher costs to develop. Blockchain is positioned as a trust anchor in the smart hospital. It creates secure and transparent flow of information when combined with IoMT. However, Blockchain must also be optimized for IoT to improve efficiency and address challenges relating to scalability and cost to achieve sustainable use.

3.5 Blockchain in Telemedicine and Virtual Healthcare

Telemedicine has become an indispensable part of the healthcare delivery system, especially after the world had to face the global health crises. Blockchain ensures that the data of telemedicine is managed through a secure and transparent system that guarantees that the consultations with patients and medical records are kept confidential and irrevocable (Hasselgren et al., 2021).

The trust in virtual healthcare is also improved as blockchain has records that are auditable in relation to consultations and treatment. Patients can confirm that their information is used in accordance with the established norms, and providers can prove that they meet the regulatory requirements (Velmovitsky et al., 2021). Furthermore, administration, billing, and insurance claim can be automated through smart contracts based on blockchain. It reduces administrative workloads and thereby enhances efficiency (Chen et al., 2024).

4. BLOCKCHAIN ARCHITECTURES AND CONSENSUS MECHANISMS IN HEALTHCARE SYSTEMS

4.1 Blockchain Architectures for Healthcare

There are several main types of blockchain systems, namely, the public, the private, and the consortium blockchain, each providing a unique set of benefits and drawbacks to the healthcare setting. Public blockchains (like Ethereum) are open and highly transparent, but due to scalability and privacy issues when dealing with sensitive medical information, they are not as scalable and transparent as they need to be (Dong et al., 2023). Single organization controlled private blockchains are more efficient and provide more privacy, but can undermine decentralization and trust (Attaran, 2022). Lying somewhere between the two is the consortium blockchains, which can be controlled by multiple institutions and offers a way to establish collaborative governance, securing their safety and transparency (Arbabi et al., 2022).

Permissioned blockchains are usually preferred in healthcare applications, as they limit someone to authorized participants. Permissioned systems give hospitals, insurers and regulators the ability to share data safely without breaching privacy laws like HIPAA and GDPR (Masood et al., 2024; Villarreal et al., 2023). Healthcare has been one of the sectors to adopt frameworks like Hyperledger Fabric because it is modular and can support customizable consensus protocols (Ngabo et al., 2021).

Figure 6. Blockchain Integration in Healthcare Data Management

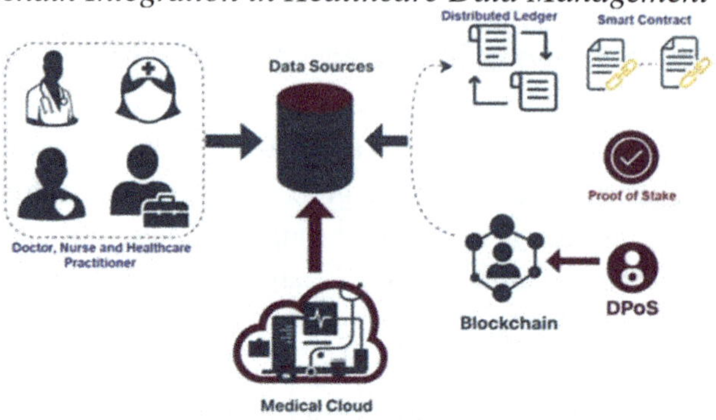

Figure 6 exhibits how to implement secure connections between healthcare data management inputs from practitioners, their patients & administrative staff into a unified area of storage an electronic lot of medical data using blockchain technology. Using distributed ledgers, and smart contracts, blockchain technology is utilized for ally providing tamper-resistance, transparency and easy sharing of electronic medical data among all parties involved. Additionally, the blockchain technology provides all stakeholders with the method of receiving realtime access having integrity and trust with respect to healthcare transactions emerging from the application of the blockchain technology in the medical and today's' digital health networks.

4.2 Consensus Mechanisms in Healthcare Blockchain

The consensus mechanisms play an important role in the verification of transaction by ensuring that blockchain systems are secure. Conventional methods like Proof of Work (PoW) are not energy efficient and cannot support healthcare-related uses that are efficient and scalable (Wenhua et al., 2023). Other alternatives like Proof of Stake (PoS) and Delegated Proof of Stake (DPoS) are more efficient and can cause the issue of centralization (Chen et al., 2024).

Practical Byzantine Fault Tolerance (PBFT) and Proof of Authority (PoA) are becoming more popular as healthcare applications because they are faster to validate transactions, and suited best to permissioned blockchains (Taherdoost, 2023). PBFT is a consensus mechanism that can tolerate malicious nodes, which is why it is best suited to healthcare networks where reliability and trust are the most important qualities (Zaabar et al., 2021). To achieve integrity and minimize computational overhead, PoA utilizes trusted validators, including hospitals or regulatory authorities(Singh et al., 2022). Upcoming consensus models, including ZeroTrust permissioned blockchain models, take the security and privacy to the next level by reducing the use of trusted sources (Thantharate & Thantharate, 2023).

4.3 Smart Contracts and Automated Governance

Smart contracts are code agreements that can execute themselves and are stored in the blockchain making it possible to automate healthcare processes including consent management, billing, and insurance claims. Smart contracts eliminate bureaucracy by incorporating rules into the blockchain and increasing transparency (Chen et al., 2024). As an illustration, data sharing may be allowed by patients using smart contracts so that their choices may be honored and tracked (Ezz et al., 2025).

Interoperability is also made possible with the help of smart contracts that allow the automatic exchange of data between institutions. Hussain et al. (2023) showed how smart contracts could be used to share data safely and not contradict the privacy regulations(Hussain et al., 2023). In the same vein, Jadav et al. (2023), put forward an effective healthcare management platform that incorporates AI and blockchain via smart contracts, which contributes to the reliability and effectiveness(Jadav et al., 2023).

4.4 Privacy-Preserving Architectures

Although blockchain provides a sense of immutability, it leaves the issue of sensitive medical data stored on public ledgers. Off-chain storage, encryption, and zero-knowledge proofs are some of the methods used in privacy-preserving architectures to reduce this challenge. Off-chain storage enables the storage of sensitive data externally and blockchain retains metadata and access logs, so that transparency but privacy is not compromised (Masood et al., 2024). Encryption allows only authorized parties to read medical records whereas zero-knowledge proofs allow verification without exposing underlying data (Ezz et al., 2025). Permissioned blockchains also improve privacy even more, as only authorized participants can access the blockchain. ZeroTrust frameworks are crucial to privacy and interoperability(Thantharate & Thantharate, 2023). These architectures are in line with the ethical considerations of healthcare and they strike a balance between immutability and patient autonomy and confidentiality.

4.5 Scalability and Performance Considerations

One of the key issues facing the healthcare blockchain systems is scalability. Healthcare produces large amounts of data, both EHRs and IoMT sensor streams, and imaging records, which can surpass the current processing capacity of blockchain(Dong et al., 2023). PBFT and PoA are consensus mechanisms that enhance efficiency, though they may experience challenges with huge deployments (Wenhua et al., 2023). The solutions will allow processing off-chain and preserve the security and immutability of blockchain (Nguyen et al., 2025). As an example, the processing of IoMT data can be performed off-chain and anchored to the blockchain periodically, which will provide integrity without overloading the system (Ghadi et al., 2024). These hybrid systems are essential in the extension of blockchain to satisfy the requirements of smart hospital systems.

4.6 Interoperability Frameworks

Blockchain-based systems facilitate exchange of data between institutions with security, consistency and reliability (Hussain et al., 2023; Tahir et al., 2024). Villarreal et al. (2023) noted that interoperability is a crucial concept in healthcare management systems, and blockchain can help address the issue of fragmentation(Villarreal et al., 2023). Interoperability standards like HL7 FHIR (Fast Healthcare Interoperability Resources) can be combined with blockchain to improve the interoperability. With the blockchain immutability and the standardized data format, healthcare systems could attain a smooth exchange of data without losing the regulatory compliance(Singh et al., 2022). These systems play a pivotal role in facilitating shared healthcare systems that place the patient at the center.

5. ROLE OF DIGITAL TWIN – BLOCKCHAIN INTEGRATION IN HEALTHCARE

The combination of blockchain technology and digital twin technology create one of the most innovative pathways forward for the smart health care ecosystem. Digital twins, or a virtual replica of a physical asset, process or state of a patient, are based upon dependable, continual and safe feeding of real-time data in order to function properly. Blockchain's decentralised, immutable and transparent architecture provides trust layer through which the authenticity and integrity of the digital twin data feeds are guaranteed and thus allows hospitals to advance towards predictive, patient-centered and resilient healthcare infrastructure (Ababio et al., 2025).

5.1 Foundations of Integration

A digital twin used in healthcare to simulate real patient physiology and hospital missions/manage use of time and resources. Thereby it achieves desired treatment outcomes based on the ingestion of real-time data from IoMT devices, EHR's and clinical data systems. However, the level of accuracy that any digital twin can provide in regards to the patient simulation is determined by the fidelity of the data that has been used to simulate the actual patient, (Badakhshan & Ivanov, 2025). Blockchain establishes immutable and auditable evidence for sensor readings, diagnostic reports and patient histories, thus facilitating the elimination of risk of altering or tampering with the data, (Ellahi et al., 2026). Through this integration, a credible digital ecosystem is established providing both the clinician using the digital twin outputs to make informed decisions and patients with confidence that the data being used to represent them is safe, secure and real time is being managed in a transparent manner (Kang, 2026).

5.2 Enhancing Predictive Analytics and Resource Optimization

Digital twins rely heavily on predictive analytics for their implementation. By utilizing models representing patient journeys, bed occupancy in hospitals or efficacy of medication, healthcare organisations can use predictive analytics to make better resource allocation decisions based on anticipated outcomes, (Khalifa & Marzouk, 2025). Blockchain technology enhances these efforts by offering long-functions longitudinal databases that feed predictive algorithms without risk of alteration from third parties; for example, through utilizing IoMT data logs to predict when a patient is likely to deteriorate and therefore would require preemptive intervention from a healthcare provider(Ramani et al., 2024). Additionally, using blockchain to secure digital twins of hospital infrastructure enables hospitals to simulate potential emergencies and develop appropriate response plans, ultimately providing improved preparedness and resiliency in their ability to handle crisis situations (Varriale, Michelino, & Godinho-Filho, 2026).

5.3 Patient-Centric Data Governance

Another major challenge associated with using digital twins in healthcare is data governance; specifically, determining who owns access to the data generated by a digital twin, whether that be a patient, an institution or otherwise, and how. Blockchain technology addresses this challenge through the use of smart contracts and permissioned ledgers, allowing patients to define specific, granular rules governing who may have access to their respective digital health profile(s)(Ezz et al.,

2025). By implementing these tools, an organisation can ensure that digital twin simulations conducted using a patient's data respect that individual's privacy and autonomy while also being transferable so they can be shared with another institution. Furthermore, in clinical trials, the use of blockchain and digital twins will allow for greater transparency in reporting of a clinical trial's outcomes, thereby increasing their integrity as well as compliance with established regulatory processes such as Good Clinical Practices(Kang, 2026).

5.4 Integration with AI and IoMT

Blockchain, Digital Twin, AI, and IoMT, when combined create a multilevel ecosystem within the healthcare system. IoMT devices produce continuous streams of patient data to the Blockchain, which allows for the securing, authentication, and verification of these inputs through the use of Digital Twin models for AI-based predictive analytics. This multilevel approach supports applications such as personalized treatment planning, remote patient monitoring, and immersive healthcare experiences in the Metaverse. Trust in recommended diagnoses will be improved due to Explainable AI models using blockchain-based verified datasets, and zero-knowledge proofs for the ethical exchange of sensitive patient data.

The use of blockchain and the development of new technologies, including AI, digital twins, metaverse, and so on widen the scope of blockchain in healthcare. Analytics based on AI take advantage of the credible datasets of blockchain to increase the validity of diagnostic and predictive models (Jadav et al., 2023). Digital twins which model the behavior of the hospital and patient results are based on blockchain-secured information to guarantee authenticity and accuracy (Nguyen et al., 2025). Explainable AI and blockchain combined with the metaverse provide patients with immersive healthcare experiences and patient data security and trust (S. Ali et al., 2023). These integrations underscore the use of blockchain as a base technology in smart hospital systems that can be harnessed to develop new applications that improve patient quality and efficiency in operations.

Blockchain is used to manage medical data in terms of security, auditing, and patient-centered data through EHRs and clinical trials, pharmaceutical supply chains, and IoMT. Its application in new technologies, including AI, digital twins, and the metaverse further increases its contribution to smart hospital infrastructures. Although there are still some difficulties, continuous research and development also make blockchain more applicable, which means that the future healthcare system will be safe, interoperable, and regulated by ethical standards (Abbas et al., 2022; Arbabi et al., 2022; Saeed et al., 2022; Yaqoob et al., 2022).

6. POLICY IMPLICATIONS OF DIGITAL TWINS AND BLOCKCHAIN IN HEALTHCARE

6.1 Evolving Landscape of Healthcare Digitalization

The combination of blockchain, IoT, AI, and digital twins is causing rapid digitalization of healthcare systems around the globe. Ecosystems that enhance trust, transparency, and immutability as the main tenets of managing medical data will shape the future of healthcare (Abbas et al., 2022; Arbabi et al., 2022). The use of blockchain is likely to be at the centre stage in facilitating secure, interoperable, and patient-centric infrastructures especially in smart hospitals with real-time data interchange and predictive analytics playing a central role (Taherdoost, 2025). The policy frameworks should also keep pace with these technological developments in order to make sure that blockchain implementation is in tandem with the ethics, regulations, and expectations of the society. Governments, healthcare organizations, and technology companies should cooperate to create the rules that will ensure a balance between innovation and patient privacy and data security (Attaran, 2022; Villarreal et al., 2023).

6.2 Enhancing Interoperability across Healthcare Systems

Interoperability is one of the most urgent issues in healthcare. The opportunities of blockchain to provide a decentralized solution to facilitate smooth exchange of data among institutions have a way forward in the future, however, it has to work on ways of integrating blockchain with current standards like HL7 FHIR (Singh et al., 2022). The implementation of interoperability frameworks that make use of blockchain immutability and at the same time adhere to regulations, including HIPAA and GDPR, should be encouraged with the use of policy initiatives (Hussain et al., 2023; Tahir et al., 2024). Future studies in this area ought to discuss the use of hybrid architectures that integrate blockchain with federated learning and off-chain storage in order to improve scalability and interoperability (Ramani et al., 2024). These strategies will facilitate the healthcare systems to process large amounts of data without affecting trust and transparency.

6.3 Privacy-Preserving Innovations

In healthcare systems based on blockchain, privacy is an essential issue. Although immutability guarantees data integrity, the use of immutability also brings into question cases of sensitive medical data being stored without breaching confidentiality. The future trends should be privacy-conscious technologies, including zero-knowledge proofs, homomorphic encryption, and permissioned blockchain (Ezz et al., 2025).

The policy frameworks are to be required to use privacy-preserving architectures in order to make sure that the adoption of blockchain does not interfere with the autonomy of the patients. One of such ways is to have patients to be in control of who has access to their data and in what cases, facilitated by a consent management system based on blockchain (Masood et al., 2024). Models of ethical governance need to incorporate transparency and accountability into the practice of sharing data and make sure privacy is maintained without compromising trust (S. Ali et al., 2023).

6.4 Blockchain and Digital Twins in Smart Hospitals

Digital twins constitute a paradigm shift of blockchain in healthcare. Digital twins can be used to predict resource distribution, patient outcomes, and emergency response by creating virtual simulations of hospital infrastructure and conditions. The blockchain makes sure that the information that supplies these simulations is original, open, and unalterable (V. Ali et al., 2023; Nguyen et al., 2025). The recent research is based on the concept of combining blockchain-secured digital twins with IoMT gadgets and AI-based analytics. This type of systems will allow smart hospitals to be highly efficient, resilient, and patient-centered (Ghadi et al., 2024; Ramani et al., 2024). These innovations have to be supported by policy frameworks through the provision of standards of authenticity of data, interoperability and ethical governance.

6.5 Blockchain in Clinical Trials and Research Governance

Clinical trials will also become more and more dependent on blockchain to guarantee the integrity of the data, its transparency, and the quality of patient confidence. The records of trial data will be immutable, and it will be impossible to manipulate it, enhancing regulatory control (Emma & Adams, 2025; Leiva & Castro, 2025). Smart contracts can be used to manage consent and, through this, patients are expected to maintain control over their information even when being part of a trial (Ezz et al., 2025). Policy frameworks should create a set of rules about research governance that is supported by blockchain and also make transparency and accountability integrated in all phases of research (Velmovitsky et al., 2021).

6.6 Pharmaceutical Supply Chain and Drug Safety

The use of blockchain in pharmaceutical supply chains is going to expand further in the future. Clear and unalterable records of drugs distribution will decrease the possibility of counterfeit drugs and increase patient safety (Akram et al., 2024). It will be supplemented by integration with IoT-enabled containers to monitor real-time when storing drugs and to ensure their safety (Kavinraja & Mithula, 2025). The policy frameworks must require the use of blockchain in pharmaceutical supply chains as a measure to improve accountability and transparency. The regulatory authorities should develop the criteria of blockchain to track drugs, and the patients should be provided with the original and safe drugs (Singh et al., 2022).

6.7 Ethical and Regulatory Considerations

One of the most important aspects of healthcare blockchain systems is governance, which includes decision-making, accountability, and ethical control. Cryptocurrency blockchains allow shared governance with many institutions taking part in the processes of decision-making (Arbabi et al., 2022). This model is where only one person does not dominate the system which promotes trust and transparency. The use of blockchain in ethical governance helps ensure that there is a record of consent and data use that is auditable (Ezz et al., 2025). Zero-knowledge proofs and smart contracts also improve compliance with ethics since selective data sharing and automated implementation of patient preferences become possible (Thantharate & Thantharate, 2023). The regulatory frameworks should be developed to meet the special issues of blockchain. The adoption of blockchains should have rules that are balanced to promote innovation and patient privacy and data security (Attaran, 2022). International cooperation will play a pivotal role in the harmonization of regulatory standards in different jurisdictions so that international operability and trust occur (Villarreal et al., 2023).

6.8 Scalability and Technological Innovation

One of the greatest obstacles to blockchain use in healthcare is scalability. Future studies must be aimed at coming up with consensus mechanisms and layer-2 solutions that are more efficient without jeopardizing the security (Dong et al., 2023; Wenhua et al., 2023). Blockchain-based hybrid architectures with off-chain storage and federated learning also provide a promising way to increase the scale (Ramani et al., 2024). The appearance of new technologies, including AI, IoMT, and the metaverse, will also be incorporated through technological innovation into blockchain. Blockchain will provide AI-based analytics with reliable datasets, whereas IoMT devices will be based on blockchain to ensure a secure communication channel and data storage (Alam et al., 2023; Khan et al., 2023). When used with explainable AI and blockchain, the metaverse will provide patients with immersive healthcare experiences and guarantee the safety and reliability of patient data(S. Ali et al., 2023).

6.9 Strategic Outlook for Smart Hospital Infrastructures

Smart hospital infrastructures and integration of blockchain into them define the strategic outlook of the blockchain in the healthcare sector. The IoMT devices, blockchain-secured digital twins, and AI-driven analytics will allow hospitals to work at a higher level of efficiency, resilience, and patient-centricity (Ghadi et al., 2024; Nguyen et al., 2025). The decentralized structure of blockchain offers the basis of international healthcare ecologies, which emphasize the importance of trust, transparency, and immutability (Saeed et al., 2022; Yaqoob et al., 2022).

The future of blockchain in healthcare is that it allows establishing trust and transparency and can establish immutability in the management of medical data. It is integrated with digital twins, IoMT, AI, and the metaverse, which places it as a foundation of smart infrastructures within hospitals. Political frameworks are to be changed in order to address the use of blockchain so that innovation should not contradict ethical principles, legal obligations, and patient rights. Blockchain may facilitate the development of resilient, trustful, and patient-centered healthcare ecosystems by solving some of the key challenges of the healthcare industry: scalability, privacy, and interoperability (Abbas et al., 2022; Arbabi et al., 2022; Saeed et al., 2022; Yaqoob et al., 2022).

7. CHALLENGES AND FUTURE DIRECTIONS

7.1 Challenges and Limitations

The adoption of blockchain in healthcare is not easy, despite its potential. Scalability is a challenge, with the healthcare system will produce large amounts of data that can be beyond the processing capacity of blockchain (Dong et al., 2023; Wenhua et al., 2023). Another reason why this cannot be widely implemented is energy consumption, latency, and storage requirements. Implementing blockchain to work with existing systems involves high costs and organization change (Atadoga et al., 2024). Privacy is another challenging issue. Blockchain makes data modification impossible, but also raises the issue of how sensitive medical data may be kept without compromising confidentiality. Among the strategies being considered to strike a compromise between immutability and privacy include off-chain storage, encryption, and permissioned blockchains (Masood et al., 2024). The application of blockchain in healthcare governance is further hampered by additional ethical concerns including informed consent and equitable access (Ezz et al., 2025).

Nevertheless, blockchain use in healthcare is not as easy as it sounds:

- ***Scalability:*** Blockchain might not be able to process large amounts of healthcare data at present (Dong et al., 2023; Wenhua et al., 2023).
- ***Integration:*** Old and regulatory systems will need to be modified to meet the decentralized nature of blockchain (Atadoga et al., 2024).
- ***Latency:*** Real-time simulation of Digital Twins would require very low latency in data exchange which could be delayed through the use of Consensus Protocols [31].
- ***Interoperability:*** Integrating Blockchain with existing Hospital Systems and the multitude of different types of IoMT Devices is complicated [17].
- ***Privacy:*** It is important to find new ways to balance immutability with confidentiality, which is achieved through encryption and permissioned access (Masood et al., 2024).
- ***Ethical Issues:*** According to Ezz et al. (2025), patient-centric governance requires informed consent and fair access(Ezz et al., 2025).

These challenges will have to be tackled to ensure maximum potential of blockchain in healthcare is achieved. Emerging Solutions toward overcoming these obstacles include utilizing Lightweight Consensus Protocols, Off-Chain Storage Methods, and Blockchain-as-a-Service Platforms help to minimize deployment complexity [31, 33]. The combination of Federated Learning with Blockchain technology appears as a promising solution to ensure all involved parties will collaborate together on training AI models at their respective institutions utilizing data provided but still will not expose any of the raw patient data [19, 24].

7.2 Future Directions

The future of blockchain in healthcare will be the incorporation of blockchain into broader digital ecosystems. The digitally twinned smart hospitals will become more and more dependent on blockchains to predict patient outcomes, streamline operations, and increase crisis-resilience(Nguyen et al., 2025; Taherdoost, 2025). The new uses of the technology in healthcare include blockchain-based federated learning, decentralized clinical trials, and drug tracking systems using IoT, among others (Kavinraja & Mithula, 2025; Ramani et al., 2024). With the maturity of blockchain, its overlap with AI, IoT, and metaverse technologies will transform the healthcare delivery model, and trust, transparency, and immutability will become the three pillars of smart hospital systems(Ahmed, 2025; Leiva & Castro, 2025). Blockchain together with digital twins create foundations for the smart hospitals of tomorrow. Future research is likely to explore the following areas:

- ***Resilience in crisis management:*** Using blockchain-secured digital twins, we will be able to simulate pandemics or mass casualties.
- ***Ethical governance:*** These networks will also allow for informed consent and equitable access to care through embedded ethical principles in the blockchain-based digital twin framework [28].
- ***Global interoperability:*** Using standard protocols will enable healthcare providers to share digital twin data across international boundaries, while complying with HIPAA and EU General Data Protection Regulation (GDPR), [14, 15].
- ***Personalization through AI:*** Digital twins will also be able to use blockchain-verified datasets together with simulations of digital twins, creating unique treatment paths for each patient [37].

The integration of blockchain and digital twins will support the transformation of hospitals into secure, patient-centric predictive ecosystems, consistent with the broader goal of digital transformation in the healthcare industry [1-3, 6].

8. CONCLUSION

The transformative potential of blockchain technology has been proven in the field of healthcare as the technology provides medical data management with trust, transparency, and immutability. In various applications, including electronic health records and clinical trials as well as pharmaceutical supply chains and IoMT, blockchain has offered secure, auditable, and patient-centered frameworks that deal with the long-standing problems of interoperability, privacy, and data integrity. It has a decentralized structure, and eliminates single points of failure through automated governance by consensus mechanisms and smart contracts, and thereby making it more accountable. The integration of blockchain with new technologies, including AI, digital twins, and IoT, extends the use of this technology to smart hospital infrastructure, allowing immersive healthcare experience, predictive analytics, and robust operational models. However, these issues of scalability, privacy, and regulatory compliance have to be resolved by new architectures and changing policy frameworks.

REFERENCES

Ababio, I. B., Bieniek, J., Rahouti, M., Hayajneh, T., Aledhari, M., Verma, D. C., & Chehri, A. (2025). A Blockchain-Assisted federated learning framework for secure and Self-Optimizing digital twins in industrial IoT. *Future Internet*, *17*(1), 13. DOI: 10.3390/fi17010013

Abbas, A. F., Qureshi, N. A., Khan, N., Chandio, R., & Ali, J. (2022). The blockchain technologies in healthcare: prospects, obstacles, and future recommendations; lessons learned from digitalization.

Ahmed, S. (2025). Enhancing Data Security and Transparency: The Role of Blockchain in Decentralized Systems. *International Journal of Advanced Engineering. Management Science*, *11*(1), 593258.

Akram, W., Joshi, R., Haider, T., Sharma, P., Jain, V., Garud, N., & Singh, N. (2024). Blockchain technology: A potential tool for the management of pharma supply chain. *Research in Social & Administrative Pharmacy*, *20*(6), 156–164. DOI: 10.1016/j.sapharm.2024.02.014 PMID: 38423927

Alam, S., Bhatia, S., Shuaib, M., Khubrani, M. M., Alfayez, F., Malibari, A. A., & Ahmad, S. (2023). An overview of blockchain and IoT integration for secure and reliable health records monitoring. *Sustainability (Basel)*, *15*(7), 5660. DOI: 10.3390/su15075660

Ali, S., Abdullah, , Armand, T. P. T., Athar, A., Hussain, A., Ali, M., Yaseen, M., Joo, M.-I., & Kim, H.-C. (2023). Metaverse in healthcare integrated with explainable AI and blockchain: Enabling immersiveness, ensuring trust, and providing patient data security. *Sensors (Basel)*, *23*(2), 565. DOI: 10.3390/s23020565 PMID: 36679361

Ali, V., Norman, A. A., & Azzuhri, S. R. B. (2023). Characteristics of blockchain and its relationship with trust. *IEEE Access : Practical Innovations, Open Solutions*, *11*, 15364–15374. DOI: 10.1109/ACCESS.2023.3243700

Arbabi, M. S., Lal, C., Veeraragavan, N. R., Marijan, D., Nygård, J. F., & Vitenberg, R. (2022). A survey on blockchain for healthcare: Challenges, benefits, and future directions. *IEEE Communications Surveys and Tutorials*, *25*(1), 386–424. DOI: 10.1109/COMST.2022.3224644

Atadoga, A., Elufioye, O. A., Omaghomi, T. T., Akomolafe, O., Odilibe, I. P., & Owolabi, O. R. (2024). Blockchain in healthcare: A comprehensive review of applications and security concerns. *International Journal of Science and Research Archive*, *11*(1), 1605–1613. DOI: 10.30574/ijsra.2024.11.1.0244

Attaran, M. (2022). Blockchain technology in healthcare: Challenges and opportunities. *International Journal of Healthcare Management, 15*(1), 70–83. DOI: 10.1080/20479700.2020.1843887

Badakhshan, E., & Ivanov, D. (2025). Integrating digital twin and blockchain for responsive working capital management in supply chains facing financial disruptions. *International Journal of Production Research, 63*(21), 1–35. DOI: 10.1080/00207543.2025.2507112

Chen, H., Wei, N., Wang, L., Mobarak, W. F. M., Albahar, M. A., & Shaikh, Z. A. (2024). The role of blockchain in finance beyond cryptocurrency: Trust, data management, and automation. *IEEE Access : Practical Innovations, Open Solutions, 12*, 64861–64885. DOI: 10.1109/ACCESS.2024.3395918

Dong, S., Abbas, K., Li, M., & Kamruzzaman, J. (2023). Blockchain technology and application: An overview. *PeerJ. Computer Science, 9*, e1705. DOI: 10.7717/peerj-cs.1705 PMID: 38077532

Ellahi, R. M., Ali, M., Ali Shah, S. A., Qureshi, M. A., Gulzar, S., Wood, L. C., & Ahmed Bekhit, A. E.-D. (2026). Harnessing digital twins: transforming livestock supply chain management: a comprehensive review. *Cogent Food & Agriculture, 12*(1), 2611196. DOI: 10.1080/23311932.2025.2611196

Emma, O., & Adams, P. (2025). Revolutionizing Clinical Trials with Blockchain: Strengthening Data Integrity and Building Patient Trust.

Ezz, M., Alaerjan, A. S., & Mostafa, A. M. (2025). Ethical AI in Healthcare: Integrating Zero-Knowledge Proofs and Smart Contracts for Transparent Data Governance. *Bioengineering (Basel, Switzerland), 12*(11), 1236. DOI: 10.3390/bioengineering12111236 PMID: 41301192

Ghadi, Y. Y., Mazhar, T., Shahzad, T., Amir khan, M., Abd-Alrazaq, A., Ahmed, A., & Hamam, H. (2024). The role of blockchain to secure internet of medical things. *Scientific Reports, 14*(1), 18422. DOI: 10.1038/s41598-024-68529-x PMID: 39117650

Hasselgren, A., Hanssen Rensaa, J.-A., Kralevska, K., Gligoroski, D., & Faxvaag, A. (2021). Blockchain for increased trust in virtual health care: Proof-of-concept study. *Journal of Medical Internet Research, 23*(7), e28496. DOI: 10.2196/28496 PMID: 34328437

Hovorushchenko, T., Moskalenko, A., & Osyadlyi, V. (2023). Methods of medical data management based on blockchain technologies. *Journal of Reliable Intelligent Environments, 9*(1), 5–16. DOI: 10.1007/s40860-022-00178-1 PMID: 35646514

Hussain, S., Rahman, H., Abdulsaheb, G. M., Al-Khawaja, H., & Khalaf, O. I. (2023). A Blockchain-Based Approach for Healthcare Data Interoperability. *International Journal of Advances in Soft Computing & Its Applications*, *15*(2).

Jadav, D., Jadav, N. K., Gupta, R., Tanwar, S., Alfarraj, O., Tolba, A., Raboaca, M. S., & Marina, V. (2023). A trustworthy healthcare management framework using amalgamation of AI and blockchain network. *Mathematics*, *11*(3), 637. DOI: 10.3390/math11030637

Kang, S. (2026). Blockchain-Secured Multi-Agent Digital Twin Framework for Distributed Manufacturing With Fuzzy PID Control. *IEEE Communications Standards Magazine*, 1–9. DOI: 10.1109/MCOMSTD.2025.3648845

Kavinraja, R., & Mithula, S. (2025). *Blockchain-Integrated Drug Tracking System with IoT-Enabled Containers.* Paper presented at the 2025 International Conference on Computational Robotics, Testing and Engineering Evaluation (ICCRTEE).

Khalifa, F., & Marzouk, M. (2025). Integrated blockchain and Digital Twin framework for sustainable building energy management. *Journal of Industrial Information Integration*, *43*, 100747. DOI: 10.1016/j.jii.2024.100747

Khan, A. A., Bourouis, S., Kamruzzaman, M., Hadjouni, M., Shaikh, Z. A., Laghari, A. A., Elmannai, H., & Dhahbi, S. (2023). Data security in healthcare industrial internet of things with blockchain. *IEEE Sensors Journal*, *23*(20), 25144–25151. DOI: 10.1109/JSEN.2023.3273851

Leiva, V., & Castro, C. (2025). Artificial intelligence and blockchain in clinical trials: Enhancing data governance efficiency, integrity, and transparency. *Bioanalysis*, *17*(3), 161–176. DOI: 10.1080/17576180.2025.2452774 PMID: 39844748

Masood, I., Daud, A., Wang, Y., Banjar, A., & Alharbey, R. (2024). A blockchain-based system for patient data privacy and security. *Multimedia Tools and Applications*, *83*(21), 60443–60467. DOI: 10.1007/s11042-023-17941-y

Ngabo, D., Wang, D., Iwendi, C., Anajemba, J. H., Ajao, L. A., & Biamba, C. (2021). Blockchain-based security mechanism for the medical data at fog computing architecture of internet of things. *Electronics (Basel)*, *10*(17), 2110. DOI: 10.3390/electronics10172110

Nguyen, T. L., Nguyen, L., Hoang, T., Bandara, D., Wang, Q., Lu, Q., Xu, X., Zhu, L., & Chen, S. (2025). Blockchain-empowered trustworthy data sharing: Fundamentals, applications, and challenges. *ACM Computing Surveys*, *57*(8), 1–36. DOI: 10.1145/3718082

Raja, G. B. (2021). Impact of internet of things, artificial intelligence, and blockchain technology in Industry 4.0. In *Internet of things, artificial intelligence and blockchain technology* (pp. 157–178). Springer. DOI: 10.1007/978-3-030-74150-1_8

Raja, G. B. (2024). Green Communication Technologies and Protocols. In *Artificial Intelligence Techniques for Sustainable Development* (pp. 86–113). CRC Press. DOI: 10.1201/9781003546382-5

Raja, G. B., Vigneashwaran, R., Rohan, M., Praveen, N., & Vijay, N. (2025). *IoT-based Sewage Atmosphere and Health Monitoring for Sanitation Workers with Alerting System.* Paper presented at the 2025 7th International Conference on Inventive Material Science and Applications (ICIMA). DOI: 10.1109/ICIMA64861.2025.11073919

Ramani, R., Mary, A. R., Raja, S. E., & Shunmugam, D. A. (2024). Optimized data management and secured federated learning in the Internet of Medical Things (IoMT) with blockchain technology. *Biomedical Signal Processing and Control*, *93*, 106213. DOI: 10.1016/j.bspc.2024.106213

Saeed, H., Malik, H., Bashir, U., Ahmad, A., Riaz, S., Ilyas, M., Bukhari, W. A., & Khan, M. I. A. (2022). Blockchain technology in healthcare: A systematic review. *PLoS One*, *17*(4), e0266462. DOI: 10.1371/journal.pone.0266462 PMID: 35404955

Sharma, A., Kaur, S., & Singh, M. (2021). A comprehensive review on blockchain and Internet of Things in healthcare. *Transactions on Emerging Telecommunications Technologies*, *32*(10), e4333. DOI: 10.1002/ett.4333

Singh, S., Sharma, S. K., Mehrotra, P., Bhatt, P., & Kaurav, M. (2022). Blockchain technology for efficient data management in healthcare system: Opportunity, challenges and future perspectives. *Materials Today: Proceedings*, *62*, 5042–5046. DOI: 10.1016/j.matpr.2022.04.998

Taherdoost, H. (2023). The role of blockchain in medical data sharing. *Cryptography*, *7*(3), 36. DOI: 10.3390/cryptography7030036

Taherdoost, H. (2025). Blockchain for security and privacy in the smart healthcare. In *Sensor Networks for Smart Hospitals* (pp. 411–433). Elsevier. DOI: 10.1016/B978-0-443-36370-2.00019-0

Tahir, N. U. A., Rashid, U., Hadi, H. J., Ahmad, N., Cao, Y., Alshara, M. A., & Javed, Y. (2024). Blockchain-based healthcare records management framework: Enhancing security, privacy, and interoperability. *Technologies*, *12*(9), 168. DOI: 10.3390/technologies12090168

Thantharate, P., & Thantharate, A. (2023). ZeroTrustBlock: Enhancing security, privacy, and interoperability of sensitive data through ZeroTrust permissioned blockchain. *Big Data and Cognitive Computing*, *7*(4), 165. DOI: 10.3390/bdcc7040165

Varriale, V., Michelino, F., & Godinho-Filho, M. (2026). The standalone and integrated value of digital twins and ancillary emerging technologies for enhancing supply chain performance. *Production Planning and Control*, •••, 1–29. DOI: 10.1080/09537287.2025.2608686

Velmovitsky, P. E., Bublitz, F. M., Fadrique, L. X., & Morita, P. P. (2021). Blockchain applications in health care and public health: Increased transparency. *JMIR Medical Informatics*, *9*(6), e20713. DOI: 10.2196/20713 PMID: 34100768

Villarreal, E. R. D., García-Alonso, J., Moguel, E., & Alegría, J. A. H. (2023). Blockchain for healthcare management systems: A survey on interoperability and security. *IEEE Access : Practical Innovations, Open Solutions*, *11*, 5629–5652. DOI: 10.1109/ACCESS.2023.3236505

Wenhua, Z., Qamar, F., Abdali, T.-A. N., Hassan, R., Jafri, S. T. A., & Nguyen, Q. N. (2023). Blockchain technology: Security issues, healthcare applications, challenges and future trends. *Electronics (Basel)*, *12*(3), 546. DOI: 10.3390/electronics12030546

Yaqoob, I., Salah, K., Jayaraman, R., & Al-Hammadi, Y. (2022). Blockchain for healthcare data management: Opportunities, challenges, and future recommendations. *Neural Computing & Applications*, *34*(14), 11475–11490. DOI: 10.1007/s00521-020-05519-w

Zaabar, B., Cheikhrouhou, O., Jamil, F., Ammi, M., & Abid, M. (2021). HealthBlock: A secure blockchain-based healthcare data management system. *Computer Networks*, *200*, 108500. DOI: 10.1016/j.comnet.2021.108500

Chapter 5
Integrating Blockchain and Digital Twins:
A Synergistic Framework for Smart Hospitals

S. Aarthi
http://orcid.org/0009-0006-9064-2091
Marwadi University, Rajkot, India

Ravikumar R. N.
http://orcid.org/0009-0009-3705-1681
Marwadi University, Rajkot, India

Shreha S. A.
http://orcid.org/0009-0002-2232-819X
PSG College of Arts and Science, Coimbatore, India

Satheesh Kumar A.
http://orcid.org/0009-0008-8182-0946
Nandha Engineering College, Erode, India

S. Srinivasan
http://orcid.org/0009-0002-0179-9849
Graphic Era (Deemed to be) University, Dehradun, India

Kavitha Bharathi S.
http://orcid.org/0000-0002-5630-7963
Kongu Engineering College, Erode, India

ABSTRACT

The integration of Blockchain and Digital Twin (DT) technologies revolutionizes smart hospital ecosystems by ensuring data integrity, interoperability, and real-time decision-making. Blockchain provides a tamper-proof infrastructure for consent management, provenance tracking, and secure IoMT communication, while Digital Twins simulate patients, assets, and operations for predictive diagnostics and optimization. This chapter presents a unified framework combining DT intelligence with blockchain's verifiability to achieve transparent, patient-centric, and adaptive healthcare operations. It discusses layered architectures, interoperability standards, and governance mechanisms that enable trustworthy automation and compliance

DOI: 10.4018/979-8-3373-8177-0.ch005

with privacy regulations. Real-world case studies on stroke-risk prediction and consent-driven patient twins demonstrate measurable improvements in auditability, latency, and accountability. The proposed model establishes a foundation for next-generation hospitals that are intelligent, resilient, and ethically governed through verifiable data ecosystems.

1. INTRODUCTION

Smart hospitals are located on the border of cyber-physical system, clinical governance, and real-time analytics. Although the volumes of the IoMT telemetry and EHR are enormous, this is not consistent, shared, and changes are not traced to jeopardize confidence and make gradual decision-making. Digital Twins (DTs) generate constantly renovating and computational depictions of patients, equipment and hospital procedures that are exploited to track, forecast and streamline them. The enhancement of DTs by blockchain is possible through provenance, the introduction of consent and access logic through smart contracts, and the sharing of data between institutions in a verifiable manner (Ranjan et al., 2023). A combination of such technologies will provide verifiable data streams between decision support and edge devices, solid functioning of key assets, and openness in interprofessional collaboration and partnership. The chapter puts a synergistic architecture into perspective, defines the requirements of interoperability (FHIR, DICOM, identity) and provides deployment patterns in the edge, cloud, and clinical application. It also establishes assessment measures that incorporate equilibrium of latency, integrity, privacy, and sustainability and determines the gaps in research on scalability, governance, ethics and safety to determine stringent and patient-centered implementation everywhere.

1.1 Motivation and Objectives

The process of healthcare decision making requires constant access to valid information amongst patients, equipment and medical procedures. However, the flows of IoMT, opaque transformations, and slow synchronization among hospitals have led to insecurity of safety, efficiency, and cooperation due to the presence of minimal auditability. Digital Twins have potential to integrate heterogeneous signals to live models of predicting a failure, customizing care, and optimization of operations but must be proven inputs and policy constrained as clinically trustworthy. Blockchain can provide evidenced provenance, programmable permission and inter-institution traceability which deal with scale-based accountability and trust. The sense of the holistic approach is provoked in this chapter because blockchain is the integrity and control over the data which is the engine of hospital twins and twins give high-frequency details providing on-chain contracts with operational semantics. The final rationale is the safe, open, and scalable smart-hospital, which is reducing the time-to-intervention, maximising asset uptime, and enhancing patient agency by verifiable use of data, limited to purpose, resilient and measurable. The Objectives are:

- Specify a reference architecture for blockchain-secured digital twins in hospitals.
- Define interoperability and governance patterns for consent, provenance, and access.
- Provide deployment playbooks across edge, cloud, and clinical applications.
- Propose evaluation metrics spanning technical, clinical, and sustainability KPIs.
- Identify open challenges and a research roadmap for scalable, ethical adoption.

1.2 Scope, Assumptions, and Contributions

The chapter establishes the scope at the level of the architectures, governance, and guidance regarding the deployment of blockchain with digital twins in the hospital environment. This consists of patient twins, the device/asset twins, and the hospital-system twins; permissioned twins; and consent, provenance, and access control smart contracts. The model assumes that it operates in controlled clinical settings, heterogeneous IoMT settings, and interoperability based on standards (e.g., FHIR, DICOM, identity frameworks). Security controls are role/purpose based and least-privilege, auditable, privacy controls are policy constrained and pseudonymized analytics, privacy controls. Some performance problems include latency budgets of edge sensing to decision support, throughput required by high frequency telemetry and resilience in the event of partial outages. These contributions involve three types such as a blueprint of reference architecture and data-lifecycle, a deployment playbook with onboarding, ModelOps twins-based, and contract governance and an evaluation framework with technical, clinical, and sustainability metrics. Delimitations are omission of consumer wearables not subject to clinical oversight, cryptocurrency mechanics and non- health care industrial twins. The reproducible and risk control patterns that are predicted in the chapter are scalable to hospital size and maturity. Assumptions are made on traceability.

1.3 Literature Review

In medicine, Digital Twins (DTs) have remained to be more than the device-level monitors and have transformed into multi-scale, cyber-physical representations, which models patients, assets and the working functionality of the hospital in real-time. Such simulators, and post hoc analytics were initially studied, and now they are utilized alongside the application of streaming signals of the IoMT, EHR situation, and learned surrogates in helping with early warnings, optimization of therapies, and situational awareness in operations (Z. Zhang, 2023). Patient flow prediction, patient-specific routes, hospital-system twins to patient flow prediction, bed capacity, energy demand and infections to staffing and logistics Physiological parameters, imaging characteristics, treatment courses have become patient-twinned, asset-twinned, to support patient flow prediction, individualized routes, hospital-system twins to patient flow prediction, bed capacity, energy demand and infections to staffing and logistics. Such strata contain fewer algorithmic bottlenecks compared to infrastructural bottlenecks and disjointed semantics, unprovable data provenance, and fragile access controls are all barriers to safe automation (Park et al., 2023).

The blockchain technologies help to eliminate this issue of lack of trust by offering provenance, programmable consent, and audit trails which can be verified by the organizational boundaries. The data-sharing policies are codified into smart contracts and are pegged by the identity of data-producers, data-analytic services and requesting applications, and off-chain storage and event-streaming and trade off at throughput and integrity guarantees respectively. Simultaneously, policy-constrained analytics support tools can be privacy-friendly, including pseudonymization, purpose binding, no raw data sprawl enclaves and cryptographic guards (Alonso et al., 2023). The intersection of DT and blockchain reconfigurations of DTs as not only the consumers of data, but the controlled data producers, the updates of their models and choice of versions to inferences, are indefinitely connected with the source proof and the justified access. Under such a change, responsible close loops: responsible telemetry required at the edge can be ensured and time stamped, state transitions in DT can only be transitioned under conditions sanctioned by the contract and transitions in state can be tracked to particular inputs, models and operators (Powell et al., 2024). It is still interoperability oriented; i.e. it must be able to map to standards of healthcare messaging and imaging, device ontologies, and credential models, to the extent that twins can subscribe to high frequency signals of different vendors and in one place or another, having similar meaning.

The new work has centered on federated and edge intelligence to twins of hospitals to de-congest central bottlenecks and to be consistent with the data-minimization principles which involves committing to on-chain promises to demonstrate the training datasets and model descent and policy compliance. Performance engineering Performance engineering Performance-engulfing IoMT deployments offer streaming rates that put a strain on DT compute protocols, tiered architectures, append-only event logs, and selective anchoring of hashes, but not on payloads (D. M. Kumar, 2024). Issues of governance, including the need to consent to renewal and emergency overrides and the responsibility of automated suggestions and sustainability of ledger activity are also present. The case studies of asset-maintenance, patient-monitoring, and supply-chain have shown that blockchain based twins can assist in time to intervention, higher equipment uptime and more data reuse to do research without responsibility. The existing state of the art accordingly indicates the composable hospital twins, coordinated by and through contracts, quantified in terms of latency-integrity-utility, integrated into learning health system where all interactions of data sharing can be verified, all model modification could be traced and all clinical decision-making could be described in the context of a managed provenance history (Quazi et al., 2024).

2. CONCEPTUAL FOUNDATIONS

The theoretical principles form the joint provision of the high-fidelity secure and operationally valuable smart-hospital systems by blockchain and Digital Twins (DTs). The blockchain provides a permissioned provenance and identity undercarriage and a policy enforcing smart contracts that are programmable. Digital twins provide the computational models of patients, devices and subsystems of the hospital that are aligned to those observed in the real world to aid in monitoring, prediction and optimization (Obodo, 2025). They are a combination of verifiable and closed loop pipelines where data creation, model development and clinical activities or operational activities are audited. Its foundations consist of three layers and are believed to be trusted data exchange; semantically consistent modeling and governance of safe, compliant automation. The idea of trust is pegged on cryptographic attestations and append-only logs, the notion of quality is given in the form of versioned twin states and validation functions, policy is implemented by policy as code, which restricts access, consent and escalation. More of the concern of this set of pillars is the interoperability with healthcare specifications, resiliency during the event of partial outage, as well as compute and storage sustainability. It will lead to integrity-saving substrate, on which scalable patient-centric hospital intelligence can be achieved (Q. Lu et al., 2023).

2.1 Blockchain Fundamentals for Healthcare

Healthcare blockchains are often permissioned blockchains, i.e. it is allowed that the institutions join, which guarantees that there is predictable performance with no risk of cryptographic security. The transactions (e.g. registering the data, changing consent or request analytics, etc.) are signed, ordered and stored forever so as to create a tamper evident audit trail. Smart contracts are made up of policy (access control, time-limited access control, revocation, levees, emergency overrides). The implementation of provenance is by repositories of off-chain the payloads based on the hash of data artifacts, model versions and transitions of a DT and anchoring the result to the blockchain but repositories of the payloads (Amofa et al., 2024). The identity and access, i.e., the control based on the public-key infrastructure, role-based and attribute-based controls and device attestation of the IoMT endpoints are founded on the controls. Data reduction involves the use of recording pointers, claims and proofs (and not contents). Event-driven patterns commit are made to the downstream services in a manner that the updates of consent and data-quality checks will immediately impact the twin workflows. Performance maintenance occurs through the form of batching, partitions / channels and selective anchoring. All these needs will provide testable descent, governance policies and religion on cross-institution must make use of information securely, intelligently and repetitively, and in saner hospitals. Table 1 Construct bridging between clinical operational requirements and blockchain opportunities and limitations.

Table 1. Blockchain Features Mapped to Healthcare Needs

Healthcare Need	Blockchain Feature	How It Helps	Constraints/Notes
Verifiable provenance	Immutable ledger + hashing	Proves data/model lineage	Anchor hashes; keep payloads off-chain
Consent enforcement	Smart contracts	Purpose-bound, time-boxed access	Requires clear policy vocabularies
Cross-site trust	Permissioned governance	Auditable multi-party exchange	Onboarding, key management, SLAs

2.2 Digital Twin Taxonomy (Patient, Device/ Asset, Hospital-System)

Digital twins are in three levels. The multimodal data of patient twins are physiological measurements, imaging patterns, laboratory patterns and history of therapy and they are being fed into state estimates and risk curves that are in a state of constant flux. They facilitate pre-emption of warning, therapy customization and path and document model version and evidence sources customization. The equipment within the device/asset twins includes MRI scanners, ventilators, and infusion pumps and consists of the data about the usage cycles, calibration drift, part wear, and cybersecurity posture and energy patterns to support predictive maintenance and compliance check (Kim et al., 2020). Hospital-system twins is cross-ward operating-theatre, sterile-supply, pharmacy and bed-management twins which models demand, personnel, infection-dynamics and resources constraints to maximize throughput and safety. The structure is also similar with twins on the lower levels, data adapters and data quality gates; state estimators and learned surrogates; intervention simulators; decision support dashboards/APIs. They need a well-defined versioning, validation data and drift monitors in order to avoid the silent performance degradation. This may be achieved through linking major transitions such as the ingestion of data, parameter updates and policy choices to a ledger, to permit attributable and reproducible operations, and permit a powerful what-if analysis and post-event inspection, without impacting on real time responsiveness. Table 2 Categorize type of data, type of methods, type of output, type of users as well as category of use case.

Table 2. Taxonomy of Digital Twins in Smart Hospitals

Twin Type	Primary Data Sources	Core Methods/ Models	Typical Outputs	Primary Users	Example Use Case
Patient Twin	Vitals, labs, meds, imaging	Temporal models, calibration, simulators	Risk score, trajectory, alerts	Clinicians	Early warning for stroke/deterioration
Asset/Device Twin	Sensor logs, maintenance, cybersecurity	Health index, anomaly detection	Failure prediction, work orders	Biomed, OT	Predictive maintenance for ventilators
Hospital-System Twin	EHR ops, bed/OR logs, energy, staffing	Queueing, simulation, optimization	Flow forecasts, staffing plans	Ops, admin	Bed turnover & OR scheduling optimization

2.3 Synergy Rationale: Integrity, Traceability, and Closed-Loop Intelligence

The combination of DT intelligence and blockchain assurance is what has created the synergy. Blockchain provides verifiable provenance, consent enforcement, and evidence that cannot be altered by any other agent of access to the material, when and why, or at all, which is the requirements of DTs. On the other hand, operationally relevant blockchains are those that are flooded with high-frequency events taking the form of DTs state updates, model inferences and interventions in such a manner that on-chain policies can be implemented. Hashing of DT inputs, parameters and outputs, traceability by linking each decision with a particular version of data and model identifier and closed-loop intelligence by using contract-driven processes (alerts, maintenance tickets, therapy checks) to write-back auditable results facilitates integrity. The feedback is exploited to ensure that the learning systems are able to compare the forecasted and measured impacts and optimize the calibration and safety (Islam & Kundu, 2019). The system minimizes uncertainty in both multi-party systems, helps in quick identification of root causes and also allows selective disclosure through the aid of cryptographic evidence. The changes made to the consent of DT subscriptions are binding, hence, it is possible to restrict or extend data streams real-time, without re-creating pipelines. All in all, the synergy offers the governance, observability, and capability of adapting, which is necessary to be trustful automation in clinical and operational settings. With the assistance of the blockchain and digital twins, as it can be observed in figure 1, the trustful automation is ensured since it guarantees the integrity of the information, the decisions traceable, the dynamic consent is controlled, and the workflows become governed by the contracts within the smart hospital systems.

Figure 1. Achieving Trustworthy Automation through Blockchain-Aligned Digital Twins

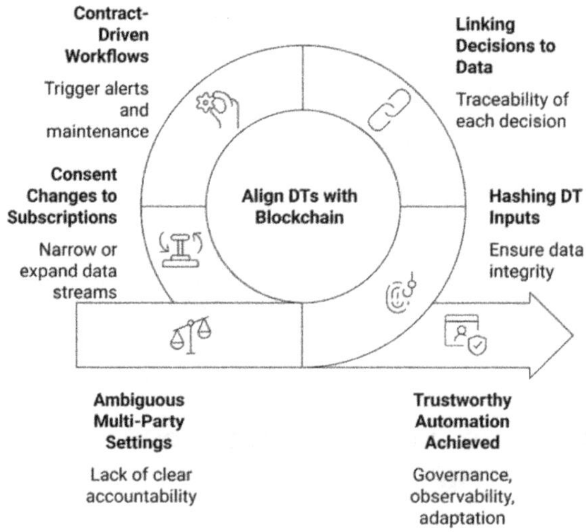

3. REFERENCE ARCHITECTURE

It has been structured in the reference architecture so that smart-hospital capabilities are implemented in loosely-coupled performance, governance, and evolvability layers. The IoMT devices generate authenticated events on the edge and penetrate quality gates and lightweight analytics. A streaming/ AI layer and the DT core are dealing with normalization, enrichment, and extraction of features and state estimation, simulation and testing of scenarios are being finalized. Consent, provenance, and policy are made available as a permissioned registry of smart contracts, decision support, coordination of maintenance, and reporting are made available in application services. Identity/access cross-cutting service, key management, observability, and twin components ModelOps and compliance tooling the data payloads are secured in safe off-chain repositories, the hashes of the claims, policy repositories and claims are stored on-chain (Gebler et al., 2025). This is achieved by the use of healthcare standards and industrial standards that make it integrate with any vendor to implement interoperability. The architecture is preoccupied with the event-based patterns, fault isolations and blue-green rollouts so that disruption is kept to a minimum. It favors the step-by-step method: begin with an asset-twin slice, to patient pathways and lastly, to hospital-system coordination, in which a steady set of objectives is to be gauged at both the governance and service-level.

3.1 Layered Blueprint: Edge/IOMT → Streaming/ AI → DT Core → Ledger/Contracts → Apps

The blue print has five layers. Edge/IoMT will validate the devices, time stamp measurements, perform sanity checks and will produce events. Streaming/AI layer unifies units, ontologies, provides context (location, clinician, procedure), and features, and inference is also provided at low latency on simple classifiers. Record of the identifiers of models and confidence ranges are stored in the DT Core, canonical states, patient trajectories, asset health and loads of the system in a hybrid of mechanistic and Markov-Lange models, and simulators. The Ledger/Contracts layer has codes of Consent, purpose, retention, and emergency access, and hashes of inputs, state deltas and outputs and workflows (e.g. an open work order, notifying a clinician) are initiated in the Ledger/Contracts layer. Applicant layer gives dashboards, alerts, ticket research, query research and reporting using the least privilege views. It is event driven and applies pub/sub, backpressure and retries as a resilience mechanism (Ziminski et al., 2020). Observability provides links/bridges between claims in the on-chain to off-chain artifacts, by tracing/metrics/logs to lineage views. The canary releases used to update the model and contract versions with blueprints are safe to evolve. The stack can be implemented both in-prem and also replicated into the cloud services through secure and audited routes. Table 3 Summarize, layers, inputs /outputs, standards, and reliability notes.

Table 3. Reference Architecture Components and Interfaces

Layer	Key Components	Inputs	Outputs	Interfaces/ Standards	Reliability Notes
Edge/IoMT	Gateways, device PKI	Sensor telemetry	Validated events	OPC-UA, MQTT	Mutual TLS, buffering, retries
Streaming/AI	ETL, feature svc	Events, metadata	Normalized streams, features	FHIR Subscriptions	Backpressure, schema checks
DT Core	State est., simulators	Features, context	Twin states, alerts	REST/Graph APIs	Canary models, rollback
Ledger/ Contracts	Permissioned nodes	Claims, policy calls	On-chain claims, triggers	Contract APIs	Channels, selective anchoring
Apps	Dashboards, tickets	Alerts, KPIs	Actions, reports	FHIR, DICOM links	Graceful degradation paths

3.2 Data Lifecycle & Provenance: Ingestion, Versioning, Lineage, Audit

The first is the authenticated ingestion the devices and systems identify keys, attest firmware and release signed records. Schema, ranges, and temporal consistency Anomalies Quality gates to quarantine. Versioning An unchanging identifier of batches of data, features, model parameters and states of DTs, semantic diffs Document changes to material are semantic diffs. To facilitate counterfactual analysis and replay, lineage graphs provide information on the relationship between each of the outputs and their inputs, model variants and transformations. Auditability is grounded on computing cryptographic digests of artifacts, lineage edges, which is grounded in the ledger and policy decisions (grants, revocations, emergency break-glass events). Content and scope are shown by access tokens; they should be renewed because of the circumstances of the consent. Retention and deletion policy enforcement is an off-chain policy and have on-chain attestations that construct an evidence of conformity but is not disclosed of the payloads. De-identification pipelines supply generated datasets, whose recipe of creation can be used to re-create datasets to offer reproducibility (Hemdan et al., 2023). Lifecycle hooks realize lifecycle maintenance or clinical behavior and document recognitions to build a loop between sensor and decision to outcome to provide audit and legal evidence of Continuous. Figure 2 illustrates the healthcare information flow, i.e. validation, versioning, lineage tracing, auditability and policy enforcement to achieve the integrity, traceability and conforming lifecycle management in digitized twin blockchain-based environments.

Figure 2. Data Lifecycle and Provenance

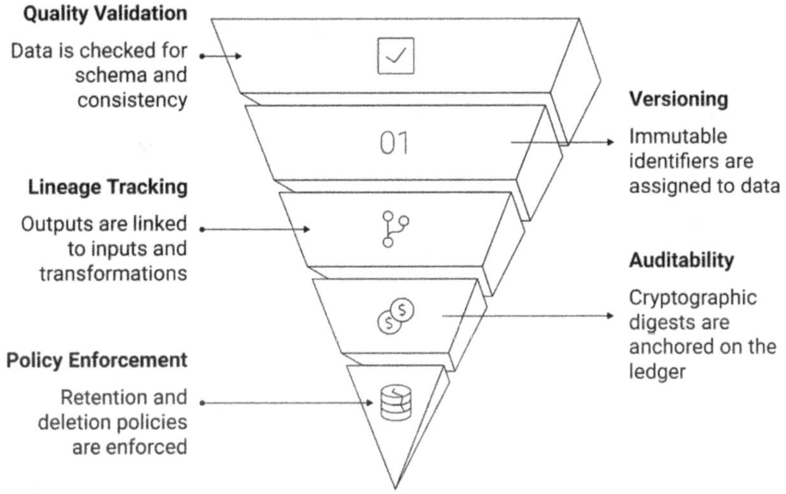

3.3 Interoperability: HL7 FHIR, DICOM, OPC-UA, Identity/Access

Interoperability guarantees consistency of meaning, routing security and inter-vendor and/or location extensibility. HL7 FHIR resources are standardized clinical units (Patient, Observation, Procedure, Consent) and may be exchanged with the help of RESTful services; FHIR Subscriptions allow making flows in DT pipelines event-based. DICOM manages the imaging objects and metadata and DTs permit updating the model to trace back to individual studies and series. The proposed industrial telemetry is compatible with the planned industrial telemetry of building systems and biomedical devices OPC-UA. Semantic drift is avoided by the help of terminologies (SNOMED CT, LOINC, ICD) and unit harmonization. Identity/Access Unites enterprise IAM and clinical functionality, identity attributes (purpose, location, time), device credentials, and is a verifiable token with consent limits (Tahar et al., 2023). The metadata of authorship and transformation is stored on the provenance resources store as a claim and a hash anchored on-chain. The interop gateways and transform documentation of legacy HL7 v2 in compatibilized feeds and proprietary feeds into standardized events are done to accomplish audit and reproducibility done with data-mapping registries. Contract template is being created in order to avoid ambiguity by consulting the test suites and conformance profiles test implementations and the standard codes. It is a standards-based approach, which eliminates vendor lock-in, enhance safety, and multi-site scaling.

4. SECURITY, PRIVACY, AND GOVERNANCE

Security, privacy and governance define the mechanisms of capabilities that are regulated and clinical risk that is safely and regulated. This security encompasses identities of a device and service, a transport and storage that is encrypted, vulnerability, and monitoring that is constant. Privacy encompasses purpose limitation and minimization, de-identification and role and context differential perspectives. Governance objectifies policy as code, which is translation of rules of law and rules of institutions into smart contracts and access controls enforced and regulated through audits and dashboards. Emergencies are addressed by break-glass procedures, algorithmic hazards or incident response and model-risk management (Phelan et al., 2024). Evidence of compliance is created by creating the claim that cannot be changed and has references to off-chain artifacts that can be proved to create them without disclosing any information. Design reviews are also included along with data-protection impact assessment and threat modeling. Sustainability is used to inform the cryptographic and infrastructure decisions in order to balance both integrity and the energy efficiency. The combination of this structure provides anticipatory, updateable and upgradable controls which keep up with evolving clinical processes and partner ecosystems not to mention regulatory imperatives and remain responsive to real-time decision support in intelligent hospitals (Boussadi & Zapletal, 2017).

4.1 Policy as Code: Consent, Revocation, Purpose-Bound Access

Institutional rules are coded in a policy as code using executable artifacts that are used in a consistent manner across systems. Consent policies specify the individuals that can access certain data, why, under what circumstances and within what period. Smart contracts carry consent grants; the purpose attribute of access tokens and immutable events as would be decisions. Revocation: the contracts are cancelled in the event that a patient rescinds the consent or scope, and notifies subscribers, the throttling or termination of streams individual streams by DT pipelines. Purpose-bound access It links queries and subscriptions to permitted scope (care, operations, research); it is impossible to treat break-glass paths as an emergency and they are not time-constrained and should be audited afterwards (Abbas et al., 2022). Contracts

Upgrades The upgrades have a controlled lifecycle, which consists of compatibility test and roll back plans. Provenance records are linked to policy decisions that are made with references to standard vocabularies in order to avoid ambiguity and are fully traced. Active consents, revocations and exceptions are displayed in the form of dashboards. Enabling policies to become executable by the institutions will reduce the mistake of manual and fast-tracking audit and ensure that the DT actions is responsive to the ethical decisions and legal requirements and bring them into effect.

4.2 Privacy-Preserving Analytics: Pseudonymization, RBAC/ABAC, Cryptographic Controls

Privacy preserving analytics is a blend of both governance and technical protection so as to promote utility with the least exposure. In pseudonymization, identifiers are removed; the linkage keys are stored in escrow and the separation of role is imposed. Role-Based Access Control (RBAC) is a minimum system, Attribute-Based Access Control (ABAC) provides a more granular system with a wider context (purpose, location, time, device posture). When it comes to the materialization of views, this is based on a role basis, hides columns, generalizes values or masking rare categories to overcome re-identification. Cryptographic controls It is an autonomous encryption, secure enclaves to perform sensitive computation, secure multi-party analytics to query cross-institutionally, and commitment schemes to commit training data without revelation (Cheng et al., 2020). Query budgets, k-anonymity tests and differential privacy can be used to limit leaking aggregate analytics. All the accesses are justified and their results documented in logs, which are linked to on-chain claims. In the case of DTs, there are no other components that are governed by privacy policies besides data inputs, but also other derivative features and model explanations, to prevent an indirect disclosure. Such interventions are supplemented by lifecycle and consent contracts in such a manner that the privacy properties can be preserved during ingestion, modeling, and decision support and responsible analytics at, at best, clinical speed become feasible (Yaqoob et al., 2023).

4.3 Compliance & Auditability: Mapping to Regulatory and Clinical Safety Standards

Compliance puts architecture and operations into agreement with the legal, ethical, and safety requirements. The controls are aligned to health data regulations and institutional policies which include consent capture, access control, breach notification, retention and cross-border transfer where necessary. Clinical safety frameworks are used to validate, manage change, and conduct post-deployment monitoring of the DT models that impact care. The auditing is implemented in a designed manner as all the critical actions, such as data receipt, data transform, data model update, recommendation, authorization are recorded with late time-stamps, identities, and evidence hash values anchored on the ledger (Agbo & Mahmoud, 2019). Monthly attestation of the off-chain repositories makes sure that there is deletion and retention policies in place and sampling audits are used to ensure that data-mapping and access-decision are correct. The model-risk management keeps a record of intended use, performance levels, drift and human-in-the-loop control with sign-offs being immutable claims. The scheduled and evidenced incident response drills, break-glass reviews, and third-party assessments are scheduled and indicated. Live posture views and machine-readable regulators reports and partners are provided by compliance dashboards. Making compliance visible and repeatable, institutions minimize legal risks, enhance trust among the stakeholders, and remain flexible to implement changes in DT and blockchain elements, without interfering with safety and accountability (Barati & Rana, 2022).

5. IMPLEMENTATION STRATEGIES

Operational pragmatism, interoperability and clinical safety are balanced with each other through effective implementation. The methodology will consist of a secure IoMT fabric: identity of devices, attestation and standardized telemetry to discourage feeble integrations. Streaming pipelines effect schema/units normalization and quality gates prior to occurrences being relayed into the services of DT. Change fidelity Change fidelity Change fidelity Change fidelity Change fidelity Change fidelity Change fidelity Change fidelity Change fidelity Consent, purpose and retention in Smart contracts are coded, i.e. policy change is automatically propagated to data subscriptions and DT behaviors (Singla et al., 2024). The three concepts which were formulated by the reliability engineering include the definition of latency, sensor-to-decision, bounds, and the presentation of graceful underperformance to partial failures and observability during triage. This is controlled by energy sensitive deployment (edge preprocessing or selective on-chain anchoring or adaptive sampling) to control cost and environmental impact. The idea to adopt a very small asset-twin/pathway slice with the security in place, governance and scale applied, deploy multi-department/multi-sites with conformance profiles and onboarding, monitoring and audit automation, etc. is suggested. It is a standards-first methodology that is tentative and generates clinical and operational profits that can be measured (O'Donoghue et al., 2019).

5.1 IOMT Integration and Secure Device Onboarding

Provision of device trust anchors and enrollment processes can be considered to be the first step towards ensuring the integrity of the IoMT concern. Every device (or gateway) is provisioned with cryptographic keys, they are certified with the integrity of their firmware and metadata (type, location, owner, calibration state) is recorded. One policy that is fully implemented in a zero-trust posture is using mutual TLS, certificate rotation and policy checks on connection time. The Telemetry has been verified at the edge-schema, unit and monotonicity of the timestamps and range and augmented with contextual tags (bed/ward, clinician, procedure) to make fine routing and provenance possible. Gateways and bursts convert the legacy protocols to standard event formats and rate control and buffering alleviate bursts and outages respectively (Götz et al., 2022). Onboarding playbooks define golden configurations, secure boot, and tamper alerts which are automatically revoked in the case of anomalies. Early minimization on data is achieved: transmit clinically significant signals of the right frequencies; compress, batch data where latency is allowable. The entries of the ledger are identically linked to the identities of devices so that downstream decisions to access and audit information can be based on a verifiable source. Finally, prior to production enrollment, there will be conformance issues and simulated failover exercise, which makes sure that the new device acceptance into production should work with DT services, consent agreements, and monitoring programs within departments and vendors (Gaddapuri, 2025) .

5.2 DT MODELOPS/MLOPS: Versioning, Validation, and Drift Management

The DT Modelops entails adoption of the processes of simulation through the use of controlled twins. It is composed of everything that is immutable with version IDs and can be reproducible with fixed dependencies and environment manifests, data schema, features, data models, simulators, calibration sets and artifacts. The deployment testing involves all the statistic performance, the calibration, robust performance in the event of the absence/noisy data and the amount of safety in the environment of its intended use. Guardrailed (rate limits, fallback policies) models are also released as shadow releases into the running traffic. Very often, the probe Discrimination/calibration measures, subpopulation, and that of the error stratification are considered and a warning against human check is given in case of exceeding limit. The performance deltas and population shift statistics introduce what the data and concept drift are and what could be the possible corrective measures to the problem, i.e. auto-recalibration, feature re-engineering or rollback (Kumari et al., 2025). On-chain provenance It can be achieved by training sets hashing, code commit, validation report and end-to-end trace sign-offs of the payloads without them being viable. Model cards and model risk registers as well as model usage are also represented by policy and code cards (some of which have been described in terms of consent and purpose). It is a dynamic science that guarantees the DT faithfulness of the time and determination pace of clinical quickness.

5.3 Reliability Engineering: Latency Budgets, Failover, and Energy Considerations

Formalisation of the objectives that are achieved at service level between sensing and decision is made possible through reliability engineering. Latency budgets give the edge processing, streaming transforms, state updates in DT, contract check, and application delivery milliseconds per second goal; budgets specify the queue size, batching point and priority lanes to priority alarms. Pattern Redundancy patterns active/active gateway, parted message broker and replicated DT are used to avoid single points of failures. Graceful degradation addresses the safety: when the ledger is unavailable temporarily hashes are computed and defaulting of the lowest priority take place; when the models are unavailable rule-based or last-known-good fallbacks. Chaos testing provides a guarantee regarding the condition of failover, back pressure and recover time. Observability brings together metrics, traces, and lineage views so that they could be in a position to offer the operators with the opportunity to correlate anomalies between device and contract (J. Lu et al., 2022). To be more precise, edge inference (decreased transportation) and adaptive sampling (entropy of signal) sampling, workload contraction during low demand intervals, and selective on-chain anchoring (hashes/claims, not payloads) are some of the energies of consideration. Only the paths that have a high sensitivity of latency are hardware accelerated, but the non-urgent analytics run on the energy-saving levels. The results of these measures, which are predetermined by the hospital capacity, are predictable responsiveness, partial resilience of failure, and long-term functionality.

6. CASE STUDY: BLOCKCHAIN-SECURED DIGITAL TWINS IN A SMART HOSPITAL

The case study details the profile of a smart hospital with tertiary-level care infrastructure that is powered by permissioned blockchain and patient and asset digital twins (DTs). The objective is the achievement of verifiability of data integrity, real-time decision support and responsible automation of the key workflows. Patient twins are multimodal (vital, laboratory, medication, imaging-based, and so on) combinations of signals offering risk patterns and recommending interventions.

Asset twins monitor high-value device wear, calibration drift and asset utilization and posture cybersecurity. Permissioned ledger ensures provenance, authorization and execution of policies by using smart contracts, with the payloads being stored in conformant off-chain stores (Ovsianko & Niemkova, 2025). Two realizations are also put into focus, i.e., a blockchain-based DT to forecast stroke-risk and a smart-contract-based patient twin that implements granular consent and purpose-bound access. The two deliver improvements in latency which are quantifiable, auditability and safety .

6.1 Deployment Context and Workflow (Patient/ Asset Twins + Permissioned Blockchain)

The hospital has zero-trust IoMT composition, which comprises of authenticated gateway that standardizes streams of devices into normal event. There is schema/ unit validation provided by a streaming layer, and provides context of telemetry (location, clinician, procedure). Risk pathways of patients, well-being of devices and predicted failures are the canonicals of patient and asset DT services. The authentication blockchain (network of hospital, vendor and regulator nodes) contains the hashed artifacts i.e. the data bursts IDs, model version, change twin state and execute the consent, purpose and retention smart contracts. The agreements are applied in the issues that are touching the areas of consent and inform subscribers about the fact that DT pipelines cut or magnify streams at the same time (Yakubu et al., 2024). To least privilege API may be implemented in clinical applications to DT; to the maintenance systems, to the work order and pattern of failure-based assets of a contract nature. The measures are also related with traces and on-chain claims to conduct sensor to decision root-cause analysis on observability. It is a cycle of audit in which the entire recommendations and maintenance measures can be trailed and recreated.

6.2 Blockchain-Enabled Digital Twin for Stroke-Risk Prediction

The stroke risk application is aimed at the early detection of neurological deterioration in high acuity wards. High frequency vitals (BP, SpO2, HRV), medication administration history, recent imaging characteristics (e.g. WMH volume proxies) and lab markers (D-dimer, CRP) are fed into patient twins to generate a 4-6-hour risk score as it rolls. The models (hybrid gradient boosting + temporal encoder) are versioned with signed manifests, calibration curve and thresholds are tested on a ward profile basis. The DT writes each scoring cycle to the ledger, in the form of a concise claim, at the end of which are input batch IDs, model version, confidence interval, and alert rationale hash. However, payloads are not on-chain, and any auditor may cryptographically reconcile a bedside notification with its accurate inputs and model state. Smart contracts provide purpose-limited access (direct care vs. research) and generate nurse/neurology alerts in case risks exceed validated levels and document acknowledgements and activities. Practically, the median sensor-to-alert latency is kept within range of budgeted, and the reduction of the false-alerts can be ensured through ward-specific calibration. The reviews of the post-event play the very evidence chain, which helps to counter the medico-legal defense and quality improvement (Fahmy, 2025). The execution of the application of DT intelligence and on-chain provenance enhances the time-to-intervention and builds trust in the validity of the alerts and governance. Table 4 One-page summary of pipeline configuration and impact seen. The figure 3 represents the workflow of a blockchain-based digital twin system to predict stroke-risk, where patient data is ingested and analyzed, verified on-chain and used to raise an alert, record an action, and after-event review to continuously improve.

Figure 3. Blockchain-Enabled Digital Twin for Stroke-Risk Prediction

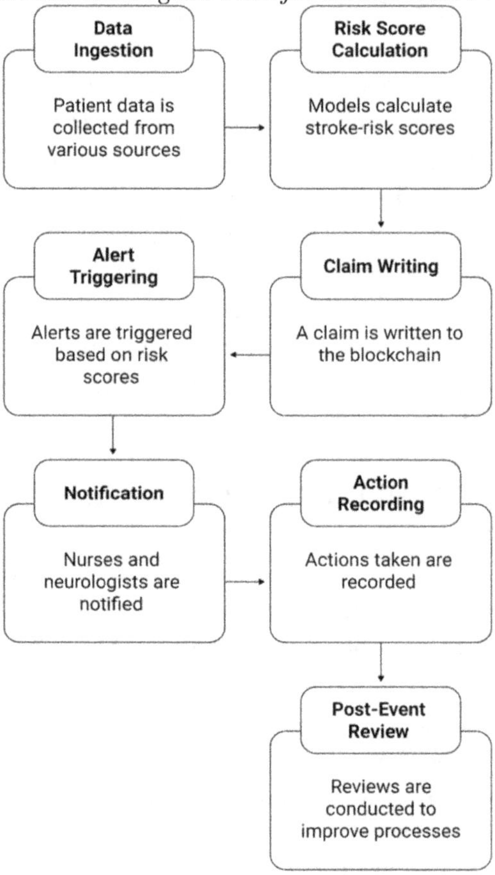

Table 4. Case Study A-Stroke-Risk DT: Inputs, Models, and Outcomes

Input Signals	Model/Version	Alert Threshold Policy	Median Latency	Precision / Recall	Operational Notes
Vitals (BP, SpO_2, HRV), labs, meds, imaging features	GBDT+Temporal Encoder v1.4	Ward-specific calibrated cutoff	5.2s E2E	0.78 / 0.72	On-chain claim per alert; off-chain payload
Vitals + labs only (fallback)	GBDT v1.3 (LKGS)	Conservative cutoff + human review	4.1s	0.70 / 0.65	Used during imaging downtime
Post-deployment (3 mo)	—	—	—	Event rate ↓ 18% false alerts	Root-cause reviews via provenance replay

6.3 Smart-Contract–Driven Patient Digital Twin for Consent and Provenance

This will be done in a way that it operationalizes granular and dynamic consent in the twin patient. The consent artifacts must be documented at the time of admission, making all of the purposes permitted (treatment, operations, research), type of data (vitals, labs, imaging), recipients, and time frames. These policies are coded in smarter contract and released as verifiable tokens, having restricted permissions as well as expirations. The only streams to which the patient DT is legally entitled to access are streams that the current tokens grant access to, revocations or rewrites of scopes are propagated immediately and throttle inputs do not incur a re-architecture of pipelines. State transitions Each twin update, which performs feature extraction, produces an explanation, hashes and policy check output anchored on the ledger, produces a non-mutable history of who accessed what, based on what consent, and why. Break-glass access is to be dual authorised and to expire and place on retrospective review queue. Such type of selective disclosure assists in research: a recorded pipeline produces de-identified derivatives, and the history of derivatives and approvals are created as on-chain claims. Clinician applications indicate the presence of active consent scopes and provenance badges to make the point of care more transparent (Pan et al., 2019). The compliance is checked by auditors with the help of reconciling claim on chains and off-chain logs and repositories that are under control. The overall outcome is patient-centered information governance - scalable, testable and completely consistent with dual functions without compromising clinical responsiveness and model fidelity. The healthcare environment that is supported by the blockchain smart contract illustrates how a patient digital twin acquires consent, issues tokens, manages data subscriptions, and provides providence and is supported by verifiable and auditable updates in a healthy and secure healthcare environment, as shown in figure 4.

Figure 4. Smart-Contract–Driven Patient Digital Twin for Consent and Provenance

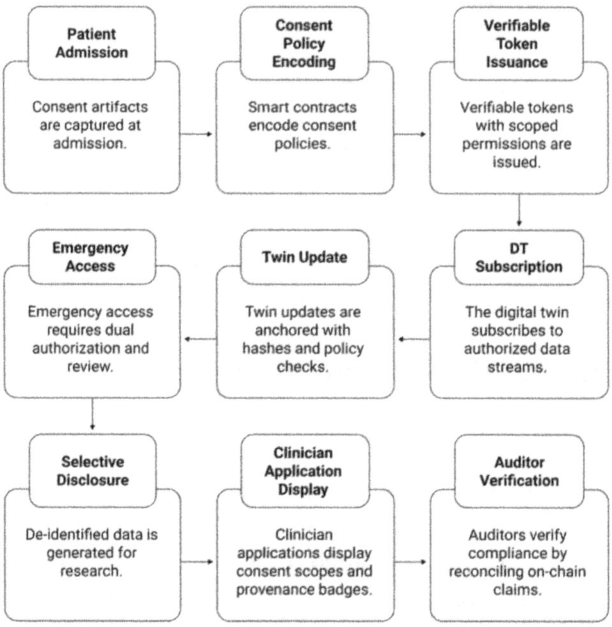

7. EVALUATION FRAMEWORK

The evaluation system balances technical, clinical and financial objectives with an aim of ensuring that Digital Twins (DTs) based on blockchain are positive outcomes that will not have adverse effects on safety, privacy and efficiency. It offers technical validation which takes into account integrity, latency, throughput, availability, and data quality of sensing, streaming, DT state updates and checking of contracts. Clinical and operational validation is a measurement of an asset-stratified time-to-intervention, reduction in adverse events, uptime and pathway compliance. Cost-energy-sustainability measures of the metrics include computation of cost-energy-sustainability, computation of storage, computation of network overheads, computation of carbon intensity, and computation of total cost of ownership at realistic loads. The methods include prospective pilot and have pre/post baseline, canary roll out, A/B testing and replay with provenance ground data (Frempong et al., 2024). The summary of the results is presented in the form of dashboards that relate the performance to the consent posture and provenance to make responsible decisions regarding scaling, replacement/refining of the policy.

7.1 Technical KPIS: Integrity, Latency, Throughput, Availability, Data Quality

End-to-end provenance of inputs, models and state deltas of a DT are proven with the ledger and verifiable by off-chain artifacts. Latency budgets feature edge processing, stream transforms, DT updates, contract checks and delivering apps; it depends on the application (e.g. alarms vs. batch analytics). Throughput includes sustained event rates, burst tolerance, including the backpressure behavior and also the loss rates. Availability of gateways, brokerage, DT services and ledger nodes are checked and have been tested with the use of chaos and failover errors. The data quality comprises of the schema conformance, unit normalization, missingness profiles, drift indicators and supervised model label fidelity. Monitoring is used to do the percentiles (P50/P95/P99), saturation and lineage coverage. The synthetic load and production shadow traffic are utilized in the de-risking (Rehman et al., 2022). The thresholds of incidents that are associated with automatic response throttle, reroute, use last known good models or increase. The effect of the consent changes, revocations, or emergency overrides on the data paths and the timeliness of the decision has been revealed by the reporting of the KPIs. Table 5 Design engineering SLOs and automatic operation upon all stages of the pipeline.

Table 5. Technical KPIs and Target Thresholds

KPI	Stage (Edge/Stream/DT/Contract/ App)	Target (P50/ P95/P99)	Measurement Method	Auto-Action on Breach
Latency	Edge→Alert (end-to-end)	≤3s/≤6s/≤10s	Traces w/ span IDs	Prioritize queue, reduce batch size
Integrity coverage	All	≥99.5% artifacts hashed	Hash audit vs. catalog	Re-ingest, flag audit
Throughput	Streaming	≥50k evts/min sustained	Broker metrics	Scale partitions, add consumers
Availability	DT services	≥99.9% monthly	SLO monitor	Failover to hot standby
Data quality pass	Ingestion	≥99% schema/ units OK	DQ rules	Quarantine, notify owner

7.2 Clinical/Operational KPIS: Time-to-Intervention, Adverse-Event Reduction, Uptime

Time-to-intervention is a ratio of time that passes between risk occurrence and its detection and immediate response by a clinician, which is further divided into sensing, analytics, alert routing and bedside response. Adverse-event reduction is an indicator of statistically significant levels of variation in rate of events (e.g., stroke development, device malfunctions, medication errors) based on risk-adjusted, seasonally controlled and confidence-interval analyses. The uptime is a measure of the performance and availability of critical assets (MRIs, ventilators, pumps) and DT services, including the accuracy/recall of predictive maintenance and the average mean time between failures (P. Zhang et al., 2018). Boardings time, bed turnover, OR schedule fidelity, is a hospital-system twin benefits measure. Human-factor indicators (acceptance of alerts, rate of overrides, clarity of explanation, work of clinician) can be used to ensure the usability and trust. To limit automated activities, KPIs are stratified into wards and shifts and represent contextual effects and a set of safety limits. Every KPI change is associated with different variants of the model, policy states, and device cohorts which can be used to tell credible causal stories. Only the clinical benefit and still meeting operation risk are sufficient, whereas privacy restrictions are also met to give the go-ahead to scale-up.

7.3 Cost, Energy, and Sustainability Metrics

The given cost and energy telemetry may be viewed as the sign of financial and environmental sustainability. The patient-day or monitored device tracing is performed following every level of the service-graph structure, i.e. compute, storage and egress. These estimations of the node and the accelerator and the carbon intensity are done on the grid measures or even using the information of the workloads with workloads assigned to such facility. Ledger overhead (consensus, anchoring frequency, block size) directs selective anchoring or channel partitioning which is successively followed by selective anchoring of blocks. These optimization levers are adaptive sampling, transport optimization through edge inference, dynamic batch sizing and tiered storage lifecycles. It is a comparison between on-prem deployment and hybrid and cloud deployment on premises of peak/average load which are part of scenario analysis and subjected to loads (Barbaria et al., 2025). The cost-of-quality lens is a relatively cheaper tool compared to the cost of operation with respect to the calculation of the savings of the avoided downtime, reduced length of stay and untoward events. Sustainability scorecards are used in the measurement of watts per event, grams CO_2e per alert and energy proportionality at the off-peak times. They will be used to purchase, make architecture right-sized and green-IT requirements and yet achieve the desired latency and integrity goals.

8. CHALLENGES AND OPEN PROBLEMS

The primary challenges can be seen in the case of a large and diverse scale and the collision of the scale with the semantics of data and institutional policies. The interoperability between vendors and sites must have powerful mappings, data-portable conformance and governance. Privacy vs utility and performance Tensions exist between rich analytics and detailed signals, consent, minimization and latency factors limit access to and compute. Blockchain has its trade-offs such as the consensus overheads, key management and upgrade choreography when DTs have the challenge of combating the model drift and reliability of explanations. Related to the algorithmic accountability are questions of trust and liability, the problem of emergency overrides and medico-legal defensibility of automated recommendations. The ethical issues include equity among subpopulations, openness during the point of care, and cryptography and compute decision-making sustainability (Ferrag et al., 2019). These gaps must be addressed by means of coordinating standards, common testbeds and multi-site and tough evidence.

8.1 Scalability and Cross-Institution Interoperability

Scaling entails complexity of assembling and managing as well. The non-uniformity of devices requires thousands of endpoints to translation of the protocols, schema merging, and automation of health checks. Data volume is imposing a burden on streaming pipelines, DT compute and ledger consensus; tiered architecture and channel partitioning are highly needed. Cross-institution processes: these various referrals, inter-centre studies need portable identities, consent objects and provenance that may have meaning across domains. There is minimal ambiguity in conformance profiles, test suites and typed contracts (D. S. Kumar, 2024). Federated discovery services support data and twin services, but give no consideration to payloads, whilst selective anchoring makes a trade-off between integrity and throughput. The version negotiation has been provided with model, policy and ontology negotiation to avoid brittle upgrades. On the operational side operation there should exist shared SLAs, incident processes and audit mechanisms that need to cross parties. The lines of conflict management and escalation are devised by the ruling powers. The impending enigma is the way to develop interoperability that is not just syntactic but is semantic and policy aware and can be safely automated across organizational boundaries without losing on performance, privacy or clarity of responsibility.

8.2 Privacy–Utility–Performance Trade-Offs

It is a strangled concept in itself that the value of the analysis should be maximized with respect to consent, minimization and latency. The smaller grains cause DT to be more vulnerable but more capable of re-identification and costly to process. Privacy protection technologies, such as pseudonymization, enclaves, differentiating privacy, secure multi-party analytics, can be useful, but also incur accuracy trade-off, or need to lead to latency. Purpose-bound access does not expose, but complicates the notion of real time subscriptions in the scenario of a varying scope. Less transport but less model complexity Edge inference; more accurate but more egress and egress control load Cloud scale. The adaptive privacy budgets which are conditioned by clinical acuity, situation with regard to the sampling and demonstrations to certify the computation and not expose the inputs lie in the open research space. The policy-as-code should be easy to comprehend by clinicians and auditors (Salunkhe et al., 2024). The analysis should be a shared frontier i.e. utility vs. privacy vs. latency, and not an individual frontier. The difficulty here, of paramount importance, is to make principled, auditable compromises, which cannot be drifted, cannot fail to emergencies, and cannot fail in adversarial situations.

8.3 Trust, Liability, and Ethical Considerations

Trust is premised on the transparency, reliability and fair influence. Clinicians must have accountable warnings, confidence which is tuned and clear escalation policies; patients must have scopes of consent which they see and provenance which are understandable. The fact that automated recommendations are already affecting care: they have to be distributed among developers, hospitals, and vendors has to conform to documented intended use, monitoring, and human-in-the-loop design implies that the liability is not resolved yet. Biased performance on under-represented groups, implicit model changes, and creep of surveillance because of repurposed telemetry are some of the ethical dangers. Stratified evaluation, fairness limitations, model cards, change logs and sunset data retention policies are some of the mitigation measures (Bian et al., 2023). Break-glass pathways should be very accountable and should be reviewed in a retrospective manner. Sustainability is moral: Decisions on cryptography and compute need to be energy-implicative. Governance boards like the clinicians, patients and ethicists should review the policies and outcomes periodically. The price of the existence of a permanent social contract of DT-blockchain systems would require demonstrable action, equitable data application, and losses in the case of harm.

9. FUTURE DIRECTIONS

The future of work is going to be centered around the concept of decentralized intelligence, composability, and networked learning health. Federated and edge AI will train and adapt the DT components to the sources of data, and on-chain attestations will assure the compliance with the lineage and policy. Micro-twins and contract-designed processes will enable rapid building of interdepartmental solutions not necessarily integrating into a custom base. The hospitals will interlink DTs to provide supply, twins of public health and community care in a manner that sets up system-of-systems that coordinate resources and shock management. Trade-offs among privacy, performance, and sustainability will be reduced with the development of privacy proofs, secure enclaves and energy-conscious consensus (Mandinyenya & Malele, 2025). Standardized conformance profiles, common testbeds, and repeatable benchmarks will also be available which will boost the fast application and generation of evidences.

9.1 Federated/Edge Intelligence and On-Chain Validation Primitives

Federated and edge learning reduce the amount of transmission of data, as well as adapting the models to the local circumstances. Patient and asset twins have the option to change their parameters depending on the distribution at the ward and the policy may decide on changing the round of aggregation, e.g. eligibility checks, fairness requirements and energy limits. Federated changes are emitted by the drift detectors as compared to retraining. Training data, hyper parameters, and validation output are attested on chain and reminders are not displayed in order to acquire verifiable lineage (Alshammari et al., 2021). The calculation and the performance on which it is based can be verified to point out that inferences or aggregation has been taken with the approved code paths. This disproportionate performance can be performed through the token less reward (reputation, credits) in which the emphasis is put on the contribution of the underrepresented cohorts. The future research directions are highly aggregated in the event of non-IID data, privacy budgets that are based on acuity and latency sensitive scheduling where clinical priorities are used (Ravikumar, Aarthi, Saparbaevich, et al., 2025). At audit-provenance, a dynamic privacy-preserving intelligence is delivered by federated/edge and on-chain attestation.

9.2 Composable Micro-Twins and Contract-Orchestrated Workflows

Micro- twins are mini-functionality like estimating ventilator compliance, predicting pharmacy stocks, even predicting bed-turnover, displaying typed events, and APIs. These units are organized in paths of contract orchestration whereby a sign of a patient degradation may activate staffing forecasts, bed and equipment checks with every decision-making action being predetermined by goal-related policies. The certified contracts and adapters libraries reduce the deployment cycles and enhance the safety via reuse. Standard vocabularies and KPI hooks are also features of versioned templates that render the similar sites to be evaluated similarly. Conformance tests and provenance attestations-based micro-twins between the vendors and the hospitals can develop (Ravikumar, Aarthi, Atamuratova, et al., 2025). The issues described above are open ones that involve prevention of policy clashes, managing global states and safe hot-swaps of components (Han et al., 2021). Composable architectures are claimed to ensure agility, maintainability and non-redundancy of verifiable governance. The 5 number refers to the ongoing cycle of generating composable micro-twins i.e. generating and setting up workflows and deploying the same, evaluating their performance and refining the same which make smart-hospital solutions modular, reusable and upgradable.

Figure 5. Composable Micro-Twins Lifecycle

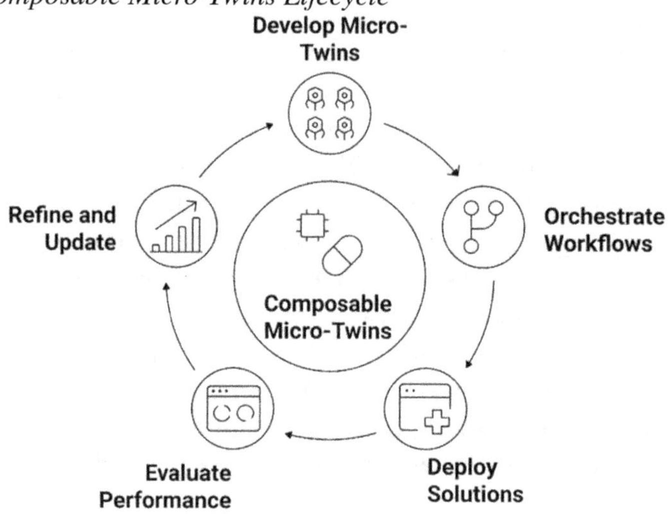

9.3 From Pilots to System-of-Systems (Hospital Networks and Public Health Twins)

To go beyond the pilot projects which focus on individual locations, it has to possess a regional coordination and strength in governance. Hospital networks can exchange insights with provenance foundations of ability, transfers and outbreaks without violating local preference and policy. Matched with the civic-health, de identified, policy-vetted, situational awareness and surge planning indicators, subscriptions are offered and in turn, hospital twin (guidelines, thresholds) feedback. The utility twins and supply-chain deliver inter-domain connectivity to enhance resilience in case of shock by matching equipment, staff and infrastructure. Interoperability is built on the basis of portable identities, templates of cross-jurisdiction contracts and of conformance testing (Nasir et al., 2022). The generation of evidence becomes multi-sited pragmatic appraisals, whose measures are typical and re-run pipelines. It is projected in respect to sustainability which develops energy sensitive timing, efficient consensus and selective anchoring on network basis. The destination is a verifiable system-of-systems of learning, audit systems where care and resource coordination between institutions are organized and facilitated by data, adaptive models and accountable policies.

10. CONCLUSION

The chapter discovered that the use of blockchains in digital twins is capable of producing verifiable, adaptive, and patient-centric smart hospital ecosystems. It has incorporated three general lessons, first, it can be seen that blockchain can be used to provide patients, assets and hospital operations with real-time, multi-scale situational awareness, second, it is possible to offer an immutable provenance, programmable consent and portable trust among departments and institutions, and the last lesson is that a combination of both can result in the closed-loop intelligence, data, models and actions that are cryptographically bound and audit-able. These principles are embodied in the proposed reference architecture and interoperability patterns and policy as code structures which are encompassed by an assessment framework employing technical and clinical and sustainability measures. Implementation guidelines have been on safe IoMT onboarding, versioned and disciplined DT ModelOps to secure drift and reliability engineering with explicit latency budgets and policies to guarantee failure.

The case studies revealed the manifestation of a tangible advantage in the prediction of risk and consent-sensitive capabilities without taking into account the loss of privacy and accountability. On-chain attestation federated/edge learning, contractual, multi-hospital system-of-systems Areas of the future that will facilitate a faster accomplishment of safe scaling are on-chain attestation federated/edge learning, composable micro-twin coordinated by contracts. Other critical areas of concern, such as semantic interoperability, trade-offs in utility performances in privacy, fairness, and liability, and the energy efficiency are also novel areas of research and governance. Nonetheless, there is a way forward that can be achieved by adoption: begin with large value cuts, high value, begin with provenance and consent, measure outcomes with rigor, and grow using standards conformant reusable building blocks. With the help of trust architecture, smart modeling can save time-to-intervention, greater asset uptime, patient agency, and eventually help hospitals to create resilient, data-verifiable care which is transparent, explainable, and continuously growing.

REFERENCES

Abbas, A. F., Qureshi, N. A., Khan, N., Chandio, R., & Ali, J. (2022). The blockchain technologies in healthcare: Prospects, obstacles, and future recommendations; Lessons learned from digitalization. [IJOE]. *International Journal of Online and Biomedical Engineering, 18*(09), 144–159. DOI: 10.3991/ijoe.v18i09.32253

Agbo, C. C., & Mahmoud, Q. H. (2019). Comparison of blockchain frameworks for healthcare applications. *Internet Technology Letters, 2*(5), e122. DOI: 10.1002/itl2.122

Alonso, R., Olivadese, R., Ibba, A., & Reforgiato Recupero, D. (2023). Towards the definition of a European Digital Building Logbook: A survey. *Heliyon, 9*(9), e19285. DOI: 10.1016/j.heliyon.2023.e19285

Alshammari, K., Beach, T., & Rezgui, Y. (2021). Cybersecurity for digital twins in the built environment: Current research and future directions. *Journal of Information Technology in Construction, 26*, 159–173. DOI: 10.36680/j.itcon.2021.010

Amofa, S., Xia, Q., Xia, H., Obiri, I. A., Adjei-Arthur, B., Yang, J., & Gao, J. (2024). Blockchain-secure patient Digital Twin in healthcare using smart contracts. *PLoS One, 19*(2), e0286120. DOI: 10.1371/journal.pone.0286120

Barati, M., & Rana, O. (2022). Tracking GDPR compliance in cloud-based service delivery. *IEEE Transactions on Services Computing, 15*(3), 1498–1511. DOI: 10.1109/TSC.2020.2999559

Barbaria, S., Jemai, A., Ceylan, H. İ., Muntean, R. I., Dergaa, I., & Boussi Rahmouni, H. (2025). Advancing compliance with HIPAA and GDPR in healthcare: A blockchain-based strategy for secure data exchange in clinical research involving private health information. *Healthcare (Basel), 13*(20), 2594. DOI: 10.3390/healthcare13202594

Bian, G., Qu, W., & Shao, B. (2023). Blockchain-based trusted federated learning with pre-trained models for COVID-19 detection. *Electronics (Basel), 12*(9), 2068. DOI: 10.3390/electronics12092068

Boussadi, A., & Zapletal, E. (2017). A Fast Healthcare Interoperability Resources (FHIR) layer implemented over i2b2. *BMC Medical Informatics and Decision Making, 17*(1), 120. Advance online publication. DOI: 10.1186/s12911-017-0513-6

Cheng, W., Ou, W., Yin, X., Yan, W., Liu, D., & Liu, C. (2020). A privacy-protection model for patients. *Security and Communication Networks, 2020*, 1–12. DOI: 10.1155/2020/6647562

Fahmy, A. M. (2025). *Exploring the role of AI in predicting chronic disease progression: Diabetes and cardiovascular diseases*. Premier Journal of Public Health., DOI: 10.70389/PJPH.100021

Ferrag, M. A., Derdour, M., Mukherjee, M., Derhab, A., Maglaras, L., & Janicke, H. (2019). Blockchain technologies for the internet of things: Research issues and challenges. *IEEE Internet of Things Journal*, *6*(2), 2188–2204. DOI: 10.1109/JIOT.2018.2882794

Frempong, D., Benson, C. E., Oyasiji, O., & Okesiji, A. (2024). Blockchain-enabled consent management in healthcare: A framework for enforcing privacy preferences and regulatory compliance. *International Journal of Multidisciplinary Research and Growth Evaluation*, *5*(3), 1059–1068. DOI: 10.54660/.IJMRGE.2024.5.3.1059-1068

Gaddapuri, N. S.Naga Srinivasulu Gaddapuri. (2025). Digital Twin Governance: IoT-driven real-time regulatory auditing in smart hospital architectures. *Computer Fraud & Security*, •••, 1462–1470. DOI: 10.52710/cfs.752

Gebler, R., Reinecke, I., Sedlmayr, M., & Goldammer, M. (2025). Enhancing clinical data infrastructure for AI research: Comparative evaluation of data management architectures. *Journal of Medical Internet Research*, *27*, e74976. DOI: 10.2196/74976

Götz, C. S., Karlsson, P., & Yitmen, I. (2022). Exploring applicability, interoperability and integrability of Blockchain-based digital twins for asset life cycle management. *Smart and Sustainable Built Environment*, *11*(3), 532–558. DOI: 10.1108/SASBE-08-2020-0115

Han, T., Ribeiro, I. de L., Magaia, N., Preto, J., Segundo, A. H. F. N., de Macedo, A. R. L., Muhammad, K., & de Albuquerque, V. H. C. (2021). Emerging drone trends for blockchain-based 5G networks: Open issues and future perspectives. *IEEE Network*, *35*(1), 38–43. DOI: 10.1109/MNET.011.2000151

Hemdan, E. E.-D., El-Shafai, W., & Sayed, A. (2023). Integrating digital twins with IoT-based blockchain: Concept, architecture, challenges, and future scope. *Wireless Personal Communications*, *131*(3), 1–24. DOI: 10.1007/s11277-023-10538-6

Islam, M. N., & Kundu, S. (2019). Enabling IC traceability via blockchain pegged to embedded PUF. *ACM Transactions on Design Automation of Electronic Systems*, *24*(3), 1–23. DOI: 10.1145/3315669

Kim, H., Park, J., Bennis, M., & Kim, S.-L. (2020). Blockchained on-device federated learning. IEEE Communications Letters: A Publication of the IEEE. *IEEE Communications Letters*, *24*(6), 1279–1283. DOI: 10.1109/LCOMM.2019.2921755

Kumar, D. M. (2024). Ethical AI design in blockchain-powered surveillance systems. *Scientific Journal of Artificial Intelligence and Blockchain Technologies*, *1*(3). Advance online publication. DOI: 10.63345/sjaibt.v1.i3.103

Kumar, D. S. (2024). GDPR compliance challenges in blockchain-based systems. *Scientific Journal of Artificial Intelligence and Blockchain Technologies*, *1*(3). Advance online publication. DOI: 10.63345/sjaibt.v1.i3.104

Kumari, S., Sowmya, K., Sharma, A. K., Kumar, A., & Goel, P. K. (2025). Blockchain and AI in rural healthcare. In *Advances in Computational Intelligence and Robotics* (pp. 191–214). IGI Global., DOI: 10.4018/979-8-3373-3241-3.ch010

Lu, J., Sattler, A., Wang, S., Khaki, A. R., Callahan, A., Fleming, S., Fong, R., Ehlert, B., Li, R. C., Shieh, L., Ramchandran, K., Gensheimer, M. F., Chobot, S., Pfohl, S., Li, S., Shum, K., Parikh, N., Desai, P., Seevaratnam, B., & Shah, N. H. (2022). Considerations in the reliability and fairness audits of predictive models for advance care planning. *Frontiers in Digital Health*, *4*(943768), 943768. DOI: 10.3389/fdgth.2022.943768

Lu, Q., Chen, L., Xie, X., Fang, Z., Ye, Z., & Pitt, M. (2023). Framing blockchain-integrated digital twins for emergent healthcare: A proof of concept. *Proceedings of the Institution of Civil Engineers. Engineering Sustainability*, *176*(4), 228–243. DOI: 10.1680/jensu.22.00073

Mandinyenya, G., & Malele, V. (2025). Post-quantum cryptographic techniques for future-proofing-blockchain-based personal data sharing. *Iraqi Journal for Computers and Informatics*, *51*(2), 109–125. DOI: 10.25195/ijci.v51i2.623

Nasir, M. H., Arshad, J., Khan, M. M., Fatima, M., Salah, K., & Jayaraman, R. (2022). Scalable blockchains — A systematic review. *Future Generation Computer Systems*, *126*, 136–162. DOI: 10.1016/j.future.2021.07.035

O'Donoghue, O., Vazirani, A. A., Brindley, D., & Meinert, E. (2019). Design choices and trade-offs in health care blockchain implementations: Systematic review. *Journal of Medical Internet Research*, *21*(5), e12426. DOI: 10.2196/12426

Obodo, O. R. (2025). Conceptualising blockchain-based consent management in multi-provider healthcare environment. International Journal of Scientific Research and Modern Technology, 116–121. DOI: 10.38124/ijsrmt.v4i9.817

Ovsianko, D., & Niemkova, E. (2025). Smart contracts as privacy-preserving mechanisms in distributed digital twin systems. Cybersecurity: Education, Science. *Technique*, *1*(29), 107–123. DOI: 10.28925/2663-4023.2025.29.867

Pan, J., Wang, J., Hester, A., Alqerm, I., Liu, Y., & Zhao, Y. (2019). EdgeChain: An edge-IoT framework and prototype based on blockchain and smart contracts. *IEEE Internet of Things Journal*, *6*(3), 4719–4732. DOI: 10.1109/JIOT.2018.2878154

Park, J., Park, E., Lee, D., Kang, S., Lee, T., Lee, S.-J., Hong, H., Kim, H., Park, Y. R., & Lee, U. (2023). Human digital twins for pervasive healthcare: A scoping review (preprint). *Interactive Journal of Medical Research*. Advance online publication. DOI: 10.2196/46012

Phelan, D., Gottlieb, D., Mandel, J. C., Ignatov, V., Jones, J., Marquard, B., Ellis, A., & Mandl, K. D. (2024). Beyond compliance with the 21st Century Cures Act Rule: A patient controlled electronic health information export application programming interface. *Journal of the American Medical Informatics Association : JAMIA*, *31*(4), 901–909. DOI: 10.1093/jamia/ocae013

Powell, W., Sultanbawa, Y., Thomson, M., Sivakumar, D., Dipu, M. A., Williams, L., Turner-Morris, C., Sigley, G., & He, S. (2024). Blockchain-enabled provenance and supply chain governance for Indigenous foods and botanicals: A design approach study. *Sustainability (Basel)*, *16*(16), 7084. DOI: 10.3390/su16167084

Quazi, F., Raju, N., Gorrepati, N., & Abdul Kareem, S. (2024). Blockchain applications in electronic health records (EHRs). International Journal of Global Innovations and Solutions (IJGIS). DOI: 10.21428/e90189c8.5043b7de

Ranjan, P. R., Yadav, A. S., Verma, A. R., Patil, A., & Gupta, D. P. (2023). Healthcare data management system using blockchain. International Journal of Scientific Research in Computer Science. *Engineering and Information Technology*, *CSEIT2390250*, 382–387. DOI: 10.32628/CSEIT2390250

Ravikumar, A. S., Atamuratova, Z., Ashirova, A., Jurayev, K., & Hayitova, M. (2025). Comprehensive evaluation of AI-driven systems in modern hospital environments. In Advances in Computational Intelligence and Robotics (pp. 61–88). IGI Global Scientific Publishing. DOI: 10.4018/979-8-3373-2787-7.ch003

Ravikumar, A. S., Saparbaevich, B. R., Kumar A., S., Jumaniyozova, M., & Toshova, S. (2025). AI-enhanced clinical decision-making through a collaborative approach. In Advances in Computational Intelligence and Robotics (pp. 249–280). IGI Global Scientific Publishing. DOI: 10.4018/979-8-3373-3311-3.ch010

Rehman, A., Abbas, S., Khan, M. A., Ghazal, T. M., Adnan, K. M., & Mosavi, A. (2022). A secure healthcare 5.0 system based on blockchain technology entangled with federated learning technique. *Computers in Biology and Medicine*, *150*(106019), 106019. DOI: 10.1016/j.compbiomed.2022.106019

Salunkhe, V., Thumati, P. R. R., Kanchi, P., Chhapola, A., & Goel, O. (2024). EHR Interoperability Challenges Leveraging HL7 FHIR for Seamless Data Exchange in Healthcare. *Darpan International Research Analysis*, *12*(3), 403–419. DOI: 10.36676/dira.v12.i3.98

Singla, D., Kumar, S., Gulzar, Y., Mir, M. S., Gupta, D., Jaziri, W., Sassi, N., & Arora, S. (2024). Designing and implementing a resilient immutability mechanism for enhanced supply chain management in E-healthcare systems. *Frontiers in Sustainable Cities*, *6*, 1403809. Advance online publication. DOI: 10.3389/frsc.2024.1403809

Tahar, K., Martin, T., Mou, Y., Verbuecheln, R., Graessner, H., & Krefting, D. (2023). Rare Diseases in hospital information systems-an interoperable methodology for distributed data quality assessments. Methods of Information in Medicine, 62(3–04), 71–89. DOI: 10.1055/a-2006-1018

Yakubu, B. M., Ali, S. M., Khan, M. I., & Bhattarakosol, P. (2024). PatCen: A blockchain-based patient-centric mechanism for the granular access control of infectious disease-related test records. *PLoS One*, *19*(9), e0310407. DOI: 10.1371/journal.pone.0310407

Yaqoob, M. M., Alsulami, M., Khan, M. A., Alsadie, D., Saudagar, A. K. J., AlKhathami, M., & Khattak, U. F. (2023). Symmetry in privacy-based healthcare: A review of skin cancer detection and classification using federated learning. *Symmetry*, *15*(7), 1369. DOI: 10.3390/sym15071369

Zhang, P., White, J., Schmidt, D. C., Lenz, G., & Rosenbloom, S. T. (2018). FHIRChain: Applying blockchain to securely and scalably share clinical data. *Computational and Structural Biotechnology Journal*, *16*, 267–278. DOI: 10.1016/j.csbj.2018.07.004

Zhang, Z. (2023). Digital twin: Application and prospect. Theoretical and Natural Science - the Open Access Proceedings Series for Conferences, 12(1), 220–226. DOI: 10.54254/2753-8818/12/20230477

Ziminski, T. B., Demurjian, S. A., Sanzi, E., Baihan, M. S., & Agresta, T. (2020). An Architectural Solution for Health Information Exchange. In *Virtual and Mobile Healthcare* (pp. 283–327). IGI Global., DOI: 10.4018/978-1-5225-9863-3.ch014

KEY TERMS AND DEFINTIONS

Asset/Device Twin: A DT of medical equipment (e.g., MRI, ventilator) to monitor health and plan maintenance.

Availability/SLO: The target level of system uptime and performance guarantees.

Break-Glass Access: Emergency access with strict time limits and automatic auditing.

Composable Micro-Twins: Small, focused twins that can be combined to build bigger workflows.

Consent Management: Recording and enforcing what data a patient allows to be used and for what purpose.

Data Lineage: A map linking outputs to their input data, processing steps, and model versions.

Data/Concept Drift: When data patterns or real-world behavior change, reducing model accuracy.

De-identification/Pseudonymization: Removing or replacing identifiers to protect patient privacy.

DICOM: The standard format and metadata for medical imaging (CT, MRI, X-ray).

Differential Privacy: Adding controlled noise so statistics can be shared without revealing individuals.

Digital Twin (DT): A live virtual model that mirrors a real patient, device, or hospital process.

Edge Computing: Processing data close to where it is generated to cut latency and bandwidth.

Federated Learning: Training models across sites/devices without centralizing raw data.

Hash/Anchoring: Creating a unique fingerprint of data and recording it on-chain to prove integrity.

HL7 FHIR: A standard for structuring and exchanging clinical data via APIs.

Hospital-System Twin: A DT of hospital operations (beds, staff, flows) to optimize efficiency and safety.

Identity & Access Management (IAM): Tools and processes to authenticate users/devices and grant access.

Interoperability: Different systems sharing data consistently using common standards and codes.

IoMT (Internet of Medical Things): Networked medical devices and sensors that send clinical data.

KPI (Key Performance Indicator): A measurable metric to track technical or clinical outcomes.

Latency/Throughput: How fast results arrive and how much data the system can handle per second.

ModelOps/MLOps: Processes to version, test, deploy, monitor, and update models safely.

On-Chain vs Off-Chain: Proofs and logs on the blockchain; actual data stored in secure external systems.

OPC-UA: A secure industrial protocol for equipment and building systems telemetry.

Patient Twin: A DT focused on an individual's health data to predict risk and support care.

Permissioned Blockchain: A private ledger where only approved parties can read/write transactions.

Policy as Code: Rules (consent, retention, purpose) written as executable logic, not manual steps.

Provenance: A verifiable history of where data came from and how it was used or changed.

RBAC/ABAC: Role-Based and Attribute-Based access controls to limit who sees what data and when.

Secure Enclave/TEE: A protected hardware area that runs sensitive code and keeps data private.

Selective Disclosure: Proving facts (e.g., "age > 18") without exposing full data.

Smart Contract: Code on the blockchain that automatically enforces rules (e.g., consent, access).

System-of-Systems: Multiple twins (hospital, supply chain, public health) working together.

Chapter 6
Digital Twin and Blockchain Integration for Smart Hospital Infrastructures Towards Personalized and Predictive Medicine

Ashok P.
http://orcid.org/0000-0002-5859-6041
Symbiosis Institute of Digital and Telecom Management, India

Vijaya Babu Burra
Koneru Lakshmaiah Education Foundation, India

Lakshmi Sridevi S.
Chennai Institute of Technology, India

Janaki N.
Vels Institute of Science, Technology, and Advanced Studies (VISTAS), India

Sarala Patchala
KKR & KSR Institute of Technology and Sciences, India

Subham Layek
Symbiosis Institute of Digital and Telecom Management, India

ABSTRACT

Digital Twin (DT) technology advances healthcare by employing real-time, data-driven virtual models of physical systems for individualized care, predictive diagnostics, and system management. DTs enhance patient outcomes, hospital efficiency, and drug research speed through applications in remote monitoring, pre-operative planning, and treatment simulation. Despite these benefits, widespread adoption is hindered by cybersecurity threats, data privacy risks, integration difficulties, high

DOI: 10.4018/979-8-3373-8177-0.ch006

deployment costs, and opaque AI decision-making. Additionally, the absence of standardized regulations remains a critical barrier. Future progress depends on developing cost-effective AI solutions, utilizing blockchain for data security, and establishing clear regulatory frameworks. By resolving these technical and operational hurdles, DTs can transform healthcare into a predictive, personalized system.

1. INTRODUCTION

The concept of smart hospitals is a significant development in the healthcare infrastructure of today. They interconnect the physical assets, patients and medical personnel using advanced digital networks. The main goal of the entire system is to improve operational efficiency and increase patient safety. This transformation is aided with the help of two main technologies, the Digital Twins (DT) and Blockchain. A Digital Twin is a virtual replica for the hospital systems. Blockchain technology is used to provide integrity and security to the data in which these replicas are based. Collectively they help hospitals anticipate and mitigate the possibility of such potential complications before they develop. This chapter discusses how these technologies can be integrated to help the advancement of personalized medicine, as well as develop intelligent infrastructure. The evolution of healthcare technologies of a past was until recently rather meagre when compared to the unleashed Digital Twin revolution that gained greater traction in the aftermath of the global covid-19 pandemic. The pandemic highlighted the need for a critical demand for remote healthcare interventions and predictive diagnostics and data-driven decision making for sustainable and effective health services. In response to this, governmental organizations, medical institutions and technology companies have accelerated their digitalization efforts aimed at improving the efficiency and productivity of resources in the healthcare sector. Digital Twin technology is particularly exceptional in promising it will be transformative with massive impacts on personalised medicine, medical research and healthcare management. As one of the latest technological advances, the development of Digital Twins has a lot of potential to revolutionise research in the pharmaceutical industry, improve the delivery of patient care and optimise how processes are managed. Digital Twins as digital replicas are physical entities simulated by highly realistic virtual models that go well beyond consumer-grade simulations in terms of their complexity and their precision. With this technology, a physical entity is always replicated digitally, automatically updated by sensors and machine learning and AI parts. Historical view, future forecast and real-time monitoring are provided by the technology. And, while Digital Twins of machinery have already been adopted for engineering purposes, digital replicas are now being adopted by medical organizations. Medical practitioners can access an extremely accurate digital representation of their patients to spot health issues sooner and predict subsequent developments to determine the best course of treatment. The technology taps into data and scientific models as its predictive mechanism to deliver healthcare-related predictions. The diagnosis system notifies doctors about upcoming bodily disturbances allowing them to start treatments ahead of patient awareness. Digital Twins (DTs) enable cardiology practitioners to simulate blood vessel problems which guides their decision-making process regarding bypass surgery procedures. Medical personnel use digital twins to prerecord cataract procedures and predict postoperative patient outcomes in eye care. Serious health effects occur because of medical equipment errors along with incorrect diagnoses and test results misreads. Digital twin systems decrease diagnostic errors and treatment accuracy. When muscle injuries get diagnosed early in treatment the patient can avoid prolonged paralysis and permanent limb loss. Cancer treatment benefits from disease progression simulation. Digital twins help cancer treatment providers provide personalized prescription medicines by allowing them to model how diseases progress within individual patients. The statement "There is no disease there is a patient" emphasizes personalized care which stands as an essential factor of digital twin applications in medical care. The latest Digital Twin technology develops personalized medical plans by uniting simulation-based analytics with both personal medical data and group epidemiological information. The investigation explores existing healthcare practices of Digital Twin technology combined with predicted healthcare applications focusing on digital patients and AI-derived pharmaceutical developments alongside optimized hospitals and medical wearables as in Fig. 1. Smart hospitals generate massive amounts of sensitive data. Digital Twins rely on this data to be accurate. However, centralized databases face security risks. Blockchain technology is providing a viable solution. It creates a system of decentralized ledgers. This ledger carefully includes each data transaction. It ensures that patient records are tamper-proof. Blockchain breeds trust between patients, doctors, and healthcare organizations. It secures the data flow from the IoT data sensors to the Digital Twin model.

Figure 1. Digital Twin Architecture Framework in Healthcare Systems

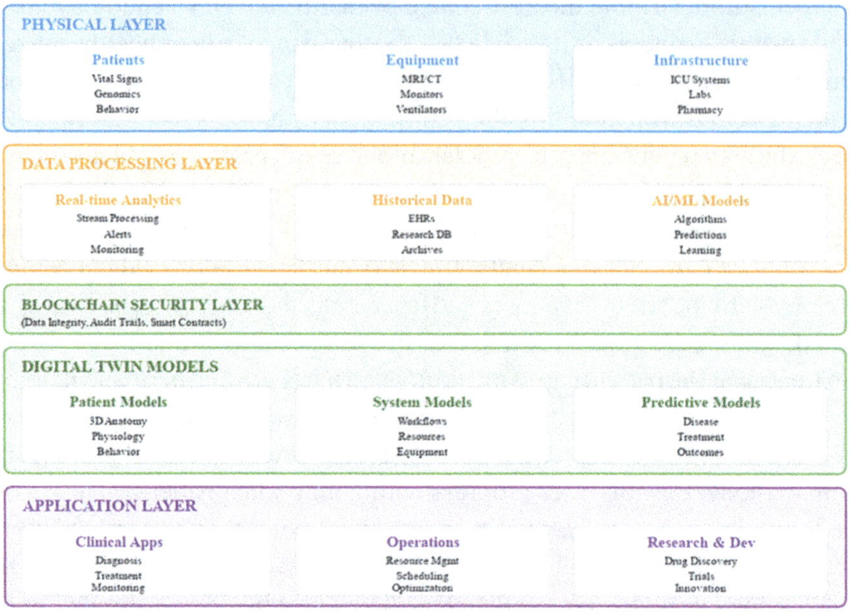

2. LITERATURE REVIEW

Digital twin technology—virtual representations of physical entities updated with real-time data—has rapidly emerged as a transformative force in healthcare, promising to revolutionize personalized and predictive medicine. By integrating data from diverse sources such as wearables, imaging, genomics, and electronic health records, digital twins enable individualized disease modelling, real-time monitoring, and simulation of treatment outcomes, thus supporting precision diagnostics and tailored therapeutics (Fischer et al. 2024; Sel et al. 2024; Katsoulakis et al. 2024; Meijer et al. 2023; Armeni et al. 2022; Adibi et al. 2024; Iliuţă et al. 2024; Delerm & Pilottin, 2024; Banoub et al. 2024). Recent advances in artificial intelligence (AI), machine learning, and the Internet of Medical Things (IoMT) have further accelerated the development and application of digital twins across a range of medical domains, including cardiology, oncology, musculoskeletal care, neurology, and hospital operations (Sel et al. 2024; D'Orsi et al. 2024; Katsoulakis et al. 2024; tefănigă et al. 2024; Jalil et al. 2024; Weerarathna et al. 2024; El-Warrak & de Farias, 2024; Narigina et al. 2024; Johnson et al. 2024). Despite their promise, digital twins face significant challenges related to data integration, privacy, regulatory frameworks, and clinical validation (Fischer et al. 2024; Meijer et al. 2023; Armeni et al. 2022; Kuriakose et al. 2024; El-Warrak & de Farias, 2024). This review provides a comprehensive overview of the current state, applications, challenges, and future directions of digital twin technology in personalized and predictive medicine. Eight unique search groups were used, focusing on foundational concepts, recent advances, alternative terminology, challenges, interdisciplinary expansion, and adjacent technologies. Digital twins originated in engineering and manufacturing but have been adapted to healthcare as virtual patient models that integrate real-time and historical data to simulate physiological processes and predict outcomes (Fischer et al. 2024; Sel et al. 2024; Katsoulakis et al. 2024; Meijer et al. 2023; Balasubramanyam et al. 2024; Delerm & Pilottin 2024). The core components include data acquisition (from sensors, wearables, and medical devices), computational modelling, and bidirectional data flow between the physical and digital entities (Sel et al. 2024; Katsoulakis et al. 2024; Delerm & Pilottin, 2024). Digital twins are being applied in various medical domains (as in Table 1):

- Cardiology: Patient-specific heart models for diagnosis, risk prediction, and treatment optimization (Sel et al. 2024; S et al. 2024).
- Oncology: Simulation of tumour progression and response to immunotherapy, including CAR-T cell therapy (D'Orsi et al. 2024; Aghamiri & Amin 2025; tefănigă et al. 2024).
- Musculoskeletal and Orthopaedic Care: Personalized surgical planning, rehabilitation, and outcome prediction (Diniz et al. 2025; Weerarathna et al. 2024).
- Neurology and Chronic Disease: Management of migraines, diabetes, and other chronic conditions through continuous monitoring and predictive analytics (Nadeem et al. 2025; Meijer et al. 2023; Subashini et al. 2024).
- Hospital Operations: Optimization of workflows, resource allocation, and patient flow (Johnson et al. 2024).

In the current health informatics environment, the convergence of artificial intelligence and machine learning, the Internet of Medical Things (IoMT), and the cloud-enabled information infrastructure has become a linchpin in the spectrum of digital twin technologies, which enables data processing at real-time with predictive analytics and monitoring of patients remotely using that data (Adibi et al. 2024; Jalil et al. 2024; Gazerani 2023). Cloud-based digital twins make possible the development of horizontal and comprehensive data-driven healthcare ecosystems (Gazerani 2023).

Table 1. Applications of Digital Twins Across Medical Domains

Medical Domain	Primary Applications	Key Benefits	Current Status
Cardiology	Heart modelling, risk prediction, surgical planning	Reduced surgical risks, personalized treatment	Clinical pilots
Oncology	Tumour simulation, treatment response prediction	Optimized therapy selection, reduced side effects	Research phase
Musculoskeletal	Surgical planning, rehabilitation monitoring	Improved surgical outcomes, faster recovery	Early adoption
Neurology	Disease progression modeling, symptom tracking	Better chronic disease management	Proof of concept
Hospital Operations	Workflow optimization, resource allocation	Increased efficiency, reduced costs	Implementation

The Key challenges include:

- Data Integration and Interoperability: Harmonizing heterogeneous data sources remains complex (Fischer et al. 2024; Meijer et al. 2023; Armeni et al. 2022; Kuriakose et al. 2024; El-Warrak & de Farias, 2024).
- Privacy and Security: Handling sensitive patient data raises ethical and legal concerns [20].
- Regulatory and Clinical Validation: Lack of standardized frameworks and robust clinical evidence limits widespread adoption (Fischer et al. 2024; Armeni et al. 2022; Kuriakose et al. 2024; El-Warrak & de Farias, 2024) as in Fig. 2.
- Scalability and Cost: High computational demands and costs hinder large-scale implementation (Fischer et al. 2024; Meijer et al. 2023; Armeni et al. 2022; Gazerani 2023).

The literature demonstrates that digital twin technology is at the forefront of a paradigm shift toward personalized and predictive medicine, offering unprecedented opportunities for individualized care, real-time monitoring, and simulation-based decision support (Fischer et al. 2024; Sel et al. 2024; Katsoulakis et al. 2024; Meijer et al. 2023; Armeni et al. 2022; Adibi et al. 2024; Iliuţă et al. 2024; Delerm & Pilottin 2024; Banoub et al. 2024). High-quality reviews and scoping studies highlight the transformative potential of digital twins, particularly when integrated with AI and IoMT, in domains such as cardiology, oncology, and chronic disease management (Sel et al. 2024; D'Orsi et al. 2024; Katsoulakis et al. 2024; tefănigă et al. 2024; Jalil et al. 2024; Weerarathna et al. 2024; El-Warrak & de Farias, 2024). However, the field is still in its early stages, with most applications limited to pilot studies, simulations, or specific clinical scenarios (Katsoulakis et al. 2024; Armeni et al.

2022; Adibi et al. 2024; Weerarathna et al. 2024; El-Warrak & de Farias, 2024). The main barriers to adoption include data interoperability, privacy, regulatory uncertainty, and the need for robust clinical validation (Fischer et al. 2024; Meijer et al. 2023; Armeni et al. 2022; Kuriakose et al. 2024; El-Warrak & de Farias, 2024).

Figure 2. Implementation Challenges and Solution Framework

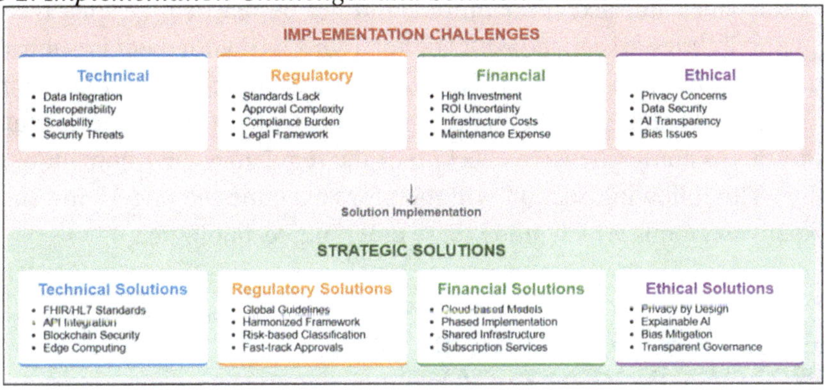

In sum, a feat of technological innovation in high-powered personalized and predictive medicine will include the advent of digital twin technology; however, thorough exploitation of its capabilities will require overcoming significant obstacles of a technical, regulatory, and ethical nature through combined and interdisciplinary investigation. According to Google Health, IBM, WHO and McKinsey together provide insights about market trends with adoption information and financial implications while showing regulatory effects in their reports. Industry adoption rates are tracked through bar charts and heatmaps whereas statistical and thematic approaches reveal data trends in the analysis. The elimination of bias requires diverse geographical studies but data dependability needs ethical attention through cross-checking and proper referencing to stop plagiarism. The analysis faces three main obstacles which consist of industry-funded publications presenting bias concerns as well as privacy regulations restricting patient data availability and the inability to access private healthcare information. The research analyses the limitations of digital twins implementation to establish essential medical applications and recommends research and legislative changes for future work.

2.1. Review Methodology

This chapter provides an in-depth analysis of the literature related to Digital Twins with Blockchain in the context of Healthcare. To this end, we used established databases such as PubMed, IEEE Xplore, and Scopus which was a systematic search of scholarship published in 2019 to 2024. Our keyword set included "Digital Twin," "Smart Hospital," "Blockchain Healthcare" and "Predictive Medicine." Emphasis was placed on peer-reviewed investigations and current reports in the industry. The inclusion protocol considered giving preference to papers providing an explanation of architectural frameworks and security considerations as well as their clinical applications, with a systematic exclusion of non English publications as well as abstracts for which full text availability could not be reached. Despite the list of technical possibilities associated with Digital Twins its deployment is often slowed down in practice by legal elements. The process of assimilating heterogeneous data sources necessarily requires compliance is stringent with data protection statutes. As a result of this, a comprehensive checkup of the regulatory environment becomes invaluable. The following section will therefore examine the underlying statutory and normative systems which guide these emerging technologies.

3. REGULATIONS FOR DIGITAL TWIN TECHNOLOGY IN HEALTHCARE

3.1. Regulations in India

India's National Digital Health Mission (NDHM) creates a safety system and standardized interface for healthcare data through digital means (Delerm & Pilottin, 2024). The Ayushman Bharat Digital Mission (ABDM) helps create secure digital health data exchange systems which support standard digital technology applications. The PDP bill is valuable because it regulates the storage and usage of patients' data and offers parameters on consent management, data storage, and also enforcement in case the privacy rules are violated. The Under CDSCO, the Medical Device Rules, 2017 provides regulations to oversee the functioning of AI-based digital health technologies and also DT applications.

3.2. Regulations in the United States

One step closer to resolving this important issue and making way for more effective provision of care is also that, To the maximum extent allowed by federal regulations, Active treatment of the consistency of data being recorded involves HIPAA privacy rule for the electronic health information. AI-powered medical devices undergo a process of FDA approval, this category includes also digital twins that help with diagnosing evaluation, and treatment planning. The 21st Century Cures Act is also advancing the efforts that are being put forth in the making of AI technology for the healthcare field alongside using real world evidence as the way for regulation and making decisions on how to use these innovations. It must comply with the Office of Management and Budget/National Institute of Standards and Technology-defined high security requirements for electronic health records.

3.3. Regulations in the European Union

DT installations are greatly influenced by rules on how to protect data in accordance with the General Data Protection Regulation (GDPR) of the European Union. GDPR mandates that DT model operators ensure they purge personally-identifiable information from datasets and ensure that they obtain direct consent from patients. Before a clinical use of DT applications, a lengthy precedent is before them, on the road to acquiring all MDR-level regulatory approval held set aside for the DT's AI-integrated healthcare solution. The artificial intelligence act introduced by the European Commission, consisting of risk-based classifications of all digital twin AI applications, have to comply with the basic safety rules and ethics of their usage.

3.4. Regulations in China

Under rules regarding cross-border flow data and digital health technologies, China's Cybersecurity Law and PIPL impose stringent restrictions that ensure that DT models meet the requirements of data localization. AI healthcare technologies are regulated by the NMPA, which defines very strict specifications as to the clinical validation required for the DT application. The 2022 Guidelines for AI-Based Medical Devices lay down the rules of transparency, explainability, and safety standards that will oversee the integration of the DT in a hospital.

3.5. Regulations in Japan

APPI and PMDA set regulations for AI and DT models regarding their work in healthcare.

3.6. Regulations in Australia

The Privacy Act 1988 serves as a governing agent of the ADHA, making it the data privacy supervisor of AI-powered medical devices.

3.7. Regulations in UK

The UK regulations for DT models remain a reference for GDPR, MHRA, and NHS AI Lab for its ethical AI standards. Table 2 contrasts national regulations, practices, and strategies for the use of digital twin technologies in healthcare. It outlines the main legislative frameworks, data security guidelines, and compliance standards that control the use of DT technology worldwide.

3.8. Blockchain as a Regulatory Enabler

Achieving compliance with the General Data Protection Regulation (GDPR) and the Health Insurance Portability and Accountability Act (HIPAA) are fair amounts to challenge to Authors among Digital Twin systems, with the two pieces of regulations imposing severe personal privacy requirements for the managing sensitive personal data. In practice, the necessity of constant protection of data integrity, confidentiality and availability makes it hard to implement advanced digital modelling technologies in healthcare environments. Blockchain technology is a potentially exciting pathway for hospitals to meet these regulatory requirements. By using the capacity of distributed ledgers to have their own traits, healthcare institutions can establish difficult mechanisms that can make sure that compliance is assured without sacrificing operational well being. With the decentralized nature of blockchain, all relevant information is stored across multiple nodes critiquing any single points of failure and strengthening the system against tampering by adversaries. One of the most salient advantages of the integration of blockchain is the process of providing an immutable audit trail. And each access event to patient data is written to as a cryptographic transaction, providing an immutable log with an unambiguous identification of actor, action performed, and exact time stamp. This granular provenance is invaluable in audit purposes as it allows both regulators and internal auditors control the data handling processes to ensure they comply with set privacy policies and legal obligations. The transparency characteristic in this approach makes it easy to implement rigorous oversight and enhance accountability over the entire healthcare ecosystem. Beyond auditability, smart contracts programmed on the blockchain can be used to autonomously enforce directives of patient consent. By storing consent preferences in programmable contracts, the system can instantly standardize and respect one's privacy preferences, thus removing the burden of manual administrative work. This automated enforcement not only makes the process of managing permissions much faster but also makes consent verification more reliable, to guarantee that patient autonomy is upheld in accordance and compliance to both the GDPR and HIPAA mandates.

Table 2. Comparison of Regulatory frameworks, data protection standards across countries

Country/Region	Regulatory Frameworks	Data Protection Standards	Approval Process for AI/DT in Healthcare	Key Challenges
India	National Digital Health Mission (NDHM), Personal Data Protection Bill (PDPB), Medical Device Rules, 2017	Data localization under PDPB, compliance with IT Act, 2000	CDSCO regulates AI-driven medical devices and DT healthcare applications	Interoperability issues, lack of standardized DT adoption guidelines
United States	Health Insurance Portability and Accountability Act (HIPAA), 21st Century Cures Act, FDA AI/ ML Regulatory Framework	Strict patient data privacy under HIPAA, National Institute of Standards and Technology (NIST) cybersecurity standards	FDA approval required for DT-integrated AI healthcare applications	Complex approval process, evolving AI regulation for healthcare
European Union	General Data Protection Regulation (GDPR), Medical Device Regulation (MDR), EU AI Act	Strongest data privacy regulations with explicit consent requirements under GDPR	MDR compliance required for DT applications, AI classified based on risk level	Stricter regulations for AI-driven healthcare, high compliance costs
China	Cybersecurity Law, Personal Information Protection Law (PIPL), AI-Based Medical Devices Guidelines	Mandatory data localization and stringent patient data privacy rules	National Medical Products Administration (NMPA) approval for AI-based medical devices, transparency in DT algorithms required	Cross-border data restrictions, complex bureaucratic process
Japan	Act on Protection of Personal Information (APPI), Pharmaceuticals and Medical Devices Act (PMDA)	APPI aligns with global privacy standards, ensuring patient data security	PMDA evaluates AI/ DT applications in medical devices	Limited regulatory clarity on AI-powered Digital Twins
Australia	Privacy Act 1988, Australian Digital Health Agency (ADHA) AI guidelines	ADHA enforces strict patient data security protocols	Therapeutic Goods Administration (TGA) oversees AI-driven DT applications	Need for enhanced DT governance framework

continued on following page

Table 2. Continued

Country/Region	Regulatory Frameworks	Data Protection Standards	Approval Process for AI/DT in Healthcare	Key Challenges
United Kingdom	UK GDPR, Medicines and Healthcare Products Regulatory Agency (MHRA), NHS AI Lab framework	UK GDPR similar to EU GDPR, ensuring strict patient data protection	MHRA requires dts in healthcare to meet risk classification standards	Challenges in adapting AI-driven dts to existing regulatory models
Global Standards	WHO Digital Health Guidelines, IEEE P2802 Standard for Digital Twins, International Medical Device Regulators Forum (IMDRF)	ISO/IEC 27701 for privacy management, interoperability standards in progress	IMDRF working on AI risk classification, standardization of DT healthcare applications	Need for harmonized global DT regulatory standards

National regulations provide a local framework, but smart hospitals operate in a global environment. Interoperability requires international cooperation. We next explore the global standards and organizations shaping this technology.

4. INTERNATIONAL ORGANIZATIONS AND STANDARDS

Digital health innovations are primarily shaped by international organizations that operate beyond the normal frameworks of nation-state regulation (Kuriakose et al. 2024; El-Warrak et al. 2024). WHO and IMDRF are responsible for formulating guidelines that will regulate the functioning of Digital Twin technology in healthcare settings. International compliance with data protection can be achieved through standardized privacy information management frameworks like ISO/IEC 27701. The IEEE P2802 Standard lays out guideline steps in developing DT models across multiple sectors, including healthcare. The Global Digital Health Partnership strives for global cooperation in establishing standard regulatory procedures that allow for easier integration of DT technology into healthcare platforms worldwide. The emergence of Digital-Twin (DT) technology in the healthcare industry is currently facing several challenges in its widespread application despite the growing awareness of safety issues and their integration into the digital health infrastructure. On a global scale, integration is still affected by a lack of strong standardisation as well as challenges related to providing interconnectivity and since then, ensuring full regulatory compliance in data exchanges across borders. Significant standardisation work still remains to be done, not least in the wake of the unfolding of digital twin technology, but in bringing clarity and adoption in the context of different national jurisdictions. In addition, it requires identifying regulating mechanisms that can provide sufficient support for medical innovation in the field of digital healthcare, which can result in the practice of clinical ethics and ensure protection of data. The implementation of digital twin technology will not limit technological innovation as it will solve its current challenges while improving patient care and data security and ethical guidelines (Fischer et al. 2024; Armeni et al. 2022). The Applications of Digital Twins in Healthcare Domain (Sel et al. 2024; S et al. 2024):

- The use of digital twins results in precise medicine when the system creates specific treatment strategies by analysing patient data including genetic information along with medical records. Cancer treatment effectiveness predictions based on algorithms helped Siemens Healthiness develop more effective medical results for patients.
- Digital Twins deploy wearable technology for ongoing disease monitoring which allows prompt medical actions toward patients with cardiovascular disease and diabetes (Adibi et al. 2024; Johnson et al. 2024). Hospital readmission rates decreased significantly because Philips developed outstanding AI-based Digital Twin systems which monitor heart diseases.
- The use of digital twins accelerates clinical trial processes through human body simulation which helps to forecast medication outcomes (D'Orsi et al. 2024; Aghamiri & Amin, 2025; tefănigă et al. 2024). The implementation of this strategy allowed AstraZeneca to reduce the costs of R&D during development by 15%. Regarding the COVID-19 vaccine. The use of AI-enhanced digital twins helps hospitals forecast their need for ICU beds alongside required staff that results in improved operational performance. The Cleveland Clinic enhanced their workflow performance through this technology which shortened patient wait times by 20 percent. The Mayo Clinic employs digital twins to let surgeons perform virtual practice on complex procedures which enhances their operational success by 25%.

5. FEATURES OF DIGITAL TWIN TECHNOLOGY

The five dimensions of DT construction form the physical entity along with the virtual model while they include connections between them together with DT data and service applications (Iliuţă et al. 2024) as in Table 3. The five dimensions interact and function together to establish the structural model of the DT as in Fig. 3. Figure 3 illustrates the five-dimensional model. It highlights the bidirectional data flow. This flow is critical for smart hospitals. The physical entity sends data to the virtual model via the connection layer. The virtual model processes this data and sends feedback. This loop enables real-time adjustments in medical equipment settings. The integration of a blockchain layer into this model would secure the 'Connections' dimension, preventing data interception during transmission. The physical entity in DT designs can represent either products or functional systems and cities that execute their assigned tasks while operating sensor devices for data acquisition. The Internet of Things enables technical observation of physical aspects through data collection capabilities including two-dimensional codes and data acquisition cards and sensors. Real-time data acquisition combined with processed information feedback is essential to enhance the design and operations through communication technology. A virtual model serves as a computerized representation of physical entities that incorporates entity capabilities together with physical properties as well as geometrical and behavioural characteristics for representation within the virtual environment. Through Virtual reality/augmented reality/mixed reality (VR/AR/MR) technology users gain access to visualization and the fusion of virtual entity data together with physical entity data.

Figure 3. Five-Dimensional Digital Twin Construction Model

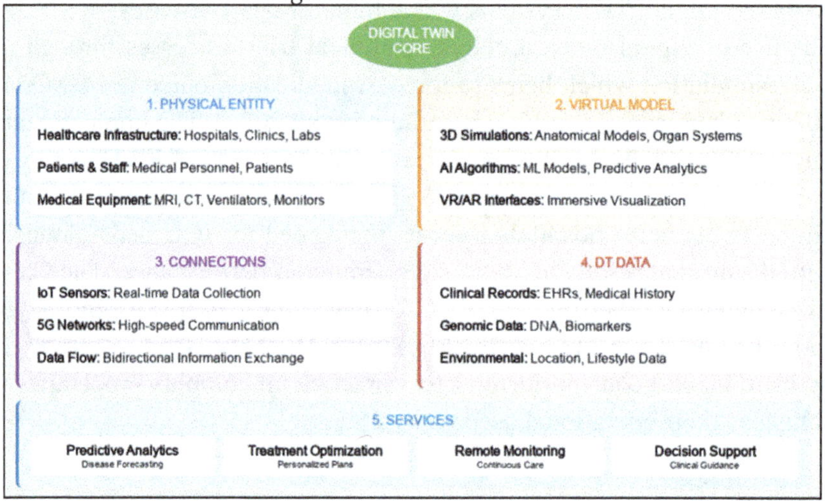

The 5G communication technology provides fast and efficient data transmission which fulfils digital twin mass data requirements. The human-virtual world interaction requires careful attention to human–computer interaction technology together with human–robot interaction and collaboration methods. Multiple information categories contained in the DT data lead to substantial model enhancement through their fusion processes. The rapid volume of obtained data enables Big Data to find useful explanations along with predictions about DT results and processes. Since the blockchain acts as an automatic safeguard to maintain data protection for the DT it also stops unauthorized modifications to dual data. DT service model supports both physical entity service along with virtual model service. Data calibration functions enable virtual models to preserve their operational integrity while maintaining their performance level. The automatic processing of twin data by AI uses optimal algorithm matching to analyse and fuse data and develop neural networks which enhances both data value and service speed and accuracy (Jalil et al. 2024; Gazerani 2023).

Table 3. Technology integration matrix showing the role and maturity of various components in Digital Twin systems.

Technology Component	Primary Function	Blockchain Role	Maturity Status
IoT Sensors	Real-time data collection	Verifies data source origin	Mature
5G Networks	High-speed data transmission	Secures Network nodes	Emerging
AI/ML Algorithms	Pattern recognition & prediction	Audits algorithm decisions	Mature
Blockchain	Data security & integrity	Core Infrastructure	Developing
VR/AR/MR	Visualization & interaction	NA	Emerging
Cloud Computing	Scalable data processing	Decentralized storage	Mature
Edge Computing	Local data processing	Secured Nodes	Emerging
Big Data Analytics	Insight generation	NA	Mature

5.1. Blockchain-Digital Twin Integration in Hospitals

The integration of Blockchain acts as a safety net for Digital Twins. In a smart hospital, devices constantly exchange data. Hackers target these connections. Blockchain secures these endpoints. It uses cryptographic hashes to lock data blocks. Should any piece of individual data in a stream of sensor data be tampered with, where the corresponding cryptographic hash will inevitably diverge, the validation mechanism will reject it instantly. Such a strict and rigorous scrutiny makes sure that the digital twin is at all times an accurate and faithful copy of its real counterpart. This integrity is not just wanted but mandatory in a safety critical deployment such as in an intensive care unit ventilator deployment or in remote patient monitoring systems (Adibi et al. 2024).

5.2 Smart Contracts for Consent Management

Smart contracts are used in smart hospitals to automate various processes. These are self-executing contracts with the terms written into code. In a Digital

Twin context, they manage patient consent. If a patient revokes consent for data sharing, the smart contract automatically locks the data. This removes the need for manual administrative work. It ensures that the hospital always complies with data privacy laws.

6. CASE STUDIES OF DIGITAL TWINS IN HEALTHCARE

6.1. GE Healthcare

Operational delays among hospitals that stemmed from broken equipment amounted to 25% of their total delays. The implementation of Digital Twins for MRI and CT equipment by GE anticipated equipment breakdowns which cut unplanned maintenance by half and simultaneously enhanced patient healthcare quality.

6.2. Boston Children's Hospital

Heart Disease in Children who had congenital heart defects needed to undergo several hazardous surgical procedures. The digital simulation of various surgical approaches led to lower unnecessary procedures by 20% along with patient survival rates that improved by 15% throughout the clinical process.

6.3. Siemens Healthiness

AI in Cancer Treatment Before implementing standard cancer treatments hospitals needed to follow strict and lengthy planning procedures. The AI-powered Digital Twins from Siemens enhanced radiation therapy performance in real-time by delivering delivering improved treatment accuracy with reduced side effects (Siemens Healthineers Case Study). Philips developed heart disease monitoring platforms to address readmission problems of heart failure patients who needed improved real-time tracking. Clinical judgment received improvement together with a 30% decrease in readmissions through Philips' development of Digital Twins which monitored health parameters and heart failure risks.

6.4. Digital Heart Models and Precise Cardiovascular Disease Management

It represents how the DT applies to cardiovascular system diagnosis (Diniz et al. 2025; Weerarathna et al. 2024). Philips used the personalized DT model to create heart models through unique CT images acquired before surgery. The tool gives surgeons immediate three-dimensional object positions that assist them with equipment selection and placement during surgical interventions. The research from Chakshu et al. applies recurrent neural networks to develop an inverse analysis method for cardiovascular DT that achieves high analysis precision. Deep learning methods enable the calculation of aortic blood pressure waveforms from blood pressure waveforms obtained from easy-accessible arteries such as radial or carotid arteries. An active DT becomes achievable because the inverse analysis method enables ongoing healthcare monitoring which detects medical developments along with their further deterioration. Biomedical applications using non-invasive or minimally invasive measurement tools have the possibility to replace complex and invasive diagnostic tools thanks to this approach. Gemalto and colleagues built a patient-specific electromechanical computer model through clinical pressure data analysis of patients who received treatment for aortic coarctation which resulted in a detailed cellular-scale model as in Table 4.

The first digital twin application in orthopaedics series began when our team developed a solution to fix the deficiencies in traditional dynamical biomechanical analysis methods (Dean et al. 2024). The system obtained human body movement status and space dynamics through human motion tracking technology. The wearable reality device and limited sensor readings calculated the actual body posture of the lower back region. The inverse kinematics system provided information alongside finite element method application which enabled establishment of the DT body of the lumbar spine allowing various human body motion postures. The AI model calculates results in real-time using obtained posture information that then uses visualization to integrate with the virtual lumbar spine. Live-time assessment of lumbar spine biomechanical properties together with real-time prediction reached its goal of monitoring and forecasting operations. A three-dimensional virtual reality system developed using Unity3D software enabled Realtime biomechanical performance recordings of the lumbar spine thus creating a new effective real-time planning solution for spine treatment. We achieved real-time prediction capabilities for intradiscal pressure and facet contact force through our method to construct the DT along with a dynamic system for digital and physical space connection. Aubert established the DT of patient fractures to evaluate four stabilization approaches and enhance operating and post-surgical management decisions for optimal surgical outcomes. The examination of repeated fracture risks focused on both bone areas under exceeding local yield strength stress and interfragmentary strain observations.

The collaboration between Pharmacy Dassault Systems and the US Food and Drug Administration approved the SIMULIA Living Heart project in 2014 to become the initial digital research on organ–drug interactions. The model constitutes a DT representation of human hearts and fulfils both researcher and educator validation criteria in medical practice. Pharmaceutical engineers and medical professionals using this technology can now observe heart tissue structure and mobility to develop more personalized medical solutions for the future. Takeda Pharmaceuticals now uses the DT technology for production purposes to make transformative therapies available worldwide. The development of DT models allows businesses to speed up pharmaceutical development while generating authentic predictions about biochemical reactions. Direct interaction between Atos and Siemens and representatives from pharmaceutical companies led to development of physical DT models that enhanced manufacturing efficiency beyond standard practices. The solution successfully operates due to support from IoT together with AI and various advanced technologies.

6.5. Secure Data Sharing in Hospital Networks (Blockchain Application)

A salient challenge in smart hospital infrastructures of the present day is in the field of secure data interdepartment communication. In recent pilot investigation, we deployed Digital Twin architecture secured to blockchain thereby harnessing a private blockchain network milieu. This configuration provided for data linkage between the radiology division and the operative unit. The patient Digital Twin received constant real-time updating and the blockchain middleware prevented any unauthorized surgeon from viewing the data, essentially preventing unauthorized data access. The result was a secure, real-time subject of operation lay that improved outcome of surgical planning all while maintaining patient privacy.

Table 4. Summary of quantitative results from Digital Twin implementation across major healthcare organizations.

Organization	Application Area	Key Metrics	Results Achieved
GE Healthcare	Equipment Maintenance	Unplanned maintenance reduction	50% reduction
Boston Children's Hospital	Cardiac Surgery	Procedure optimization	20% fewer procedures, 15% improved survival
Siemens Healthineers	Cancer Treatment	Radiation therapy accuracy	30% improvement in treatment precision
Philips	Heart Disease Monitoring	Readmission rates	30% reduction in readmissions
Mayo Clinic	Surgical Training	Operational success rates	25% improvement
Cleveland Clinic	Workflow Optimization	Patient wait times	20% reduction

7. DIFFICULTIES IN HEALTHCARE DIGITAL TWIN IMPLEMENTATION

Digital twins demand significant money because their development relies on extensive cloud service investments together with IoT infrastructure and Artificial Intelligence technology expenses (Nadeem et al. 2025; Meijer et al. 2023; Subashini et al. 2024). Hospital facilities face financial strain due to significant implementation costs associated with cloud and IoT infrastructure. Real-time patient data makes digital twins vulnerable to cyberattacks and associated security threats (Banoub et al. 2024) as in Fig. 4.

Figure 4. ROI Analysis and Implementation Timeline

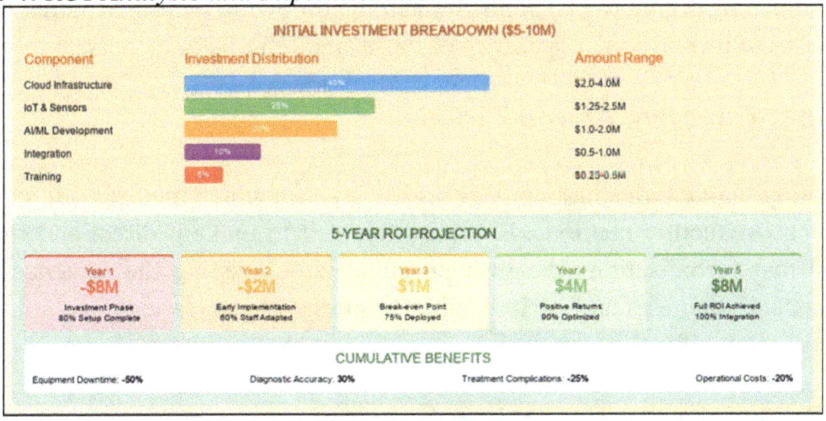

The 2024 HIMSS study demonstrates that cybersecurity represents an important barrier to medical professionals through their survey results which found 70% of the respondents adopting this view. Healthcare operations become substantially harder because HIPAA and GDPR along with NDHM require strict data protection compliance (Katsoulakis et al. 2024; Armeni et al. 2022). The inability to achieve universal regulatory standards creates administrative delays which become legal obstacles for patient care approval. The inconsistent nature of local laws commands 40% of AI-based healthcare applications to undergo extended regulatory procedures. The medical use of Digital Twins needs to properly interact with existing hospital systems including EHRS databases and IOT equipment. The issue arises because fifty percent of institutions claim technical incompatibility between systems which hinders AI progress. The question arises when computers give incorrect instructions to doctors about who bears responsibility for such mistakes. Being led to an unusable destination reflects the current situation. Judging these self-learning AI models poses a challenging task to officials who draft regulations and guidelines because of their autonomous development. Approximately 30% of doctors are opposed to AI making decisions since, let's be honest, these algorithms can be confusing. It's similar to that intelligent friend who never shares how they know things. Thus, they continue to use human judgment.

8. THE FUTURE OF DIGITAL TWINS IN HEALTHCARE

Digital twins unlock new healthcare applications which include individual medicine programs and proactive disease forecasting methods (Fischer et al. 2024; Meijer et al. 2023; Armeni et al. 2022; Gazerani 2023). We need to navigate through multiple technological along with regulatory along with public support hurdles before establishing digital twins' applications. The following section explores several approaches to increase the popularity of these small digital assistants.

8.1. Cost-Effective AI and Clouds

Creating digital twins harbour significant expense which requires our attention to find cost reduction methods. Rephrase this text to make it direct and flowing with normal verbalization whenever possible while keeping the sentences easy to understand. Siemens and various other businesses have started developing less expensive straightforward versions.

8.2. Blockchain for Protecting Secrets

Everyone has become familiar with both cybersecurity breaches and digital attacks in the news media. Application of blockchain technology will establish completely secure medical record storage. A digital vault works just like this system where only approved users can access its contents while also enforcing honesty from everyone involved.

8.3. Interoperability and Standardization

Different countries, different rules. WHO and FDA together with other prominent entities should form global AI health care guidelines that all nations can follow. Through this system each person understands what things are acceptable and unacceptable. Digital Twins need systems which can exchange data with other devices using FHIR and HL7 protocols. Digital Twins require the ability to exchange information with ehrs but they must do it without causing system problems. FHIR and HL7 provide healthcare organizations with a specialized linking system that functions as a secret code to maintain proper communication between systems.

8.4. AI That Talks Your Language

Medical staff need to comprehend the explanations behind AI recommendations because they desire to see the rationale for which treatments the AI system proposes. We are developing methods to increase AI transparency because it should explain its decisions to enable everyone to understand its information.

8.5. Digital Twins in the Drug Game

There exists a possibility to preview drug effects via digital versions of patients before giving medications to actual patients. AI-Powered Genomic Modelling brings revolutionary capabilities to customized medicine according to its mission. Such clinical trials could save both time and financial resources according to available evidence.

8.6. Uniting for Ethics in AI

Experts demonstrate the best capability to develop necessary regulations that AI in healthcare will require. The examination of medical-professional-technology-government alliances for fairness purposes looks at the Google DeepMind-NHS UK partnership as an example.

8.7. Personalised Medicines

Personalized Medicine using Digital Twins The health and care sector together with many other industrial fields has achieved significant benefits from IoT (Dixit 2025). Real-time data collection from clinical and health sensors along with additional environmental or other sensors constitutes one aspect together with systems that facilitate communication between people machines and equipment. Digital patient data becomes accessible through the integration of patient-generated reports and remote monitoring as well as diagnostic procedures and electronic medical records. Cloud computing and artificial intelligence including machine learning represent two fundamental emerging technologies that are developed successfully at the same time. These technologies have evolved into necessary instruments to both process huge volumes of (IoT) data and discover new knowledge as well as perform these processes in real time. Computer models of the SARS-coronavirus 2 spike protein along with the angiotensin converting enzyme 2 receptors of assorted human and animal species in silico simulations enable researchers to conduct virtual comparisons of protein receptor binding affinities which can lessen reliance on conventional land-based laboratory work. Researchers face numerous challenges when developing complete and effective human digital twins because of extensive physiological relationships between body systems. Laboratory medicine could achieve great progress by developing the ability to create even small human tissue components like receptors or specific subcellular elements. Several scientific studies provide foundation for digital human twin development through large-scale data collection from both patients and healthy people in terms of biochemical and genomic information. Recent research has focused heavily on digital twins in healthcare, which have the potential to change predictive management and tailored medication. New applications have been made possible by the combination of digital twin-based engineering and data-driven healthcare methodologies.

The ability of digital twin technology to produce virtual representations of real objects is a crucial feature that makes it possible to simulate interventions and do predictive maintenance. This approach is comparable to in-silico clinical evaluations, which use dynamic human models to evaluate the effectiveness of medical treatments. Lehrach and associates. Proposed an individualised care system based on 'virtual twins' to model patients' biological states using diverse datasets, including clinical and imaging data. Big data technologies and increasing computer capability have made such customized digital models more feasible, enabling doctors to replicate potential treatments before actual application, hence improving patient care and lowering costs. Several research have examined the use of digital twins in specific medical diseases (Roopa 2023). Digital twins in orthodontics demonstrated their worth according to Cho et al.'s findings through three-dimensional imaging combined with facial scans that produced precise models which led to improved patient results. Digital twins have been used for management of chronic diseases like multiple sclerosis when dealing with complicated heterogeneous medical information. Modern appliances known as digital twins unite clinical genomic information and environmental factors with medication-related information to show prediction possibilities regarding disease initiation and medication performance. Medical professionals use digital twin models as an imitation of the circulatory system to support cardiac illness diagnosis and treatment. Through its 'Living Heart' program the company achieves this innovative change by transforming two-dimensional images into three-dimensional heart models suitable for accurate medical procedures.

Precision public health receives substantial advancements because of the implementation of digital twins. Public health programs improved through COVID-19 because it brought attention to more efficient disease monitoring and outbreak control practices. Medical research confirms that digital twins unite patient information with artificial intelligence situational technologies through cloud systems to track diseases instantaneously. The combination of digital twins and blockchain technology operates to protect medical data security through transparent systems that allow healthcare facilities to distribute resources properly. In urban health planning, digital twins have been instrumental in developing 'smart healthy cities' (Li et al. 2024). Geographic information systems (GIS) and digital twin models are utilised to monitor urban conditions, predict environmental health impacts, and inform policy decisions. For instance, the Boston digital twin project allows urban planners to visualise the effects of new infrastructure on public health, such as the impact of high-rise buildings on sunlight exposure, which is linked to seasonal affective disorder.

8.8. Healthcare and Life Sciences

The manufacturing sector and other industries had already adopted digital twin technology before it advanced into life sciences and healthcare applications. This technology offers numerous possible uses across this sector. COVID-19 pandemic speedup digital transformation thus boosting the adoption levels of these digital tools. Central health institutions operate with enhanced efficiency requirements as patients seek better care standards. New solutions such as Digital Twins are now under investigation by the industry because they show promise to enhance process optimization and result enhancement. The life sciences field witnesses growing use of Digital Twins mostly dedicated to drug discovery programs and development projects. Blood flow and mechanical operations and electrical signals of the human heart can be studied in detail because a software company produced a virtual heart model. Through the application of this method drug testing as well as medical device development continues to advance. Several healthcare operations and medical devices alongside infrastructure and patient models utilize digital twin technology for digital duplication. Virtual models enable tracking and analysis and forecast of variables such as personalized care plans along with proactive infrastructure maintenance and research and development expense management.

8.9. Drug Development

Because they can replicate the effects of novel drugs, digital twins are essential to drug testing (Attaran et al. 2024). Large volumes of data are produced during the drug development process, and digital twins aid in efficiently organizing and analysing this data. Clinical trials can go more quickly with the use of these virtual models, requiring fewer participants but preserving accuracy. It enables researchers to choose the best antigen and speed up development through virtual simulations. The technology is integral to vaccination research.

8.10. Clinical Research

Digital twins have the potential to revolutionize clinical research today as they enable study investigators to predict the treatment response before the drug is tested in the patient, thus eliminating the need for large in vivo tests (Narigina et al., 2024). The methodology provides safe and efficacious experimental evaluation for evaluation of all developmental stages. Therefore, researchers can leverage the virtual patient models to ingest large sets of data and understand significant patterns and, in turn, improve the treatment methods step-by-step. Such an approach promises to bring healthcare delivery systems to a degree of precision that is finely granulated as well as individually tailored. The significance of digital twins is in the ability to recreate human disease trajectories in a controlled environment - animal-based - to bridge a critical translational gap. Broader access to this technology is launching personalized medicine into new unreachable realms. Using enormous data bank repositories clinicians can make exhaustive simulations for therapeutic interventions, such as implantation of cochlear implants, carried out in patient cohorts, without any disproportionate costs.

8.11. Operational and Educational Optimization

Digital twin technology along with augmented and virtual realities leverages medical education (Li, 2022). Training simulates a risk-free capability, empowering medical personnel to perform any procedure once again as per need while improving patient security and hands-on, abilities gaining. Medical schools have been adding these simulations to their curricula to provide their students with hands-on experiences to learn from. With virtual models of human anatomy, specialists and trainees are able to practice their skills, before going in for real-life treatments. Digital twins are the driving force in the automobile sector for innovation. Car manufacturers have a gift for behavioural data collection. They connect with consumers through interactive dashboards and by specialized tools. Manufacturers use Digital Twin technology for performance evaluations, safety and efficiency evaluations, when developing the vehicle. Digital twins are being used for failure detection, flight state analysis, weight inspection and aircraft maintenance in aviation, mainly. Despite these advancements, however, data quality, as well as data integration, remains big challenges. For the digital twin models to generate valid and reliable output, they shall be constructed out from defined and good quality data. Digital twin systems must establish user trust by removing the potential issues related to explainability and bias linked with any AI. But as technologies improve, industry, academia and lawmakers must collaborate to ensure that new technologies are developed and used in an ethical way. Typically, digital twins have the power to bring healthcare back to life by first, using predictive analysis, second, personalizing pharmaceuticals, and third, spreading awareness through public health campaigns. Despite the challenges that remain, research and developments will allow for the creation of the groundwork for wide-scale adoption, thus resulting in a better quality and efficiency of patient care across the different healthcare systems. The implementation of digital twin technology proves to be very promising for the development of clinical operations across healthcare systems. By recreating physical infrastructures within a virtual world and linking them with real-time data streams, these virtual representations give rendering healthcare providers unprecedented analytical capabilities and streamline the optimization of workflows, into the efficient allocation of resources, for overall operational efficiency. The digital twins of the clinical workflow allow the health care provider to assess the process and to make improvements. Through data taken from various sources such as electronic medical records (EMR), medical devices, and administrative systems, digital twins identify bottlenecks, inefficiencies, and improvement opportunities. Digital twins are also helping to reduce the capacity planning process, making it easier for health institutions to better anticipate the future for everyone. Algorithms based on the predictive analytics concept and machine learning analysis of the data collected from the EHRs, medical devices and administrative systems can also play a role in decisions on day-to-day operations. By predominantly looking at patient flow, staff levels, and equipment use, and comparing with historic data of operation, they can forecast a crisis scenario in the near future which empowers healthcare organizations to proactively adjust staffing schedules, assign optimal bed assignments, or delay treatments for better patient experience and care. Digital twin technology can be integrated fairly easily with real-time data, monitoring, and analysis derived from wearables, medical sensors, and Internet of Things devices, making continuous monitoring possible across the operations of healthcare services. By tracking key performance indicators, patient flow, and operational parameters, digital twins can quickly recognize deviations from the projected norms and sound alerts.

Digital twins can be of aid in the simulation of complex clinical scenarios for healthcare practitioners to polish and enhance their clinical decision-making skills. By using patient data, medical history, and information gathered from real-time monitoring, digital twins can help healthcare practitioners gain access to realistic instances to analyse and diagnose, as well as developing a treatment regimen. This is an interactive simulation that can serve as a good learning process for healthcare professionals to develop their ability to make an appropriate diagnostic reason, consider options for treatment of various diseases, and make a decision in a risk-free environment. Any identification twin technology has the potential to create quality improvement programs, which can be utilized to increase patient safety in clinical practice. Things that went wrong, close calls, or differences that are creating a problem can be a good way of getting to finding opportunities for further improvement. The ability to see evidence and protocols enable effective evidence-based practices and compliance with protocols. This creates a culture of continual improvement, which is itself an error - and patient safety - reducer in any clinical process. A digital twin can make it easier for other, different departments and healthcare professionals to come together and communicate with one another on a single, common platform. This technology allows for real-time data sharing, joint creation of patient care plans and efficient communication. Furthermore, a virtual platform offers a resource for data sharing and advancements with caregivers and patients in real time, as well as a means to communication and assess care plans. Combined, this improves care communications with other teams, reduces handovers, and increases collaboration to help drives clinical workflows more effectively and improve patient outcomes.

Real-time monitoring of the clinical process and a mechanism for continuous improvement using digital twins. The ongoing process of amassing data that is fed into the digital twin allows managers to continually assess long-term excellence of the clinic. Following this, immediate feedback means healthcare practitioners can identify trends and understand the repercussions of any changes in process while continuing to put preventive measures into decisions that help optimization of processes. This way, by responding to cues as they are encountered, companies can address inefficiencies and otherwise make ongoing refinements in clinical operations. Digital twins are under the help of health providers to practice various medical aspects. Digital twins allow to simulate procedures, from invasive to non-invasive health care practitioners have to undergo. Digital twins make it possible for multiple healthcare professionals to collaborate on a shared virtual platform. Digital twins will facilitate communication between different professional groups and enable healthcare professionals to work together and coordinate the care for patients. This allows for an overall better understanding of each profession within the interprofessional process, which in turn allows for better cooperation and the ability to increase a patient's health through thorough and integrated treatment. Digital twins can be further used to create a platform for professional development for those working in the field of healthcare. Via digital twins, practitioners can remain open to new developments, develop new expertise, and gain further specialized knowledge from case studies, simulations, and virtual training. Self-paced learning and ongoing training is the vehicle to gain life-long learning and professional growth for healthcare practitioners and ensure they are able to deliver quality care. Digital twin technologies can also be used for research and development. They can be used for testing theories, analysing data, and performing experiments. In order to offer insights that may drive evidence-based practices and innovation in the healthcare field, these tools are being used to model different demographics, treatment methods and illness scenarios for patients as in Fig. 5.

8.12. Convergence of Blockchain and Digital Twins for Trusted Ecosystems

The future of smart hospitals lies in the union of DT and Blockchain. Digital Twins provide the simulation. Blockchain provides the trust. Future systems will use "Tokenized Digital Twins." This allows patients to own their medical data. They can grant access to researchers via tokens. This convergence solves the data silo problem. It creates a trusted ecosystem where data flows freely but securely. Research must focus on the speed of these transactions to handle real-time hospital data (Katsoulakis et al. 2024).

Figure 5. Healthcare Outcomes Comparison Analysis

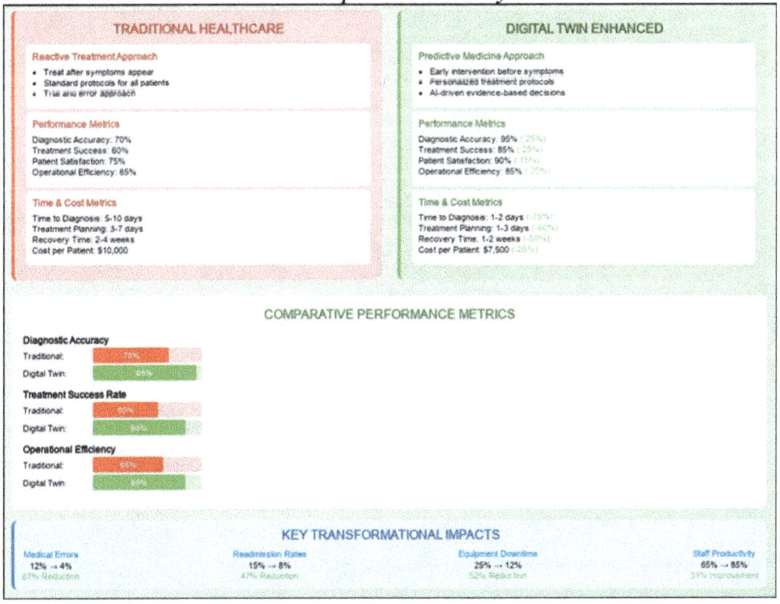

CONCLUSION

Digital Twin technology is a cornerstone of the smart hospital infrastructure. It moves healthcare from reactive to predictive. However, the success of Digital Twins depends on data trust. This is where Blockchain integration is critical. Blockchain ensures security, interoperability, and data integrity. It protects patient privacy while enabling efficient hospital workflows. The combination of these technologies addresses key challenges in modern healthcare. Future developments must focus on standardizing these integrations. This will create a secure, efficient, and patient-centric smart hospital ecosystem.

REFERENCES

Adibi, S., Rajabifard, A., Shojaei, D., & Wickramasinghe, N. (2024). Enhancing healthcare through sensor-enabled digital twins in smart environments: A comprehensive analysis. *Sensors (Basel)*, *24*(9), 2793. PMID: 38732899

Aghamiri, S. S., & Amin, R. (2025). The potential use of digital twin technology for advancing CAR-T cell therapy. *Current Issues in Molecular Biology*, *47*(5), 321. PMID: 40699720

Armeni, P., Polat, I., De Rossi, L. M., Diaferia, L., Meregalli, S., & Gatti, A. (2022). Digital twins in healthcare: Is it the beginning of a new era of evidence-based medicine? A critical review. *Journal of Personalized Medicine*, *12*(8), 1255. PMID: 36013204

Balasubramanyam, A., Ramesh, R., Sudheer, R., & Honnavalli, P. B. (2024). Revolutionizing healthcare: A review unveiling the transformative power of digital twins. *IEEE Access : Practical Innovations, Open Solutions*, *12*, 69652–69676.

Banoub, R. G., Sanghvi, H., Gill, G. S., Paredes, A. A., Bains, H. K., Patel, A., & Patel, A. (2024). Enhancing ophthalmic care: The transformative potential of digital twins in healthcare. *Cureus*, *16*(12). PMID: 39840199

D'Orsi, L., Capasso, B., Lamacchia, G., Pizzichini, P., Ferranti, S., Liverani, A., & Lo Presti, E. (2024). Recent advances in artificial intelligence to improve immunotherapy and the use of digital twins to identify prognosis of patients with solid tumors. *International Journal of Molecular Sciences*, *25*(21), 11588. PMID: 39519142

Dean, M. C., Oeding, J. F., Diniz, P., Seil, R., & Samuelsson, K.ESSKA Artificial Intelligence Working Group. (2024). Leveraging digital twins for improved orthopaedic evaluation and treatment. *Journal of Experimental Orthopaedics*, *11*(4), e70084. PMID: 39530111

Delerm, F., & Pilottin, A. (2024). Double edged tech: Navigating the public health and legal challenges of digital twin technology. *European Journal of Public Health*, *34*(Supplement_3), ckae144–1510.

Diniz, P., Grimm, B., Garcia, F., Fayad, J., Ley, C., Mouton, C., & Seil, R. (2025). Digital twin systems for musculoskeletal applications: A current concepts review. *Knee Surgery, Sports Traumatology, Arthroscopy : Official Journal of the ESSKA*, *33*(5), 1892–1910. PMID: 39989345

Dixit, P. (2025). Exploring the Role of Digital Twins in Revolutionizing Healthcare: Opportunities and Challenges. *International Journal of Advanced Research*.

El-Warrak, L., & de Farias, C. M. (2024). The State of the art of digital twins in health—A quick review of the literature. *Computers*, *13*(9), 228.

Fischer, R.-P., Volpert, A., Antonino, P., & Ahrens, T. D. (2024). Digital Patient Twins for Personalized Therapeutics and Pharmaceutical Manufacturing. *Frontiers in Digital Health*, *5*, 1302338. Advance online publication. DOI: 10.3389/fdgth.2023.1302338 PMID: 38250053

Gazerani, P. (2023). Intelligent digital twins for personalized migraine care. *Journal of Personalized Medicine*, *13*(8), 1255. PMID: 37623505

Iliuţă, M. E., Moisescu, M. A., Pop, E., Ionita, A. D., Caramihai, S. I., & Mitulescu, T. C. (2024). Digital twin—A review of the evolution from concept to technology and its analytical perspectives on applications in various fields. *Applied Sciences (Basel, Switzerland)*, *14*(13), 5454.

Jalil, M. S., Arafat, M. S., Islam, R., Rafi, S. S., Jony, M. A. M., & Hossen, F. (2024). AI and Digital Twins in Healthcare: Revolutionizing Remote Patient Monitoring and Precision Medicine.

Johnson, Z.. (2024). Digital Twins for Healthcare Using Wearables. *Bioengineering (Basel, Switzerland)*. PMID: 38927842

Katsoulakis, E., Wang, Q., & Wu, H.. (2024). "Digital Twins for Health: A Scoping Review." *npj. Digital Medicine*, *7*(1), 77. Advance online publication. DOI: 10.1038/s41746-024-01073-0 PMID: 38519626

Kuriakose, S. M., Joseph, J., & Kollinal, R. (2024). The rise of digital twins in healthcare: A mapping of the research landscape. *Cureus*, *16*(7). PMID: 39184791

Li, T., Shen, Y., Li, Y., Zhang, Y., & Wu, S. (2024). The status quo and future prospects of digital twins for healthcare. *EngMedicine*, *1*(3), 100042.

Li, Z. (2022). *Digital-twin Healthcare: A Gateway to Future Medicine*. Preprint.

Meijer, C., Uh, H. W., & El Bouhaddani, S. (2023). Digital twins in healthcare: Methodological challenges and opportunities. *Journal of Personalized Medicine*, *13*(10), 1522. PMID: 37888133

Nadeem, M., Kostic, S., Dornhöfer, M., Weber, C., & Fathi, M. (2025). A comprehensive review of digital twin in healthcare in the scope of simulative health-monitoring. *Digital Health*, *11*, 20552076241304078. PMID: 39777066

Narigina, M., Romanovs, A., & Bruzgiene, R. (2024, May). Digital twin technology in healthcare: A literature review. In 2024 IEEE 11th Workshop on Advances in Information, Electronic and Electrical Engineering (AIEEE) (pp. 1-8). IEEE.

Roopa, M. S. (2023). A systematic review: Digital twin in healthcare. *International Journal for Research in Applied Science and Engineering Technology*, *11*(5), 4818–4825.

Sel, K., Osman, D., Zare, F., Masoumi Shahrbabak, S., Brattain, L., Hahn, J. O., & Jafari, R. (2024). Building digital twins for cardiovascular health: From principles to clinical impact. *Journal of the American Heart Association*, *13*(19), e031981. PMID: 39087582

tefănigă, S. A., Cordo , A. A., Ivascu, T., Feier, C. V. I., Muntean, C., Stupinean, C. V., & Bolboacă, S. D. (2024). Advancing precision oncology with digital and virtual twins: A scoping review. *Cancers (Basel)*, *16*(22), 3817. PMID: 39594772

Subashini, R.. (2024). Digital Twin - An Innovative Strategy in Healthcare Transformation: An Extensive Review. *Journal of Research in Applied Sciences.*

Weerarathna, I. N., Kumar, P., Verma, P., Raymond, D., Luharia, A., & Mishra, G. (2024, November). Leveraging digital twin technology to combat cardiovascular disease: A comprehensive review. In 2024 2nd DMIHER International Conference on Artificial Intelligence in Healthcare, Education and Industry (IDICAIEI) (pp. 1-6). IEEE.

Chapter 7
Distributed Ledger-Powered Digital Twin Models for Intelligent Hospital Infrastructure Management

S. Tamilselvi
http://orcid.org/0000-0002-1330-9248
Kongu Engineering College, Erode, India

Satheesh Kumar A.
http://orcid.org/0009-0008-8182-0946
Nandha Engineering College, Erode, India

Ravikumar R. N.
http://orcid.org/0009-0009-3705-1681
Marwadi University, Rajkot, India

S. Aarthi
http://orcid.org/0009-0006-9064-2091
Marwadi University, Rajkot, India

Duggirala Aravind
http://orcid.org/0009-0005-4362-7684
ASET College of Science and Technology, India

Tamilarasi Rajamani
http://orcid.org/0000-0001-5606-8133
Villa College-QI Campus, Malé, Maldives

ABSTRACT

The integration of Distributed Ledger Technologies (DLTs) with Digital Twin (DT) systems is transforming smart hospital infrastructures by facilitating secure, transparent, and real-time operational intelligence. As healthcare settings rely more on IoMT devices, AI analytics, and automated processes, it's crucial to ensure that the data shared between real and virtual systems is reliable and accurate. DLT provides decentralized validation, immutable storage, and automated smart-contract governance, ensuring trustworthy Digital Twin updates for predictive maintenance,

DOI: 10.4018/979-8-3373-8177-0.ch007

patient-flow optimization, and resource management. By strengthening interoperability, enhancing cybersecurity resilience, and supporting transparent data-sharing mechanisms, DLT-enabled Digital Twins offer a robust foundation for next-generation intelligent hospital ecosystems. This chapter looks at different design models, real-life examples, performance details, and future research directions that are important for making healthcare changes that are scalable, secure, and ethical.

1. INTRODUCTION

The E-health (Electronic Health) revolution is transforming the hospital infrastructures using smart, data-driven technologies to improve clinical, operational, and administrative performance. To achieve responsive environments that can be relied upon to make real-time decisions, smart hospitals have come to be intelligent with sensory devices, autonomous workflow and data analytics that guarantee the integration of these elements. Digital Twin (DT) technology has become one of the key ideas of this transformation, facilitating virtual interactions of physical systems, processes, and patient pathways (Vallée, 2023). These virtual models are helpful in making proper simulations, predictive maintenance, risk assessment and optimizing workflow. Nevertheless, with the growth of interrelated systems in hospitals, such as IoMT devices, electronic records, and intelligent elements of the facility, secure, reliable, and transparent data ecosystems are essential. Distributed Ledger Technologies (DLTs) provide a decentralized system of infrastructure with enhanced data integrity, privacy, and interoperability in these complicated networks. By combining DLT with DT systems, it is possible to securely synchronize real-time hospital data, increase its traceability, and make the decisions tamper-proof, which makes DLT-powered Digital Twins the foundation of the next generation intelligent hospital setting (Ricci et al., 2022).

1.1 Evolution of Smart Hospital Ecosystems

The simple digital record systems have been developed into smart hospital ecosystems with high levels of interconnectedness that are pervasively sensed, automated, and artificially intelligent (AI-assisted) decision support. The initial hospital systems were more geared towards the digitization of administrative and clinical documentation with EHRs and PACS. Gradually, IoT improvements, wireless connection, and miniaturization of medical equipment allowed collecting data in real-time about patients, equipment, and infrastructure of the facility. This change preconditioned the emergence of IoMT-powered hospitals that are able to conduct ongoing monitoring and automatic alert (Saratkar et al., 2025)s. Cloud and edge computing combined to amplify processing capacity, which made it possible to conduct fast analytics and make localized decisions with little latency. With the implementations of AI-based triage systems, predictive analytics, digital workflow engines, and autonomous logistics (including robot-assisted delivery), the definition of a smart hospital grew to the level of complete digital coordination. The next-generation hospitals today target continuous interoperability, foresight intelligence, and dynamic operations. This development points to the necessity of safe, stable, and reliable data flows, which Distributed Ledger Technologies can support the reliability and accountability of the widening ecosystem. The figure 1 demonstrates the technological development of early digital hospital systems up to the modern smart hospital ecosystems facilitated by the use of IoT, AI, cloud-edge computing, and next-generation operational intelligence.

Figure 1. Evolution of Smart Hospital Ecosystems

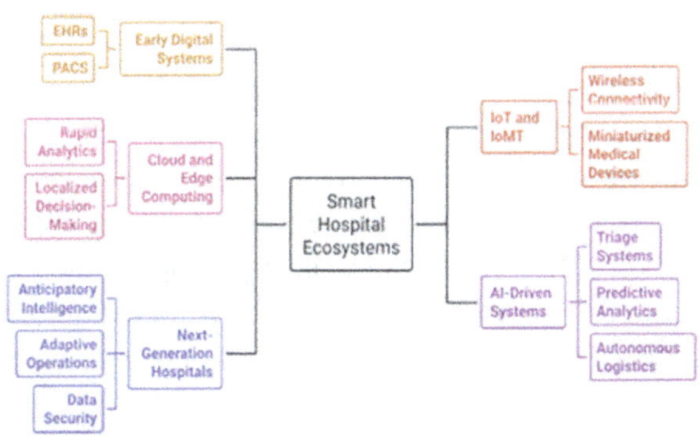

1.2 Role of Digital Twins in Modern Healthcare

The Digital Twin technology is a transformative technology in the contemporary world of healthcare because it has provided dynamic, real-time virtual images of patients, medical equipment, clinical procedures, and hospital facilities. These digital models reflect the condition, actions and interactions of the physical system and allow constant observation, simulation of scenarios, and predictive modeling. To apply in the medical field, personalized twins will enable individualized treatment plans, prognosis of rehabilitation, and risk identification. Operationally, DTs maximize bed capacity, emergency traffic, energy consumption, equipment, and allocation of resources by analyzing different situations and ensuring they are implemented (Sun et al., 2023). Simulation of disruptions, e.g., equipment malfunction, unexpected patient arrival, or outbreak of infections will enable the hospital administrators to make a decision based on data in advance. In addition, sensor data, IoMT devices, and AI algorithms intertwining will guarantee that the DT model will be constantly updated with the correct information. The success of Digital Twins, however, relies on the reliability, traceability and integrity of the data that sustains these virtual systems that forms an organic synergy with Distributed Ledger Technologies.

1.3 Need for Distributed Ledger Technologies in Secure Hospital Operations

Distributed Ledger Technologies are designed to mitigate the basic security and trust issues, which appear in very interconnected hospital environments. As the amount of real-time data across the IoMT devices, clinical information systems, and Digital Twin platforms continues to rise, the hospitals are exposed to greater risks associated with data manipulation, unauthorized access, and system breaches. The conventional central databases are prone to single point of failures and do not have clear procedures of ensuring data authenticity. DLT is a decentralized format In which every transaction or data update is cryptographically hash and time-stamped and permanently stored in several nodes (Wang et al., 2023). This guarantees that the Digital Twin models are run based on trusted information which cannot be tampered with by anyone and thus enhances the reliability and accuracy of simulations and automated decisions. The smart contracts also simplify the process of consent, identity checks, secure devices onboarding, and audit trails in hospitals. DLT helps to improve the interoperability of heterogeneous systems and makes all stakeholders accountable by allowing transparent data governance. In line with this, the use of DLT in the hospital workflow enhances the cybersecurity level, aids in enforcing the regulations, and offers a reliable basis of intelligent infrastructure powered by DT.

2. BACKGROUND TO THE STUDY

The intricacy of the current healthcare processes requires strong digital systems that can handle large amounts of clinical, administrative, and infrastructural data. Nevertheless, the conventional hospital information systems are usually siloed with low interoperability, poor data quality and low real time functionality. This brings about huge loopholes in decision making, patient safety and performance. The rise of IoMT devices, cloud computing, and edge computing has helped overcome some of these shortcomings by bringing in pervasive sensing, distributed analytics, and an exchange of data in a high velocity (Kamel Boulos & Zhang, 2021). However, these developments lead to cybersecurity vulnerabilities, privacy issues, data validation and traceability challenges. When the Digital Twin models are used to predict analytic health and manage smart facilities in hospitals, the integrity and reliability of underlying data is critical. The solution to these problems is offered through Distributed Ledger Technologies that offer decentralization and impossibility of tampering with data, as well as transparent data governance and safe synchronization across multi-stakeholder and complex hospital ecosystems.

2.1 Limitations of Conventional Hospital Information Systems

Traditional hospital information systems are mainly configured to support administrative processing, clinical records and record management but not real-time decision-making or predictive analytics. These systems are normally deployed in discrete modules, e.g. EHR, billing, radiology and lab systems, which mean that data flows will be fragmented and interoperability will be limited. Absence of centralized data governance causes discrepancies and overlap of information across departments as well as slowness in information transfer. In addition, traditional systems are also dependent on centralized structures which ensure they are likely to fail when there is downtime and also due to cyberattacks that can cripple the running of a hospital (Peng et al., 2020). They have a lower scalability level that limits their capacity to handle the high frequency data produced by the current IoMT devices and constant monitoring systems. Traditional systems can hardly accommodate the data velocity, granularity and real-time timing needed as hospitals strive to adopt AI and Digital Twin technologies. With these limitations, predictive maintenance, operational forecasting and automated decision making are difficult. All these restrictions highlight the importance of more secure, transparent, and interoperable infrastructures, opportunities that Distributed Ledger Technologies are capable of providing.

2.2 Emergence of IOMT, Edge Computing, and Real-Time Health Data

Internet of Medical Things (IoMT) devices have revolutionized real-time health monitoring because the sensors, medical devices, wearable and diagnostic devices are connected to one data ecosystem. These devices continuously generate physiological information, operating rates, and information regarding the environment, which is essential in the care of patients, as well as the management of the facility. This ecosystem is complemented by edge computing, where information is processed closer to the source and reduces the latency, as well as, reduces the bandwidth constraint associated with cloud-based architecture. This local processing allows real-time analytics, real-time anomaly detection and real-time updates to Digital Twin models at the cost of performance (Vasiliu-Feltes et al., 2023). Meanwhile, cloud computing assures the capability to expand and storage of extensive amounts of historical data on long-term health data. Data-intensive and dynamic settings where predictive diagnostics, personalized medicine, and autonomous clinical procedures can be implemented will be achievable with IoMT and edge-cloud solutions. Despite these advancements, there are certain data integrity, secure synchronization and trust issues and this is especially so when multiple systems and stakeholders are involved. These concerns indicate the timeliness of Distributed Ledger Technologies as a concept to ensure the secure and verifiable exchange of data in real time.

2.3 Data Integrity, Traceability, and Cybersecurity Challenges in Hospitals

Hospitals are targeted with sensitive patient data, equipment data that is mission critical and operational metrics in real-time, and they form one of the ideal targets of cyberattacks and data manipulation. Medical device telemetry can be tampered with, unauthorized access, insider threats, and ransomware are all risky. It is necessary to ensure data integrity because inaccurate or distorted information may cause misdiagnosis, malfunctioning of operation, or the loss of patient safety. Conventional security controls are usually not transparent and do not provide audit trails which are immutable and help in tracking the data provenance. Moreover, sophisticated hospital networks imply high numbers of vendors, systems, and devices, which causes problems in end-to-end traceability (Agbo et al., 2019). These concerns are further intensified by the introduction of Digital Twin systems, where the responsibility of making decisions based on Digital Twin is based on reliable and proven information. Distributed Ledger Technologies can solve these issues by offering cryptographically secured entries, decentralized validation and tamper resistant audit controls. DLT improves trust, in that each update of data, be it made by IoMT sensors, clinical systems, or equipment in the facilities, is authentic, time-stamped and traceable. This enhances the resilience of cybersecurity and regulatory conformity towards more digital hospital settings.

3. RESEARCH OBJECTIVES

The major objective of the chapter is to explore the application of Distributed Ledger Technologies to improve the design, implementation, and performance of Digital Twin systems employed in intelligent hospital infrastructure management. With the shift in the hospital environment towards more interconnected environments with the help of IoMT tools, AI-based analytics, and predictive modeling, Digital Twins cannot operate without the reliable, secure, and transparent data exchange. This chapter is thus devoted to the analysis of DLT-enabled DT architectures, discussion of the technical issues related to interoperability, scalability, and system reliability, and an assessment of the benefits and limitations of decentralized ledger mechanisms integration with the virtual twin models in general. The purposes cover both operational and technological aspects, which allow a holistic.

- To design and analyze DLT-enabled Digital Twin architectures for smart hospital management.
- To examine interoperability, scalability, and reliability challenges in DLT-DT integration.
- To evaluate security, privacy, and data governance improvements enabled by DLT.
- To assess the impact of DLT-powered DTs on predictive maintenance and hospital workflow optimization.
- To identify implementation barriers, ethical concerns, and future research directions for scalable DLT-DT solutions.

4. CONCEPTUAL MODEL

The conceptual model is a combination of Distributed Ledger Technologies and Digital Twin systems that allows developing a digital hospital infrastructure management digital ecosystem based on security, transparency, and real-time. It demonstrates how the operational and clinical data is constantly generated by physical hospital equipment, IoMT devices, and clinical processes and entered into the Digital Twin environment. In order to be trusted, every transaction of data is authenticated and stored in an immutable manner using DLT mechanisms to form a valid and irreducible audit trail. Smart contracts process automation and fulfill particular functions, which include the confirmation of devices, verification of consent, predictive maintenance onboarding, and alerts (Mishra & Mehra, 2025). The model focuses on a smooth alignment of the physical and the virtual components in a decentralized validation method such that the DT simulations and predictions can be launched in the accurate and reliable data. In general, the conceptual architecture will offer an overview of the way decentralized technologies can be used to improve the performance, security, and reliability of Digital Twins in smart hospitals of the next generation (Ravikumar, Aarthi, Saparbaevich, et al., 2025). The digital twins and distributed ledger collaboratively generate, validate, store, synchronize, automate, and improve hospital operational data and performance via a continuous cycle, as shown in figure 2.

Figure 2. Digital Twin and DLT Integration Cycle

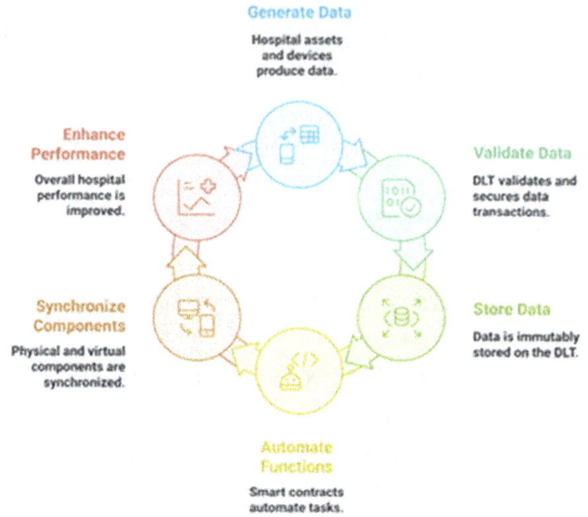
Generate Data
Hospital assets and devices produce data.
Validate Data
DLT validates and secures data transactions.
Store Data
Data is immutably stored on the DLT.
Automate Functions
Smart contracts automate tasks.
Synchronize Components
Physical and virtual components are synchronized.
Enhance Performance
Overall hospital performance is improved.

4.1 Proposed DLT-Powered Digital Twin Framework

The suggested framework will integrate Digital Twin layers with Distributed Ledger layers to create a unified, safe and autonomous hospital management ecosystem. The physical layer produces constant feeds of real-time data on the condition of patients, equipment status, and environmental parameters at the IoMT devices, sensors, medical equipment, and facility systems. Such streams are sent to the Digital Twin layer which models the behavior and the state of actual assets in virtual form, which allows continuous monitoring and predictive simulation (Ravikumar, Aarthi, et al., 2025). The Distributed Ledger layer works simultaneously with the validation, timestamping, and permanent acquisition of important transactions and data updates. Through decentralization aspects of consensus, the framework renders that no individual can compromise data, enhancing the aspect of trust and audit (Arbabi et al., 2022). The processes automated by smart contracts are implemented into the DLT layer, including the scheduling of equipment maintenance, access to the premises, and data-sharing deals. The interoperability modules support the sharing of verified information between clinical systems, functional platforms, and other external stakeholders. This framework will promote transparency, minimise inconsistencies in data, and facilitate smart decisions throughout the work of the hospital. Table 1 Maps major layers of the combined architecture and their contribution to work.

Table 1. Integrated DT–DLT Architectural Components and Functional Roles

Architecture Layer	Components	Functional Role	Output
IoMT Layer	Sensors, RFID, devices	Data generation	Continuous telemetry
DT Layer	Models, simulations	Real-time updates	Predictions & analytics
DLT Layer	Nodes, ledger	Validation & immutability	Verified data blocks
Smart Contract Layer	Rules, triggers	Automation	Actionable events

4.2 Data Flow, Synchronization, and Consensus Mechanisms

The DLT- DT ecosystem starts with data generation through medical devices, environmental sensors, and clinical processes and facility systems on a continuous basis. These are data points that are directed to the Digital Twin where they update the virtual representations in real-time. At the same time, critical data updates, i.e., patient identity, equipment logs, or workflow events are sent to the DLT layer to be verified. The blockchain consensus mechanisms allow synchronization of the updates and guarantee that the updates achieved are verified, authentic, and consistent between all the participating nodes (Aarthi et al., 2025). Based on the operational requirements of the hospital, consensus can be based on a Proof of Authority, Byzantine Fault Tolerance, or a lightweight hybrid approach to ensure efficiency and integrity at the same time. The coordinated information is used to guarantee that only credible information is sent to the Digital Twin to reduce mistakes and discrepancies in predictive modeling (Gordon & Catalini, 2018). Bidirectional flow can also be provided: knowledge created by the DT may include some suggested device failures or workflow plans, which are recorded on the DLT using smart contracts to execute them transparently. This collective synchronization enhances value of precision and reliability of hospital operations which are driven by DT.

4.3 Trust, Access-Control, and Smart-Contract Layers

In the Digital Twin model based on the DLT, trust is generated via cryptographic validation, decentralized governance, and uneditable records of data. Each device, system and stakeholder is given an identifiable identity to ensure authenticated participation. The access-control layer defines the access control of certain data elements, whether by reading, writing, or updating, based on role-based access control, the principles of zero-trust, and decentralized identity management systems. This will keep unauthorized access at bay and will guarantee that the sensitive clinical and operational data will only be distributed to authorized entities. Smart contracts are the foundation of automation of the system and they are used to implement a set of rules without a human operator. They are patient consent management, equipment maintenance triggers, workflow authorization and emergency response coordination (Tuli et al., 2020). The enforcement of data-sharing agreements between departments, vendors, and regulatory bodies also takes place in real-time with the help of smart contracts. The trust and access-control layers ensure compliance, security and transparency by integrating logic into an environment that cannot be compromised. The two offer a secure base upon which there can be a harmonious communication between Digital Twins and decentralized hospital ecosystems.

5. RESEARCH METHODOLOGY

Research methodology is based on the multi-layered approach which involves simultaneous systematic literature review, architectural review and validation of the research using real-life examples. To find out the trends, gaps, and thematic patterns, a systematic literature review is carried out to find out the existing studies on Digital Twins, Distributed Ledger Technologies, and smart hospital infrastructures. Then, the current technological frameworks are analyzed and compared with models through the methods of architectural analysis and evaluation of their appropriateness to the integration of the DLT and DBT. These analyses help in the formulation of the conceptual models and indicate the advantages and disadvantages of different design options (Roy et al., 2025). Lastly, the case-study-based approach will confirm the suggested ideas based on the recent practical application of the ideas in the world hospital settings. With this triangulated methodology, there is thoroughness because of the combination of theoretical evidence, technical assessment, and practice. The synthesis makes the findings of the chapter more reliable and relevant.

5.1 Systematic Literature Review and Thematic Mapping

The systematic literature review is based on structured procedures to determine academic articles, technical reports, standards documentation, and case studies in the area of Digital Twin, Distributed ledger technologies, and smart healthcare systems. High-quality sources are collected with the help of databases like IEEE Xplore, SpringerLink, Scopus and PubMed. Defined keywords and Boolean combinations are used to conduct searches in order to do a broad but targeted search. Inclusion and exclusion criteria enable the filtering of publications with the help of relevance, recency, and methodological rigor. Then, thematic analysis is used to classify the findings into the main themes that include data governance, interoperability, cybersecurity, real-time analytics, and DT-driven optimization (Dimitrov, 2019). The thematic mapping helps to have a consolidated picture of the research sphere that currently exists and to point to the main challenges, opportunities, and gaps. The acquired insights will be used as the basis of conceptual model and research objectives development. The methodological nature of the research makes this transparent, less biased, and increases the validity of evidence given in the later paragraphs.

5.2 Architectural Analysis and Model Comparison

Architectural analysis looks at the structural elements, communication channels, data management plans and security measures of available Digital Twin and DLT systems. This evaluation considers reference models, industrial designs and healthcare-oriented designs to determine their strengths and weaknesses as well as applicability to integrated deployment within a hospital setup. Alternative architecture comparison Model comparison techniques are applied to compare architectures on factors like latency performance, scalability, modularity, consensus efficiency and interoperability between the heterogeneous systems (Margheri et al., 2020). A particular focus is made on the way various architectures can synchronize real time data, integrate sensors, and provide secured access. The comparative knowledge can guide the creation of an ideal conceptual framework of the DLT-powered Digital Twins. Another trade off identified during this analysis process is the choice of different blockchain models Hyperledger Fabric, Ethereum based solutions or hybrid permissioned ledgers to use them in the application of hospital infrastructure. Generally, the architectural comparison would mean that the proposed structure is anchored on real-life practicability and technological suitability (Brogan et al., 2018).

5.3 Case-Study-Driven Validation Approach

The validation method is based on the case-study approach and includes real-life examples of hospitals and healthcare organizations that have applied Digital Twin models, blockchain systems, or a combination of both technologies. The parameters used in the analysis of each case study include system architecture, deployment challenges, operational outcomes, and quantifiable predictive maintenance, workflow, and cybersecurity improvements. The strategy will focus on the latest applications in technologically developed healthcare settings to make them relevant in terms of practicality (Zhang et al., 2023). Technical reports, research publications, industry documentation are analyzed to obtain data that help to comprehend how DLT improves reliability, transparency, and trust in the operations driven by DT. The comparative assessment of various cases enables detection of shared success variables, technical and contextual variables that affect adoption. These results reinforce the pragmatism of the suggested conceptual model and prove that it has some practical implementation. The case-study validation can be also taken to be actionable by the hospital administrators, system designers and researchers who wish to use decentralized and intelligent infrastructure management solutions.

6. LITERATURE REVIEW

The intersection of Digital Twin (DT) technologies and Distributed Ledger Technologies (DLTs) has become an issue of great interest over the last several years as they are likely to revolutionize healthcare data management, its operational efficiency, predictive analytics, and cybersecurity. Literature indicates that the two areas have achieved a lot in their own right but when it comes to combining them, the area has only reached its nascent stages. This section summarizes existing research trends, gaps that have been identified as critical and evaluations of technical feasibility of combined DT-DLT systems in intelligent hospital infrastructures (Gupta et al., 2025). The review is divided into three thematic areas in line with research objectives of the chapter (1) Digital Twins in healthcare, (2) Blockchain-enabled data governance, and (3) integrated DT-DLT architecture research centered around interoperability, scalability, and performance.

6.1 Digital Twins in Healthcare: Trends, Gaps, and Current Models

Digital Twins have become an essential part of future healthcare systems by facilitating real-time digitalization of patients, devices, processes and healthcare settings. The existing models are physiological Digital Twins that can model organ behavior and disease progression and operational twins applied to bed allocation, emergency management, optimization of surgical workflow, and smart facility maintenance. Recent research points to the growing merging of AI, machine learning, and IoMT sensor data in order to increase the accuracy and responsiveness of Digital Twins (Rajab et al., 2024). The research trends are directed to focus on predictive maintenance of medical equipment, personalized treatment with simulation, and optimization of resources in a virtual hospital. Regardless of this development, there are still a number of gaps. The current implementations of DT are based on central databases, that create vulnerabilities in terms of data manipulation, lack of traceability and single points of failure. Also, the issue of interoperability is still in the limelight since healthcare systems generally work with disparate devices and vendor-specific data standards (Bathalapalli et al., 2024). The integrity of data, particularly where there is constant monitoring, poses the question of the credibility of the recommendations made by DT. The other most popular restriction is the lack of trusted data-sharing between clinical departments, external service providers, and regulatory authorities. These issues point to the necessity of decentralized, secure infrastructures that would enable transparent, verifiable, and scalable Digital Twin operations, in which case the area of the DLT is no longer viewed as a groundless option (Amofa et al., 2024). Table 2 Overviews some of the major Digital Twin applications in clinical and operational environments.

Table 2. Comparison of Digital Twin Applications in Healthcare

Application Area	Purpose	Benefits	Examples
Patient-Specific Simulation	Models physiological processes	Personalized treatment	Cardiac DT, rehabilitation DT
Predictive Equipment Maintenance	Monitors device behavior	Reduces downtime	MRI/CT DT models
Emergency Workflow Optimization	Simulates congestion scenarios	Faster triage, reduced wait time	ED DT models
Facility & Energy Management	Tracks environmental conditions	Energy efficiency	Smart ICU/ward twins

6.2 Role of Blockchain/DLT in Healthcare Data Governance

Other DDTs, blockchain in particular, have received significant levels of interest as facilitators of safe, auditable, and privacy-preserving healthcare data ecosystems. Studies have shown that, DLT provides the necessary security of immunities, integrity and resistance to tampering by decentrally utilizing consensus to ensure that essential medical records are not compromised. Checking the capabilities of the systems based on DLT, it is possible to note secure patient identity management, decentralized EHR sharing, authentication of IoMT devices, pharmaceutical supply-chain verification, and oversight of audit trails of clinical activities. Smart contracts also automate consent processes, access and use of research data as well as regulatory compliance mechanism (Chhinal et al., 2025)s. Nevertheless, in literature, there are also constraints related to the implementation of DLT in healthcare. The IoMT generates high volumes of transactions which raises scalability issues and the latency issues can affect time-sensitive clinical services. Although alleviated in permissioned blockchains, this energy consumption and storage overhead is still a design concern. Furthermore, the implementation of DLT into the legacy hospital systems and cloud platforms, as well as the current interoperability frameworks, presents further architectural difficulties (Chakilam, 2025). Regardless of these constraints, scientists always say that DLT offers a solid base towards enhancing trust, accountability, and security within the distributed healthcare systems. As a result, DLT is also becoming a subject of discussion as a critical enabler of enhancing the trustworthiness of Digital Twin ecosystems. Table 3 Comparisons critical DLT capabilities that facilitate safe hospital data activities.

Table 3. Key Features of Distributed Ledger Technologies for Hospital Data Governance

DLT Feature	Function	Hospital Benefit	Example Framework
Immutability	Prevents data tampering	Reliable audit trails	Hyperledger Fabric
Decentralized Validation	Multi-node verification	Removes single point of failure	Quorum
Smart Contracts	Automated workflows	Consent & scheduling automation	Ethereum
Permissioned Access	Controlled visibility	Compliance-oriented sharing	Corda

6.3 Integrated DT–DLT Systems: Interoperability, Scalability, and Performance Studies

Recent research suggests hybrid DT–DLT systems to resolve insecure and unreliable security concerns in single Digital Twin solutions. The frameworks normally combine IoMT sensing, edge computing, cloud analytics and blockchain layers to facilitate consistent and verifiable data streams. It is suggested in the literature that DLT enhances the reliability of DT through the unalterable documentation of sensor scans, equipment conditions as well as workflow incidents, thus minimizing the chances of tainted or distorted data affecting DT simulations. It is also observed that interoperability is improved, since DLT has the capability of interconnecting data sharing among heterogeneous devices and platforms, using standardized validation and consensus regulations (Hemdan & Sayed, 2025). The performance studies have shown both positive and negative results with respect to the blockchain set-up.

Hyperledger Fabric and Quorum are two permissioned blockchains with lower latency and increased throughput, which is more appropriate in the hospital setting than a public blockchain network. They also propose edge-assisted consensus mechanisms which can allow them to reduce the computational overhead but preserve the integrity of the data. Although yielding promising results, studies admit that unresolved issues regarding real-time synchronization of DT and DLT layers remain a problem, particularly in high frequency monitoring. Moreover, the architecture involving predictive analytics, machine learning pipelines, and automation to use smart contracts needs considerable design thoughtfulness to resolve the security/

durability versus computation efficiency dilemma (Abhimanyu Gupta et al., 2025). In general, the research literature demonstrates the increased appreciation of the advantages and issues of mixed DT-DLT systems. Although there are promising prototypes available, there are still limited large-scale hospital-wide implementations, which indicates the potential of significant possibilities in the field of further research and practical confirmation.

7. CASE STUDIES: REAL-WORLD IMPLEMENTATIONS OF DLT-ENABLED DIGITAL TWINS

The latest developments in the field of healthcare digitization have allowed some of the major hospitals to implement integrated Digital Twin and Distributed Ledger solutions to enhance operational efficiency, predictive analytics, and cybersecurity. These practical applications can offer useful insights into the practical validity, performance results, and difficulties of integrating DT systems and decentralized ledger systems (Tiwari & Kumar, 2025). The two cases studies below consider two large deployments, namely Mayo Clinic Blockchain-Integrated Digital Twin to predictive equipment maintenance, and the Digital Twin with DLT of the National University Hospital (NUH) Singapore, patient flow and emergency optimization. Both illustrate that Data integrity, traceability, and real-time synchronization can be improved with the help of DLT and allow Digital Twins to perform reliably in complicated hospital settings. The cases also present significant factors like interoperability, latency issues, employee education, and regulatory issues, which provided a balanced view of the preparedness and scalability of the DLT-enabled DT systems in the next generation smart hospitals. Table 4 Gives reported improvements realized in actual deployments of DLT to DT.

Table 4. Comparative Performance of DLT-DT Hospital Implementations

Case Study		Performance Gains	Security Improvements	Operational Outcomes
Mayo Clinic (2024)		40–60% improved device uptime	Tamper-proof logs	Faster maintenance cycles
NUH Singapore (2023–24)		Reduced triage wait times	Verified patient identity	Optimized patient flow
General Findings		Higher prediction accuracy	Strong access control	Improved resource allocation

7.1 Case Study 1: Mayo Clinic's Blockchain-Integrated Digital Twin for Predictive Equipment Maintenance (2024)

Mayo Clinic proposed a Digital Twin system using blockchain to enhance predictive maintenance of such essential imaging devices as MRI, CT, ultrasound, and others. The architecture included IoMT-enabled sensors on the elements of the equipment that continuously sent the operational metrics of temperature, vibration, coil current, and device usage to the Digital Twin model. The blockchain validation nodes running in the hospital network validated every update of data in the network and recorded the maintenance logs that cannot be modified, which guarantees that the historical records will remain unaltered. The hybrid system had various advantages in operation (Lu et al., 2023). The Digital Twin identified anomalies earlier and more accurately because of trusted sensor data, which was carried out by predictive models. Smart contracts automatically activated maintenance requests and thus minimized manual intervention and downtime. The benefits of cybersecurity improved considerably: blockchain helped to remove unauthorized changes in machine logs, avoid manipulations with maintenance history, and enhance the authentication of device access. Although it was successful, its deployment issues were the inability to integrate with older maintenance software, latency associated with consensus when loading large amounts of data, and the necessity to train personnel with specialized skills. However, the system has proved that blockchain-supported Digital Twins can be used to guarantee the reliability of equipment and operational resilience (Alzubi et al., 2023). The figure 3 represents the interaction of the IoMT sensors, Digital Twin analytics, and blockchain validation in detecting anomalies, automating maintenance, improving cybersecurity, and making systems reliable.

Figure 3. Mayo Clinic's Blockchain-Integrated Digital Twin Workflow for Predictive Maintenance

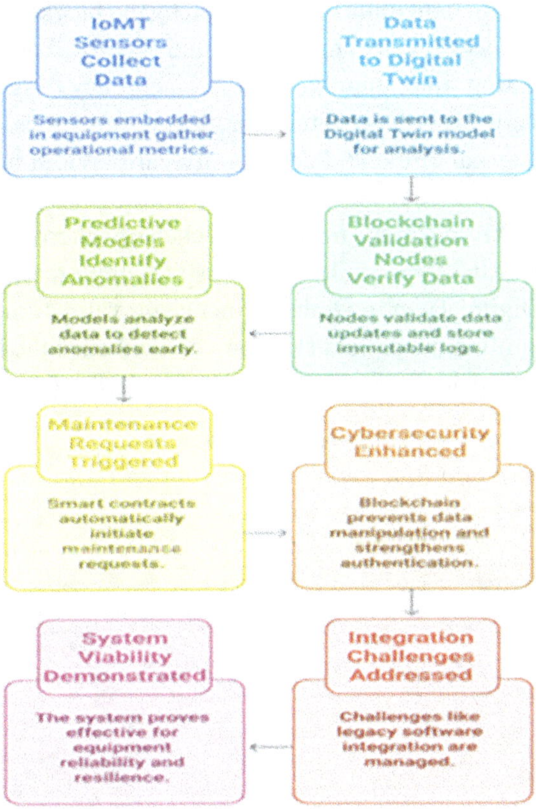

7.2 Case Study 2: Singapore National University Hospital (NUH) – Digital Twin + Distributed Ledger for Patient Flow & Emergency Optimization (2023–2024)

To improve the coordination of patient flow, the emergency triage, and interdepartmental work, NUH Singapore developed an integrated Digital Twin and Distributed Ledger that could improve real-time patient flow. Patient movement, bed availability, triage priority, and diagnostic workflow states were mentioned in the Digital Twin model. The DT was revised due to the constant data obtained by means of IoMT devices, RFID tags, and hospital information systems. Equally, a trusted blockchain level ensured patient identity, consent, and workflow actions and ensured a safe interdepartmental synchronization (Fatokun et al., 2021). The coordinated network made it possible to make dynamic decisions during times of peak demands. DT-based simulations predicted ED congestion and recommended the optimal resources allocation. The sharing of consent-based data between radiology, emergency, and inpatient units were handled by the blockchain-managed smart contracts, and the delays were also minimized and speedy diagnostics was offered. Reduction in the waiting time, improvement in emergency triage and transparency in the patient routing processes were the quantitative outcomes. Scalability testing was positive; not external clinic and community-care system integration was still problematic (Kamruzzaman et al., 2022). The trends the NUH identified in the predictive triage of AI and cross-hospital blockchain interoperability will make the model a pattern of the large-scale smart hospital implementation. The figure 4 demonstrates that Digital Twin modeling/ blockchain validation was put into practice in NUH to streamline the patient flow process, enhance the accuracy of triage, share data safely, and scale the system to new levels in the future.

Figure 4. Digital Twin and Blockchain Integration Workflow at NUH

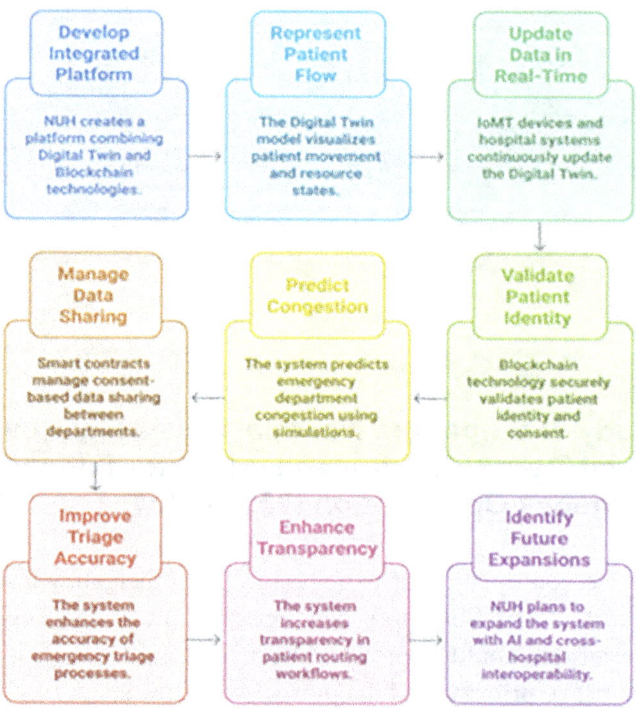

8. RESULTS AND DISCUSSION

The analysis findings suggest that the combination of Distributed Ledger Technologies and Digital Twin systems can greatly improve the reliability, security, and operation intelligence of smart hospital systems. Architectural evaluation proves that decentralized validation enhances data integrity and avoids manipulation of vital telemetry to ensure that Digital Twins will be used on verifiable, trusted information. The analysis of data flow indicates that there are fewer challenges in the synchronization of IoMT devices, edge systems, and DT models with the help of permissioned ledger mechanisms. According to comparative observations based on case studies, predictive maintenance accuracy, workflow efficiency, and optimization of the workflow have been quantitatively enhanced when the DLT protects the DT data pipelines (Zheng et al., 2019). There are however trade-offs that are more computational overhead, latency related with consensus and difficulty with integrating with existing systems. In general, the DTL-based DT architectures have good prospects of scalable, secure and automated hospital management, in cases where technical constraints are alleviated by designing and policy alignment.

8.1 Insights From Architectural Evaluation and Data Flow Analysis

As an evaluation in architecture has shown, DLT–DT ecosystems must be layered seamlessly, which means that physical sensors, Digital Twin model, distributed ledgers, should be made to work together. Authorized blockchain systems assist in an effective data validation and also ensure the adherence to clinical data processing care. The analysis of the data flow indicates that real time synchronization can be enhanced through pre-processing sensor output edge nodes prior to transactions to the ledger which minimizes congestion and latency. This hybrid architecture is necessary so that Digital twins are always fed with validated and high-fidelity data that is vital in predictive analytics and operational forecasting. The other lesson is on fault tolerance: decentralized nodes of the ledger remove the points of failures, allowing the ongoing DT activity even with the partial network outages (Kuo & Zhang, 2023). Moreover, irretrievable data records promote transparency and audit functionalities in clinical and facility operations. Nevertheless, it depends on the consensus algorithms, the amount of data created by the IoMT, and network capacity. Lightweight consensus, optimized batching, and selective logging strategies are some of the key design considerations to implement to make them always responsive to real-time and ensure a high data integrity level.

8.2 Impact on Latency, Security, Interoperability, and System Resilience

There are both beneficial and adverse impacts of the integration of DLT on the latency that can improve the security of data at the price of validation. Supported by consensus mechanisms, such as PBFT or Proof of Authority, the latency issue can be eradicated, and Digital Twins can be updated in real-time without being deprived of cryptographic security. Regarding security, DLT is highly beneficial since it does not require tampering, unauthorized access, and other fraudulent updates of devices (Coorey et al., 2022). Efficient incident forensics and compliance reporting will also be assisted by irrefutable records. Standardized data-exchange logic is also a factor that improves interoperability by being enforced by smart contracts and allows an easier integration of IoMT devices, EHR platforms, and facility systems. This consistency reduces inconsistency of the inputs of DT that gives power to predictive validity ultimately. The system resilience is enhanced by decentralization to ensure that the DT operations are sustained in case the specific servers or departments are out (Hulsen, 2024). Despite these benefits, there are some challenges, including overhead of blockchain storage, control of network traffic, and integration with the old systems of clinical use. These are some of the issues that must be addressed to achieve the optimal performance when deploying massive hospitals.

8.3 Comparative Assessment of DLT-DT Implementations in Hospitals

Comparative study of actual implementations of DT and DLT shows that there is a high degree of performance improvement without mentioning that there is also diversity in terms of the implementation scale, density and the presence of digital infrastructure. The hospitals that employ the Digital Twins with the assistance of DLT note the rise in the accuracy of predictive maintenance, a decrease in the downtime of equipment, and the increase of the workflow transparency (Abdullah et al., 2023). Triaging routing and predicting of emergencies When the prediction of eliminating a blockchain-guaranteed data pipeline is confirmed, emergency departments have gained faster access to triage routing and greater coordination. Nevertheless, the implementations vary in consensus choice, integration architecture and policies in operation. The good latency and throughput of systems using edge-assisted permissioned blockchains are upon a pair with those using cloud-only. Smaller hospitals have a lower technical complexity with limited scalability and large multispecialty centers have higher integration difficulties. The results on security are always good regardless of the deployment but performance optimization involves delicate balancing of block size, frequency of transactions, and complexity of smart-contracts (Kumari et al., 2025). Altogether, comparative results approve the feasibility of the concept of integration of DLT and DT but note the necessity of standardized platforms and scalable consensus models.

9. FUTURE RESEARCH

Further studies are required to investigate scalable and lightweight consensus schemes that would allow real time Digital Twin functionality without reducing security. Another potential direction that can be pursued in the future is the integration of predictive models based on AI and decentralized data infrastructure to ensure autonomous DT decision-making with credible ledger data. Research should also look into the area of ethical and regulatory concerns especially in sensitive hospital settings where identity management, patient consent, and data transparency demands rigid adherence systems. It has been observed that emerging trends, including federated ledgers, cross-hospital blockchain networks, and zero-trust architectures, suggest ways to develop interoperability security further (Ratta et al., 2021). Besides this, it will be significant to test energy-efficient blockchain models, privacy-sensitive smart contracts, and decentralized identity systems to adopt them on large scale. These ideas are to be proven in future research by conducting longitudinal deployments of hospitals to evaluate the effect in the long term (Ravikumar, Renukadevi, et al., 2025). Table 5 Provides details of the emerging research areas and the challenges that they pose in their future development.

Table 5. Future Research Directions and Corresponding Technical Challenges

Research Direction	Opportunity	Technical Challenge
Lightweight Consensus	Real-time DT updates	Reducing validation latency
Federated Ledgers	Cross-hospital sharing	Privacy-preserving interoperability
Zero-Trust Models	Stronger cybersecurity	Continuous authentication overhead
AI-Driven Predictive Twins	Autonomous operations	High computational demand
Privacy-Preserving Analytics	Secure data use	Complex cryptographic methods

9.1 Lightweight Consensus Models for Healthcare DT Systems

The ability to run Digital Twin systems in hospitals requires lightweight consensus mechanisms to make them real-time responsive. The conventional blockchain consensus protocols like Proof of Work or Proof of Stake do not suit because of their computational load, latency, and energy expenses. Studies are thus shifting to other effective systems like Practical Byzantine Fault Tolerance (PBFT), Proof of Authority (PoA), Raft-based consensus, and Directed Acyclic Graph (DAG) structure. These models provide the opportunity to validate DT updates rapidly and ensure a high level of security. The other direction, which is also emerging, is hybrid edge ledger consensus where the edge gateways are local verification of IoMT data and then they send aggregated transactions to blockchain (Riascos et al., 2022). This has a great impact on minimizing network traffic as well as improving throughput. Also, tunable consensus schemes depending on workload trends and criticality of hospital operations can dynamically tune the strictness of validation. To identify the best settings, future research should conduct benchmarking of these models with different workload in the hospitals, device densities, and emergencies to achieve the best settings. Weightless but sturdy consensus has been on the list of preconditions of the implementation of the Digital Twin based on DLT.

9.2 Integration of Ai-Driven Predictive Twins With Federated Ledgers

Digital twins that are based on AI are strongly dependent on machine learning models, real-time analytics, and predictive forecasting. Combining these abilities with federated ledger networks opens up possibilities of secure collaborative analytics within various hospitals, research units and device ecosystems. An example of a federated ledger is where various institutions can share legitimate knowledge, without having to reveal uncoded patient information, which can solve vital privacy and interoperability issues. It is possible to use AI models integrated into Digital Twins to make predictions, which can be verified by using immutable ledger logs (e.g., equipment failure, patient deterioration, or workflow congestion). With smart contracts, risk warnings can be automated, maintenance orders dispatched, and clinical guidelines implemented when the DT predictions go above the threshold values (Mammadova & Ahmadova, 2023). Future studies are encouraged to examine the interactions between federated learning structures and multilayer ledgers so that decentralized AI training can be applied using validated hospital data. The other space is privacy-saving methods like the different privacy, zero-knowledge proofs, and homomorphic encryption, which can be used to maintain confidentiality in the pipeline of DT2-DLT. Such integration will offer more precise, scalable, and safe predictive healthcare systems.

9.3 Ethical, Regulatory, and Zero-Trust Security Enhancements

One of the biggest issues facing the implementation of DT-DLT in hospitals can be ethical and regulatory compliance. Digital Twins deal with sensitive data on patients, operational data and predictive analytics and this necessitates a compliance with laws. Future studies are encouraged to explore ways through which smart contracts can write regulatory stipulations related to consent, data sharing and retention (Onwubiko et al., 2023). A potentially successful approach to securing DT-DLT networks is a zero-trust architecture in which there are no trusted devices or users. This solution involves constant authentication, dynamic authorization and micro-segmentation in the hospital systems. Ethical issues are fairness of AI-based DT predictions, disclosure of automated decision-making, and efforts to reduce the algorithmic influence. The studies should also touch upon the cross-border data exchange, right to digital identity, and long-term storage of immutable medical records. Privacy enhancing technologies, like secure multi-party computation and confidential computing, are to be analyzed to facilitate ethical policy compliant DT -DLT ecosystems. Ethical and regulatory alignment will be an important factor in large scale adoption.

10. MANAGERIAL IMPLICATIONS

Combining the use of Distributed Ledger and Digital Twin technologies can introduce hospital administrators with strategic opportunities to increase the efficiency of operations, the safety of data and make decisions that are predictive. DLT-based Digital Twins can be used by managers to enhance equipment reliability, streamline patient traffic, minimize operational delays, and enhance audit preparedness (Vazirani et al., 2020). These technologies bring about transparency in all departments, aid in making evidence-based decisions, and reduce the risks of data manipulation or system failure. Administrators should also be ready to undertake new governance duties such as developing data sharing practices, investing in employee training, and enforcing regulations. The implementation will need a systematic roadmap that will include selection of technology, infrastructure preparation, risk analysis and involvement of the stakeholders. When well directed, the integration of DLT-DT can make a massive improvement in the performance and resilience of hospitals.

10.1 Strategic Benefits for Hospital Administrators

The adoption of Digital Twin systems that are powered by DLT brings various strategic benefits to the hospital administrators. The operations can be seen in real-time, and effective management of resources can be performed proactively, eliminating the bottlenecks in emergency, diagnostic, and inpatient processes. The downtime of equipment is reduced by blockchain-ensured predictive maintenance that can be verified, and the critical medical equipment should be available at all times (Daraghmi et al., 2019). Unchangeable audit trails will improve accountability and facilitate regulatory audits and make compliance less risky. The adoption of DLT helps to build confidence between the internal units and external partners by aligning data validation between hospital programs. Administrators can also use DT-based simulation models to test the policy changes, staffing strategies, or facility redesigns prior to their implementation (Ravikumar & Aarthi, 2025). Increased cybersecurity measures help in the prevention of ransomware and unauthorized access of data, providing institutional resiliency. All in all, these advantages help in a better quality of care to patients and operational excellence.

10.2 Policy, Compliance, and Governance Requirements

The Digital Twin systems based on the use of DLT are to have a robust governance structure to guarantee legal, ethical, and operational adherence. Policies should clarify the ownership of data, rights of access, retention time and means of revocation of permissions. The patient consent rules, cross-departmental data sharing policies, and automated compliance audits should be encoded using smart contracts. The architectures of hospitals should be consistent with the regulations, e.g., HIPAA, GDPR, or local health-data protection regulations, and the data-handling processes are transparent and traceable (Götz et al., 2022). The governance systems must comprise risk assessment boards, cybersecurity team, and multi-stakeholder decision boards to govern the adoption of technology. Continuous monitoring, incident reporting, as well as immutable logging of the forensic analysis should be implemented in compliance workflows. Interoperability standards, including HL7 FHIR, are other standards that administrators should consider to enable integration with EHR and IoMT systems. Good governance means ethical use, reduced legal risks and building institutional trust.

10.3 Implementation Roadmap for Digital-Health Decision Makers

Implementation of the Digital Twin systems that are enabled by DLT requires a developed implementation roadmap to ensure its success. The first stage is an assessment of readiness, which includes electronic infrastructure, data maturity, and level of cybersecurity. The decision makers will then have to name the high-impact use cases like predictive equipment maintenance, emergency workflow optimization or secure patient identity management. The choice of technology must be with regard to blockchain type (public, private, or consortium), consensus mechanisms, interoperability layers, as well as cloud-edge configurations(Bokolo, 2022) . Pilot Deployments: Pilot deployments are needed to test performance, latency and integration issues. After the successful assessment, it is possible to gradual scale across the departments using suitable change-management strategies. Adoption is mainly played by staff training, stakeholder awareness and cross-functional communication. Constant monitoring and benchmarking on performance achieve long-term success. This roadmap allows expanding the capabilities of the DLT-DT with data-driven, secure, and sustainable growth.

11. CONCLUSION

The combination of the Distributed Ledger Technologies and Digital Twin systems is a breakthrough in the development of the intelligent hospital infrastructure management. This chapter revealed that the results of DBT are a safe, clear, and unreadable environment that guarantees the integrity, reliability, and credibility of the data utilized by Digital Twins. Based on architectural analysis and real-world example, it can be seen that using decentralised validation with real-time digital modelling allows hospitals to gain accuracy in predictive maintenance, patient flow, data governance, as well as operational resilience. The value offered by the chapter goes as far as to introduce a systematic conceptual framework, define technical conditions of interoperability and scalability, and demonstrate how smart-contract automation and a decentralized identity system facilitate safe and efficient clinical operations. The chapter also takes the field of knowledge of DLT-based Digital Twins as a revolutionary pillar of the modern hospital ecosystems further by compiling the information available in the literature, modern technologies, and practical applications. The discussion also provides insight into the current problems of latency, consensus performance, legacy system integration and regulatory compliance which promotes the required lightweight consensus protocols, privacy-preserving architectures and robust zero-trust security models. It is anticipated that in the future, the next-generation healthcare systems will be more dependent on decentralized, intelligent and autonomous infrastructure architectures that are capable of supporting the predictive, adaptive and patient-centric operational functions. With more interconnected IoMT devices, AI-founded analytics, and federated data platforms, Digital Twins based on DLT are going to be important in building resilient, interoperable, and ethically administered digital health settings. The chapter therefore puts the integrated DLT-DT paradigm as a technology pathway that is future ready, secure, and sustainable to realize smart infrastructures in hospitals.

REFERENCES

Aarthi, S., Aravinthan, K., Ravikumar, R. N., Sivakumar, N., & Wanglen, S. (2025). Cryptography securing data in motion within Blockchain, internet of everything, and Federated Learning. In *Convergence of Blockchain, Internet of Everything, and Federated Learning for Security* (pp. 39–78). IGI Global., DOI: 10.4018/979-8-3373-1424-2.ch002

Abdullah, S., Arshad, J., Khan, M. M., Alazab, M., & Salah, K. (2023). PRISED tangle: A privacy-aware framework for smart healthcare data sharing using IOTA tangle. *Complex & Intelligent Systems*, *9*(3), 3023–3041. DOI: 10.1007/s40747-021-00610-8

Abhimanyu Gupta, A. V., Tejal Shah, K. D., & Sandeep Raghuwanshi, S. J. (2025). Blockchain-enabled digital twins for secure and transparent health data management. Economic Sciences, 21(03(S) September), 206–222. DOI: 10.69889/2wyxmw53

Agbo, C. C., Mahmoud, Q. H., & Eklund, J. M. (2019). Blockchain technology in healthcare: A systematic review. *Healthcare (Basel)*, *7*(2), 56. DOI: 10.3390/healthcare7020056 PMID: 30987333

Alzubi, J. A., Alzubi, O. A., Singh, A., & Mahmod Alzubi, T. (2023). A blockchain-enabled security management framework for mobile edge computing. *International Journal of Network Management*, *33*(5), e2240. Advance online publication. DOI: 10.1002/nem.2240

Amofa, S., Xia, Q., Xia, H., Obiri, I. A., Adjei-Arthur, B., Yang, J., & Gao, J. (2024). Blockchain-secure patient Digital Twin in healthcare using smart contracts. *PLoS One*, *19*(2), e0286120. DOI: 10.1371/journal.pone.0286120 PMID: 38422025

Arbabi, M. S., Lal, C., Veeraragavan, N. R., Marijan, D., Nygard, J. F., & Vitenberg, R. (2022). A Survey on Blockchain for Healthcare: Challenges, Benefits, and Future Directions. *IEEE Communications Surveys and Tutorials*, •••, 1–1. DOI: 10.1109/COMST.2022.3224644

Bathalapalli, V. K. V. V., Mohanty, S. P., Kougianos, E., Iyer, V., & Rout, B. (2024). PUFchain 3.0: Hardware-assisted distributed ledger for robust authentication in healthcare cyber-physical systems. *Sensors (Basel)*, *24*(3), 938. DOI: 10.3390/s24030938 PMID: 38339656

Bokolo, A. J. (2022). Exploring interoperability of distributed Ledger and Decentralized Technology adoption in virtual enterprises. *Information Systems and e-Business Management*, *20*(4), 685–718. DOI: 10.1007/s10257-022-00561-8

Brogan, J., Baskaran, I., & Ramachandran, N. (2018). Authenticating health activity data using distributed ledger technologies. *Computational and Structural Biotechnology Journal, 16*, 257–266. DOI: 10.1016/j.csbj.2018.06.004 PMID: 30101004

Chakilam, P. K. (2025). Interoperability in healthcare: Leveraging enterprise Integration Architecture for seamless data exchange. *European Modern Studies Journal, 9*(4), 652–661. DOI: 10.59573/emsj.9(4).2025.63

Chhinal, S., Khanal, B., Singh, M., & Ansari, M. S. A. (2025). A blockchain framework for ensuring medical data security in Internet of Medical Things. *Transactions on Emerging Telecommunications Technologies, 36*(10), e70271. Advance online publication. DOI: 10.1002/ett.70271

Coorey, G., Figtree, G. A., Fletcher, D. F., Snelson, V. J., Vernon, S. T., Winlaw, D., Grieve, S. M., McEwan, A., Yang, J. Y. H., Qian, P., O'Brien, K., Orchard, J., Kim, J., Patel, S., & Redfern, J. (2022). The health digital twin to tackle cardiovascular disease-a review of an emerging interdisciplinary field. *NPJ Digital Medicine, 5*(1), 126. DOI: 10.1038/s41746-022-00640-7 PMID: 36028526

Daraghmi, E.-Y., Daraghmi, Y.-A., & Yuan, S.-M. (2019). MedChain: A design of blockchain-based system for medical records access and permissions management. *IEEE Access : Practical Innovations, Open Solutions, 7*, 164595–164613. DOI: 10.1109/ACCESS.2019.2952942

Dimitrov, D. V. (2019). Blockchain applications for healthcare data management. *Healthcare Informatics Research, 25*(1), 51–56. DOI: 10.4258/hir.2019.25.1.51 PMID: 30788182

Fatokun, T., Nag, A., & Sharma, S. (2021). Towards a blockchain assisted patient owned system for electronic health records. *Electronics (Basel), 10*(5), 580. DOI: 10.3390/electronics10050580

Gordon, W. J., & Catalini, C. (2018). Blockchain technology for healthcare: Facilitating the transition to patient-driven interoperability. *Computational and Structural Biotechnology Journal, 16*, 224–230. DOI: 10.1016/j.csbj.2018.06.003 PMID: 30069284

Götz, C. S., Karlsson, P., & Yitmen, I. (2022). Exploring applicability, interoperability and integrability of Blockchain-based digital twins for asset life cycle management. *Smart and Sustainable Built Environment, 11*(3), 532–558. DOI: 10.1108/SASBE-08-2020-0115

Gupta, S., Mehra, P., Nandy, B., Mohammed, P. R., Pradhan, P. K., Duseja, S., Sharma, N., & Pujari, P. R. (2025). Blockchain in health care, evolutionary or revolutionary - an evidence-based review. *Journal of Pharmacy & Bioallied Sciences*, *17*(Suppl 1), S63–S65. DOI: 10.4103/jpbs.jpbs_672_24 PMID: 40511197

Hemdan, E. E.-D., & Sayed, A. (2025). Smart and secure healthcare with digital twins: A deep dive into blockchain, federated learning, and future innovations. *Algorithms*, *18*(7), 401. DOI: 10.3390/a18070401

Hulsen, T. (2024). Applications of the metaverse in medicine and healthcare. *Advances in Laboratory Medicine*, *5*(2), 159–165. DOI: 10.1515/almed-2023-0124 PMID: 38939198

Kamel Boulos, M. N., & Zhang, P. (2021). Digital twins: From personalised medicine to precision public health. *Journal of Personalized Medicine*, *11*(8), 745. DOI: 10.3390/jpm11080745 PMID: 34442389

Kamruzzaman, M. M., Yan, B., Sarker, M. N. I., Alruwaili, O., Wu, M., & Alrashdi, I. (2022). Blockchain and fog computing in IoT-driven healthcare services for smart cities. *Journal of Healthcare Engineering*, *9957888*, 1–13. Advance online publication. DOI: 10.1155/2022/9957888 PMID: 35126961

Kumari, S., Sowmya, K., Sharma, A. K., Kumar, A., & Goel, P. K. (2025). Blockchain and AI in rural healthcare. In *Advances in Computational Intelligence and Robotics* (pp. 191–214). IGI Global., DOI: 10.4018/979-8-3373-3241-3.ch010

Kuo, T.-T., & Zhang, P. (2023). Editorial: Blockchain and distributed ledger technology—enabled architectures for improving healthcare. *Frontiers in Blockchain*, *6*(1275474), 1275474. Advance online publication. DOI: 10.3389/fbloc.2023.1275474

Lu, Q., Chen, L., Xie, X., Fang, Z., Ye, Z., & Pitt, M. (2023). Framing blockchain-integrated digital twins for emergent healthcare: A proof of concept. *Proceedings of the Institution of Civil Engineers. Engineering Sustainability*, *176*(4), 228–243. DOI: 10.1680/jensu.22.00073

Mammadova, M. H., & Ahmadova, A. A. (2023). Development of digital twin ecosystem and ontology in medicine. *Technology Transfer Fundamental Principles and Innovative Technical Solutions*, *21–23*, 21–23. Advance online publication. DOI: 10.21303/2585-6847.2023.003203

Margheri, A., Masi, M., Miladi, A., Sassone, V., & Rosenzweig, J. (2020). Decentralised provenance for healthcare data. *International Journal of Medical Informatics*, *141*(104197), 104197. DOI: 10.1016/j.ijmedinf.2020.104197 PMID: 32540775

Mishra, D. K., & Mehra, P. S. (2025). Exploring blockchain-based patient-centric healthcare: A comprehensive review. *Concurrency and Computation*, *37*(12–14), e70124. Advance online publication. DOI: 10.1002/cpe.70124

Onwubiko, A., Singh, R., Awan, S., Pervez, Z., & Ramzan, N. (2023). Enabling trust and security in Digital Twin management: A blockchain-based approach with Ethereum and IPFS. *Sensors (Basel)*, *23*(14), 6641. DOI: 10.3390/s23146641 PMID: 37514938

Peng, Y., Zhang, M., Yu, F., Xu, J., & Gao, S. (2020). Digital Twin hospital buildings: An exemplary case study through continuous lifecycle integration. *Advances in Civil Engineering*, *2020*(1), 1–13. DOI: 10.1155/2020/8846667

Rajab, R. M., Abuhmida, M., Wilson, I., & Ward, R. P. (2024). A review of IoMT security and privacy related frameworks. Proceedings of the ... *European Conference on Information Warfare and Security*, 23(1), 733–743. DOI: 10.34190/eccws.23.1.2239

Ratta, P., Kaur, A., Sharma, S., Shabaz, M., & Dhiman, G. (2021). Application of Blockchain and Internet of Things in healthcare and medical sector: Applications, challenges, and future perspectives. *Journal of Food Quality*, *2021*, 1–20. DOI: 10.1155/2021/7608296

Ravikumar, A. S., Atamuratova, Z., Ashirova, A., Jurayev, K., & Hayitova, M. (2025). Comprehensive evaluation of AI-driven systems in modern hospital environments. In Advances in Computational Intelligence and Robotics (pp. 61–88). IGI Global Scientific Publishing. DOI: 10.4018/979-8-3373-2787-7.ch003

Ravikumar, A. S., Saparbaevich, B. R., Kumar A., S., Jumaniyozova, M., & Toshova, S. (2025). AI-enhanced clinical decision-making through a collaborative approach. In Advances in Computational Intelligence and Robotics (pp. 249–280). IGI Global Scientific Publishing. DOI: 10.4018/979-8-3373-3311-3.ch010

Ravikumar, R. S., Manujakshi, Aarthi, S., Urazbaeva, Y., & Tamilselvi, S. (2025). Navigating data privacy, security, and regulatory challenges in healthcare AI ensuring fairness, bias mitigation, interpretability, and trust. In Transformative Role of Transformer Models in Healthcare (pp. 25–54). IGI Global Scientific Publishing. DOI: 10.4018/979-8-3373-2038-0.ch002

Ravikumar, R. N., & Aarthi, S. (2025). AI-powered synergistic robotics and IoT ecosystems for predictive and preventive healthcare. In *Robotics and IoT Synergy in Next-Generation Healthcare* (pp. 1–32). IGI Global Scientific Publishing., DOI: 10.4018/979-8-3373-5447-7.ch001

Riascos, R., Ostrosi, E., Sagot, J.-C., & Stjepandić, J. (2022). Conceptual approach for a Digital Twin of medical devices. In *Advances in Transdisciplinary Engineering*. IOS Press., DOI: 10.3233/ATDE220661

Ricci, A., Croatti, A., Mariani, S., Montagna, S., & Picone, M. (2022). Web of Digital Twins. *ACM Transactions on Internet Technology*, *22*(4), 1–30. DOI: 10.1145/3507909

Roy, P., Sherazi, S. H. T., Delda, M. J. M., Maqsood, M., & Ahmad, M. (2025). Secure data sharing in healthcare. In *Advances in Healthcare Information Systems and Administration* (pp. 255–286). IGI Global., DOI: 10.4018/979-8-3693-4199-5.ch011

Saratkar, S. Y., Langote, M., Kumar, P., Gote, P., Weerarathna, I. N., & Mishra, G. V. (2025). Digital twin for personalized medicine development. *Frontiers in Digital Health*, *7*, 1583466. DOI: 10.3389/fdgth.2025.1583466 PMID: 40851640

Sun, T., He, X., & Li, Z. (2023). Digital twin in healthcare: Recent updates and challenges. *Digital Health*, *9*, 20552076221149652. DOI: 10.1177/20552076221149651 PMID: 36636729

Tiwari, K., & Kumar, S. (2025). Accelerating healthcare data access: A blockchain and decentralized indexing approach. *Concurrency and Computation*, *37*(15–17), e70172. Advance online publication. DOI: 10.1002/cpe.70172

Tuli, S., Tuli, S., Wander, G., Wander, P., Gill, S. S., Dustdar, S., Sakellariou, R., & Rana, O. (2020). Next generation technologies for smart healthcare: Challenges, vision, model, trends and future directions. *Internet Technology Letters*, *3*(2), e145. DOI: 10.1002/itl2.145

Vallée, A. (2023). Digital twin for healthcare systems. *Frontiers in Digital Health*, *5*, 1253050. DOI: 10.3389/fdgth.2023.1253050 PMID: 37744683

Vasiliu-Feltes, I., Mylrea, M., Zhang, C. Y., Wood, T.-C., & Thornley, B. (2023). Impact of blockchain-Digital Twin technology on precision health, pharmaceutical industry, and life sciences: Conference proceedings, Conv2X 2023. *Blockchain in Healthcare Today*, *6*(2). Advance online publication. DOI: 10.30953/bhty.v6.281 PMID: 38187956

Vazirani, A. A., O'Donoghue, O., Brindley, D., & Meinert, E. (2020). Blockchain vehicles for efficient Medical Record management. *NPJ Digital Medicine*, *3*(1), 1. DOI: 10.1038/s41746-019-0211-0 PMID: 31934645

Wang, E., Tayebi, P., & Song, Y.-T. (2023). Cloud-based digital twins' storage in emergency healthcare. *International Journal of Networked and Distributed Computing*, *11*(2), 75–87. DOI: 10.1007/s44227-023-00011-y

Zhang, P., Kelley, A., Schmidt, D. C., & White, J. (2023). Design pattern recommendations for building decentralized healthcare applications. *Frontiers in Blockchain*, *6*(1006058), 1006058. Advance online publication. DOI: 10.3389/fbloc.2023.1006058

Zheng, X., Sun, S., Mukkamala, R. R., Vatrapu, R., & Ordieres-Meré, J. (2019). Accelerating health data sharing: A solution based on the Internet of Things and distributed ledger technologies. *Journal of Medical Internet Research*, *21*(6), e13583. DOI: 10.2196/13583 PMID: 31172963

KEY TERMS AND DEFINITIONS

Blockchain: A type of DLT that organizes data into cryptographically linked blocks, ensuring immutability, transparency, and tamper resistance.

Consensus Mechanism: A protocol used in DLT to validate transactions and maintain data consistency across distributed nodes.

Data Provenance: The traceable record of data origins, transformations, and movement, ensuring authenticity and regulatory compliance.

Decentralized Identity (DID): A secure identity framework that enables users and devices to control their credentials without reliance on centralized authorities.

Digital Twin (DT): A real-time virtual replica of a physical asset, process, or system used for monitoring, simulation, and predictive analytics in healthcare environments.

Distributed Ledger Technology (DLT): A decentralized data management framework where records are securely stored, validated, and shared across multiple nodes without a central authority.

Edge Computing: Localized processing at or near the source of data generation to reduce latency and support real-time DT synchronization.

Interoperability: The ability of systems, devices, and applications to exchange, interpret, and use data consistently across heterogeneous healthcare environments.

IoMT (Internet of Medical Things): A network of connected medical devices, sensors, and clinical systems that continuously collect and exchange patient and operational data.

Permissioned Blockchain: A private blockchain where only authorized participants can validate transactions and access specific data.

Predictive Maintenance: A data-driven approach that uses DT models and sensor analytics to anticipate equipment failures and schedule timely maintenance.

Smart Contract: A self-executing program on a blockchain that automates rules, workflows, and agreements without manual intervention.

Zero-Trust Security: A cybersecurity model that assumes no device or user is inherently trustworthy and enforces continuous authentication and authorization.

Chapter 8
Blockchain-Enabled Identity and Patient Record Management for Secure and Smart Hospital Systems

Rahmath Nisha A.
http://orcid.org/0009-0001-5146-2411
Saveetha School of Management, Saveetha Institute of Medical and Technical Sciences, Chennai, India

R. Pooja
Saveetha School of Management, Saveetha Institute of Medical and Technical Sciences, Chennai, India

M. Radhakrishnan
Saveetha School of Management, Saveetha Institute of Medical and Technical Sciences, Chennai, India

ABSTRACT

The accelerated digitalization of healthcare has compounded data fragmentation, interoperability, cybersecurity, and patient-centered governance issues in the information systems of hospitals. This chapter suggests a systemic approach, which is a blockchain-enabled identity and health record management together with digital twin technologies to facilitate safe, smart, and interoperable smart hospital processes. Blockchain technology is framed as a trust and governance layer that can support self-sovereign identity-based consent, immutable data provenance, and auditable

DOI: 10.4018/979-8-3373-8177-0.ch008

access control, and digital twins can offer real-time, predictive models of patients, hospital operations, and infrastructure. The chapter presents a blockchain-digital twin governance infrastructure and a maturity model that describes the levels of adoption at smart hospitals, starting with safe digital records, the next level as intelligent and autonomous digital twin ecosystems.

1.0. INTRODUCTION

Rapidly increased digitalization of healthcare systems has brought large-scale use of electronic health records (EHRs), networked medical devices and data-driven clinical applications. Despite these improvements, healthcare information infrastructures are still experiencing ongoing challenges of data fragmentation, low interoperability, and cybersecurity threats. Patient records tend to be spread across institution-specific systems, which are unable to communicate and, thus, create incomplete medical histories, duplicated diagnostics, and slow clinical decision-making (Roehrs et al., 2017). Moreover, the use of centralized EHR systems has exposed the vulnerability to cyber-attacks since centralized repositories are single point of failure. A number of massive data breaches have affirmed that traditional health information systems find it difficult to guarantee confidentiality, integrity, and trust in scale (Kuo et al., 2017). These constraints can be used to underscore the importance of other digital architectures capable of enabling secure, interoperable, and resilient healthcare data management. The new technology like blockchain and digital twins promise to address these issues. Decentralized data governance, audit trails that cannot be altered, and controlled identity management are supported by blockchain, whereas digital twins are used to support real-time system modeling, predictive analytics, and optimization of the operation (Agbo et al., 2019; Fuller et al., 2020; Jones et al., 2020). Nevertheless, they are not well developed when used together as integrated smart hospital systems. The chapter discusses how identity and record management as a blockchain-enabled solution can be functionally connected to the digital twin system to make smart hospitals secure, intelligent, and interoperable. Although some promising solutions to such challenges are proposed by the emerging technologies like blockchain and digital twins, their implementation in a hospital setting is still disjointed. Justifying the necessity of an integrated approach, the next section discusses the structural constraints of the current hospital information systems and determines particular gaps in research that prompt the given study.

2.0. PROBLEM CONTEXT AND RESEARCH GAP

Although the digital health technologies are increasingly being adopted, the existing hospital information systems are not integrated, institution-focused, and not sufficiently governed. Patient data is shared amongst heterogeneous platforms that are run by hospitals, labs, pharmacies and insurers and this inhibits interoperability and care continuity. The latter is also complicated by the centralized data storage models that increase cybersecurity risks and provoke the ethical issues associated with the privacy, consent, and data ownership (Kuo et al., 2017). Even though blockchain and digital twin technologies have been widely researched in the healthcare sector, the current body of knowledge analyses the two technologies as standalone answers. The research on blockchain has been mostly concentrated on decentralized security, auditability, and identity management (Agbo et al., 2019; Dunphy and Petitcolas, 2018), and the research on digital twin is centered on the real-time modeling, simulation, and predictive decision support in order to optimize clinical and operational processes (Fuller et al., 2020; Jones et al., 2020).

A rich literature on a systematic description of data flows, identity controls, and trust mechanisms that need to ensure blockchain security to operate reliable digital twins in hospitals is still missing. It is possible to define several research gaps. To start with, there are limited researches on the ways in which blockchain can authenticate and provide irrevocable provenance to the real-time data flows that supply digital twin models. Second, self-sovereign identity (SSI) and other patient-centric identity management strategies are the topics that have hardly been considered with regard to hospital-scale digital twins (Dunphy and Petitcolas, 2018). Third, common interoperability standards, including HL7 FHIR, are rarely examined in the integrated blockchain-digital twins' systems in smart hospitals (Hylock & Zeng, 2019). Lastly, governance, regulatory compliance, and ethical oversight are not always brought up in the context of cyber-physical hospital ecosystems but rather as single elements. It is of vital importance to fill these gaps to achieve the potential of smart hospitals. In this chapter, the research addresses these challenges by suggesting a comprehensive conceptual architecture that makes blockchain a trust and governance layer of digital twin-based operations of a hospital.

Table 1. Recent period of review of literature (2023-2025)

S No	Main Focus	Healthcare Setting	Blockchain x Digital Twin Coverage	Author
1	**Blockchain-secure patient Digital Twin** — concept design and prototype examples; smart contracts to regulate the DT updates.	Client-oriented concepts of DT; illustrative examples (PLOS ONE open access).	Clearly combines blockchain and patient DTs; shows smart-contract-based update/consent processes.	Amofa et al., 2024.
2	Effects of blockchain-DT tech-workshop/ proceedings overview, conceptual implications of precision health.	High-level arguments that blockchain can support DT ownership/monetization; no operational architecture or hospital pilot; general discussion	High-level precision-health context Broad activity; blockchain may support ownership/monetization of an asset but not operational architecture or hospital pilot.	Garg et al., 2023
3	Digital twins in healthcare: Scoping / review Scoping of digital twins Scoping in healthcare methods, applications, challenges, Systematic mapping of applications.	Cross-domain DT systems (cellular - organ - hospital systems).	Extensive coverage of DTs but less of blockchain as a governance/trust layer to DTs (says could be synergistic)	Katsoulakis et al., 2024.
4	IoT healthcare Scalable blockchain integration-- prototype/Hyperledger Fabric simulation; IoT metadata on-chain, off-chain in IPFS.	IoT / device ecosystem, simulated scenario (prototype-level).	Good at IoT data provenance and scalability patterns (parallel chains, Hyperledger); lacks DT model implementation as such.	Mohammadi et al. (SCALHEALTH), 2024
5	Improved multi-layer blockchain security model- MLBSM to solve IoT/blockchain latency and scalability	General IoT / real-time systems (security model evaluation).	Pay attention to the latency mitigation (clustering, parallelism) and privacy; it applies to DTs that require low latency but does not depend on the DT under consideration.	Elomda et al., 2025 (MDPI Information).

3.0. CONTRIBUTION OF THE CHAPTER (Author, 2026)

The chapter is more than just a descriptive review of the blockchain and digital twins' technologies because it presents an integrated and hospital-specific contribution that has not been adequately captured in extant literature. In contrast to the previous literature that discusses blockchain or digital twins as independent enablers, this paper directly situates blockchain as a governance and trust infrastructure of digital twin-oriented smart hospital activities.

The main original input of this chapter is the introduction of a Blockchain-Digital -Twin Governance Architecture of Smart Hospitals that systematically brings together self-sovereign identity (SSI), interoperable health data standards and real-time digital twin intelligence to a single cyber-physical system. Blockchain is not viewed as a secure data store in this architecture, but as a policy enforcement and provenance layer that regulates the creation, updating, access, access, and auditing of digital twins among the hospital stakeholders. To be more precise, the chapter contributes in four areas that are novel,

3.1. Integrating Blockchain and Digital twins Governance-Centrically

The current healthcare paradigms utilize blockchain or digital twins to provide security of records or to simulate and optimize. One of the earliest chapters to introduce the idea of blockchain as a dynamic layer of governance that controls the ingestion of digital twins' data, update of the model, and access control is based on smart contracts and SSI-based consent interactions.

3.2. Hospital Architectural Perspective at the scale of a hospital

Previous research on digital twins is typically either patient-level or device-level models, whereas blockchain research is concerned with data exchange or identity management. This is also the first chapter to go beyond the scope of cyber-physical systems at the hospital scale, combining patient, equipment, and operational digital twins within one blockchain-secured system.

3.3. Interoperability-Aware Design

In contrast to most conceptual frames, the suggested architecture includes the healthcare interoperability standards (e.g., HL7 FHIR) as the mediator layers between outdated hospital systems, blockchain networks, and digital twins. The design option is a direct response to the integration difficulties in the real world that are highly ignored in other designs.

3.4. Evidence-Based Positioning of Research Gaps

The chapter presents its framework as a reaction to reported empirical and architectural gaps, not a generic conceptual offering by synthesizing recent (2023-2025) literature and systematically mapping unresolved limitations - including the absence of performance benchmarks, the non-existence of SSI-enabled consent in DT systems, and limited governance models.

Put collectively, these contributions transform the convergence of blockchain and digital twins into a technological possibility and convert it into a governable, interoperable, and scalable smart hospital paradigm.

4.0. THE BLOCKCHAIN-DIGITAL TWIN MATURITY FRAMEWORK OF SMART HOSPITAL

The chapter offers a novel Blockchain-Digital Twin Maturity Framework on Smart Hospitals to curb this issue of absence of a formalized guidance to integrate blockchain and digital twins (DTs) into hospital settings. This framework differs with the fact that unlike previous research that talks about blockchain or DTs individually, this framework conceptualizes their co-evolution through progressive stages of hospital digital transformation, focusing on governance, trust, and operational intelligence. In healthcare information system studies, maturity models are a common method of advising a gradual adoption, capability evaluation, and strategic planning. In the same spirit, the suggested framework introduces five levels of maturity each with a depiction of a deeper level of integration, technological maturity, and organizational maturity to implement blockchain-secured DT (Agbo et al., 2019; Katsoulakis et al., 2024).

Level 1: The Integrity of Digital Records: The first tier is where hospitals implement blockchain in order to guarantee electronic health records (EHRs) and audit logs are intact and irreversible. The secure data governance mechanism, blockchain, is utilized, and the DT capabilities are low or do not exist. This tier is concerned with compliance, traceability, and trust in underlying hospital data systems in line with initial blockchain healthcare implementations (Roehrs et al., 2017).

Level 2: Asset and Process Digital Twins: At this step, hospitals implement DTs of discrete assets and processes, e.g., personal equipment monitoring, inventory management, or workflow modeling. The Blockchain ensures sensor feeds and maintenance records are secured so that DT models can be run on valid and sensitive data. The integration is still localized, and the operational advantages like predictive maintenance and optimization of processes are starting to appear (Fuller et al., 2020; Kherbache et al., 2021).

Level 3: Digitally Twinned Patients with Blockchain Security: This tier refers to the assimilation of blockchain and patient-level DTs. DTs are constantly simulating patient physiological conditions based on real-time information and blockchain control's identity, consent, and provenance by smart contracts and self-sovereign identity (SSI). The step allows reliable predictive clinical decision support analytics, especially in an emergency and intensive care setting (Amofa et al., 2024; Dunphy and Petitcolas, 2018).

Level 4: Hospital Operational Digital Twins: At Level 4, DTs are extended outside individuals and represent hospital-wide activities, such as bed and staff scheduling, and resource use. Blockchain acts as a governance foundation that coordinates the DT updates within departments and holds accountability to the working decisions. The level helps with simulation of scenarios and plans of the surge in the case of pandemics or large-scale emergencies (Jones et al., 2020)

Level 5: Smart and Self-Sufficient Digital Twin Ecosystems: The utmost level of maturity is envisioned as smart hospital systems where DTs are enhanced with artificial intelligence and machine learning that help with predictive and prescriptive decision-making. Blockchain makes it possible to establish decentralized trust, automated policy enforcement, and auditable AI governance, and privacy-preserving methods may include zero-knowledge proofs. Such a level promotes independent optimization of hospital work without acute ethical and regulatory control (Mittelstadt, 2017; Elomda et al., 2025). AI digitalization has defined the importance of organization which focusing on current tactics while exploring the new market potential timely basis (Rao et al., 2023).

5.0. CONCEPTUAL AND THEORETICAL FOUNDATIONS

The transformation of healthcare with the assistance of blockchain, digital identity model, interoperability model, and digital twin system requires a foolproof conceptual foundation. These pillars entirely rely on distributed computing, information governance, cyber-physical systems and data ethics. Together, they create the intellectual framework, based on which safe, open-minded, and forward-thinking smart hospital patterns can be structured. This part illustrates on each of these pillars in detail.

5.1. Decentralized Ledger Technology (DLT)

DLT is an example shift in the conventional centralized data management approach, wherein a disseminated architecture can only mean that the presence of multiple nodes, can store copies of a common, append-only synchronized ledger. This architecture is particularly advantageous in healthcare since medical information is often utilized by a diverse team of stakeholders, clinicians, laboratories, pharmacies, insurers and regulators. Therefore, a mechanism that permits creating certain immutability, tamper-proof recording, and end-to-end auditability is non-negotiable. The crucial part of DLT is consensus algorithms, which indefinitely chooses how the participants of the network should agree on the validity of transactions. The most common consensus model called Practical Byzantine Fault Tolerance (PBFT) allows the system to accomplish an agreement due to the malicious or unpredictable behavior of a certain portion of nodes (Kuo et al., 2017). PBFT is efficient enough to make it especially relevant in permissioned healthcare settings, in which actors are authenticated and trusted to different levels.

Additionally, industry reports by (Agbo et al., 2019) emphasizes the paramount significance of disseminated validation that can be utilized along with blockchain to eradicate limitations present in the centralized electronic health record (EHR) databases and minimize the threats associated with tampering of data, voluntary alteration of data, or cyber-attacks.

5.2. Self-Sovereign Identity (SSI)

Self-Sovereign Identity (SSI) offers a fundamental change to the way digital identities are managed: institutions do not own and control identities but the individuals themselves do. In conventional identities, hospital IDs, insurance IDs and national health number are allotted by centralized authorities. Arrangements like these have the inclination of creating fragmented identities, interoperability and serious privacy threats. SSI lifts these restrictions since it allows patients to exercise control over their identity attributes using decentralized identifiers (DID) and digitally signed verifiable credentials (VCs). As shown by (Dunphy and Petitcolas, 2018), the prospect of SSI is that it provides greater privacy due to the ability of users to show evidence of certain identity attributes (e.g., age, insurance validity) without disclosing the personal information.

Moreover, according to (Tobin and Reed, 2017), SSI enhances trust, security, and autonomy because it does not rely on a single provider, but instead, identity verification is decentralized over distributed systems.

Table 2. Creative Comparison of Blockchain Consensus Mechanisms for Hospital Systems

Consensus	Latency	Throughput	Energy Use	Hospital Suitability
PoW	High	Low	Very High	Not Suitable (Public, Slow, Energy Intensive)
PoS	Medium	Medium	Low	Partially Suitable (Public/Consortium)
PBFT	Low	High	Low	Highly suitable (Permissioned hospitals)
RAFT	Very Low	High	Low	Highly Suitable (Permissioned hospitals)

Based on these theoretical bases, the chapter now shifts of conceptual discussion into system design. The following section outlines the suggested blockchain-digital twin solution, which would convert the principles into a feasible framework adapted to smart hospital settings.

5.3 Interoperability Standards (HL7 FHIR and Global Health Informatics)

One of the most important issues in healthcare digital transformation is still interoperability. Health systems have to interact effectively across platform, gadgets, and organizations. In the absence of standardized data formats and exchange formats, integration of blockchain would create silos of data instead of ensuring the connectivity of systems. One of the most powerful standards that are aimed at resolving this issue is HL7 FHIR (Fast Healthcare Interoperability Resources). FHIR divides clinical data into modular resources which can be shared safely through APIs. A study conducted by (Hylock and Zeng, 2019) reveals that the integration of FHIR with blockchain enhances the data consistency, longitudinal record keeping, and transparency of access in real-time. Also, the research of the global health informatics puts emphasis on the standardized data models, metadata formats, and security frameworks. According to (Roehrs et al., 2017), to achieve an effective integration of personal health records (PHRs), EHRs, and mobile health systems, the health information systems should employ consistent terminologies and exchange structures in interoperability.

5.4. Digital Twin Frameworks in Healthcare

Digital twin concept has become astonishingly popular in the contemporary healthcare systems as an approach to developing high-fidelity virtual simulations of physical clinical settings, patient conditions, and workflow in hospitals. These computational replicas work in parallel with the physical ones as they continuously receive real- time information with the IoT devices, EHR inputs, and monitoring equipment. According to (Jones et al., 2020), digital twins are dynamic structures that can develop together with the systems on which they are based. In contrast to the case of static simulations, digital twins constantly change according to the new information, which could offer insights into predictive maintenance, resources optimization, and simulations of patient-specific treatment.

(Fuller et al., 2020) also show that digital twins can streamline healthcare processes by indicating equipment malfunctions, congestion in the patient process, and experimenting with various treatment outcomes before they are deployed. Digital twins are further enriched with blockchain and become more integrity- and trust-filled. Blockchain will guarantee the information entering the virtual model is correct, legitimate and cannot be altered easily which is crucial in simulations that must be made during high-stakes clinical decision-making.

The use cases of blockchain-secured digital twins are:

- Forecasting ICU occupancy
- Optimizing surgical scheduling.
- Modeling the trajectory of COVID-19 spread or outbreaks.

Dynamically predicting surgical robot or imaging device downtime. Therefore, smart hospitals consist of computational intelligence in the form of digital twins.

5.5. Data Ethics and Privacy Theories

Ethical standards and data privacy concepts cannot be overlooked in facilitating transformation in the field of digital healthcare. With an increasingly widespread use of AI, IoT and blockchain in systems, patient rights protection is no longer a matter of bargain. GDPR and HIPAA set the pillars of principles regarding:

1. Informed consent
2. Openness in information processing
3. Data minimization
4. Accountability
5. Secure storage and transfer

(Mittelstadt, 2017) points out such emerging ethical hazards of algorithm-based health systems as the lack of transparency, the possibility of bias, and the abuse of sensitive personal data. Blockchain is in line with these principles because it maintains unaltered records of access to their data, and patients can monitor their data usage. According to Radanović and Likic (2018), blockchain enables patients to be empowered by a verifiable audit trail, which increases wholeness in digital care models. The ethical and privacy theories are thus utilized in the wise deployment of blockchain and digital twins such that technological advancement does not undermine the dignity and autonomy of patients.

6.0. DIGITAL HEALTH TRANSFORMATIONS AND DATA CHALLENGES

Digital health technologies have extensively revolutionized the healthcare delivery process, permitting it to be more data-driven and focused on remote monitoring and more coordinated treatment pathways. The emerging importance of electronic health records (EHRs), mobile health (mHealth) applications, wearables, and telemedicine platforms has amplified the area of patient-centered care and enhanced clinical decision-making (Cuff, 2023).

(Roehrs et al., 2017) suggested that, a scarcity of standardized and interoperable health information exchange leads to numerous unwanted tests and unfinished patient history, as well as the delay in coordinated care. Such interoperability limitations can destabilize the health philosophy and disrupt the smooth clinical processes. The COVID-19 pandemic also emphasized the susceptibility of a disconnected health information system. As (Manteghinejad and Javanmard, 2021) point out, the crisis revealed the necessity to share data that is reliable and timely to aid the surveillance, triage, and population-level decision-making.

However, numerous healthcare institutions failed because they had incompatible systems and were unable to find one single platform that could handle large-scale flows of health data safely and in the most transparent way. There is also the issue of privacy and ethical issues. Patients have no idea with which data they operate, how it is processed, and disseminated through the digital environment. The argument presented by (Kostkova, 2015) is that a large proportion of the users agree to share the data without knowing the risks involved, which brings concerns of the concept of informed consent, data autonomy, and the long-term analysis of personal health information. Wearables and mobile applications also contribute to a further blurring of this landscape, where user-created information is not necessarily subject to existing health privacy laws, and thus there are no clear delimiters of how it is safeguarded and those held responsible. The issue of cybersecurity is also a serious problem. With the increase in digital health data, the risk of breach, ransomware, and unauthorized access also increases.

According to (Kuo et al., 2017), centralized EHR infrastructures result in a single point of vulnerability to cyber threats. Violations like these not only put sensitive patient information at risk, but eventually leads to a reducing level of institutional trust and interruption of the continuity of clinical care. An amalgamation of these problems points to one clear contradiction: Although digital health technologies are meant to enhance connectivity and the level of intelligence, the prevailing infrastructure is still disjointed, insecure, and also ethically doubtful.

7.0. BLOCKCHAIN PRINCIPLES FOR HEALTHCARE IDENTITY AND RECORDS

The blockchain technology is demonstrated as a disorderly resolution to a protected and clear decentralized management of health data. In principle, blockchain is a distributed registry where transactions are stored in cryptographically anchored and unalterable blocks stored on many nodes. In such a decentralized structure, there is no reliance on the authority and the threat of tampering, unauthorized changing, or data loss is greatly minimized (Kuo et al., 2017). The transactions in each of the blocks are authenticated and its cryptographic connectivity to the block is obligatory to guarantee the integrity of the data in the entire chain (Javed et al., 2021).

(Dwivedi et al., 2020) identified that smart contracts can amplify the process of multi-site research, automating the data verification process, enhancing traceability, and reducing administrative overhead. Regarding the clinical settings, smart contracts can be utilized to permit controlled access to patient records and allow autonomous audit without even using centralized intermediaries. Healthcare systems that are structured based on blockchains have a numerous benefit in terms of identity validation and health records.

As (Dunphy and Petitcolas, 2018) demonstrated, all of the decentralized identity models are entirely based on blockchain that can provide safe patient authentication along with reducing the threats of centralized identity repositories. The audit trails are immutable and allows healthcare personnel to establish the time and method by which patient records were opened, which holds them accountable to regulatory standards. These features play a crucial role in justifying cybersecurity and privacy risks that prevail in the conventional electronic health record (EHR) solutions. The assurance of blockchain in healthcare can be also reinforced by real-world implementations. Similarly, MedRec prototype, engineered in MIT, is entirely based on blockchain-based architecture that achieves longitudinal records of patients where the medical information can be visible and controlled by the patient. Though it remains an experimental system, it demonstrates how decentralized models can be used to increase privacy, data provenance, and interoperability (Azaria et al., 2016).

Compatibly, government introduced programs like the blockchain-based health infrastructure in Estonia emphasize the promise of distributed registries in securing the health records of the citizens at the same time providing controlled access to the authorized parties (Mettler, 2016).

8.0. SELF- SOVEREIGN IDENTITY MANAGEMENT AND BLOCKCHAIN

SSI model is a digital identity model that is facilitated by distributed ledger technologies, e.g. blockchain. It is not like the traditional account-based models since it operates like real identities. This model creates a direct connection between the parties who would like to communicate or exchange data through so-called VCs (Zhuang et al., 2023). Another study published in Cell shows the importance of the use of Self-Sovereign Identity (SSI), a user-centric model of providing individuals with full authority over and approving of their identities being governed in a decentralized way.

The cryptography used to generate SSI credentials makes users pseudo anonymous and checkable anywhere at any time (through blockchain) instead of being registered with a third-party login service using credentials they stored and confirmed by a centralized authority (as required with popular identity management models such as the centralized and federated model), which is a federation of centralized models (Cocco & Tonelli, 2024). The SSI model consists of a holder, or a person with a specific credential, an issuer, or a person who issued the credential, and a verifier, or a person who receives the presented credential and has to verify the validity of the credential. The data stored in an SSI system is stored in user-owned digital wallets as opposed to being stored in a centralized system and the user retains their keys (Zhuang et al., 2023). The overall architecture has four modules:

(1) The Creation Module, which allows the creation of tokens of blockchain,
(2) Linkage Module, attaching the patient token to the patient account of every health system,
(3) Authentication Module, that is, allowing patients to give medical experts access to their token in order to obtain their medical records at numerous different healthcare facilities and areas of specialization, and
(4) Exchange Module, which encompasses the HIE procedure and token validity check (Zhuang et al., 2023).

The potential revolutionary changes in healthcare processes introduced by blockchain include the ability to develop a patient with a history of consent audit and a self-sovereign identity. These identity systems are primarily used to authorize and authenticate. Most of the digital identities are no longer given to the user, but the business does it and maintains control over the identity. This enables the service provider to control the identity and related services without the customer having any idea and control (St Clair et al., 2020).

9.0. INCORPORATION OF BLOCKCHAIN WITH DIGITAL TWINS IN SMART HOSPITALS

Digital twin is a recent technology that has gained significance in contemporary healthcare, and it delivers the virtual image of patients, medical equipment, and hospital functions in real-time. Digital twins continuously update the models of their models unlike the static simulation which relies on fixed data points. This provides a dynamic system which is capable of supporting prediction, surveillance and decision making in the clinical settings. According to (Jones et al., 2020), digital twins are adaptive models that develop with the physical counterparts, allowing a more accurate analysis and operational forecasting. Digital twins are useful in a number of applications in hospital settings. Digital twins, as (Fuller et al., 2020) observe, are able to streamline patient traffic, simulate treatments, anticipate equipment malfunctions, and real-time assess the use of resources.

To give an example, intensive care units can rely on digital twin-based forecasting to predict the number of occupied beds or available ventilators, and surgical departments can test various scheduling options and apply them. Digital twins improve operational delays and increase the effectiveness of clinical processes by making them proactive in planning. In the case of patient specific application, a digital twin will combine physiological, laboratory, imaging, and wearable sensor data to generate a personalized, computational model.

This type of model has the ability to model disease progression, access medication responses, or test different treatment plans without putting patients at risk. As stated in (Amofa et al., 2024), virtual experimentation capability allows precision medicine and enables clinicians to make more informed decisions, depending on continuously changing patient data. Adaptability, modularity, connectivity, and programmability are some of the important properties of digital twins that ensure their functionality. Adaptability guarantees the model to evolve with the entry of new data; modularity divides various functional or physiological aspects into independent sub-models; and connectivity helps to integrate the model with IoT devices and hospital systems.

9.1. Blockchain–Digital Twin Convergence Architecture for Smart Hospitals

Layered architecture: The integrated architecture illustrated in Figure 1 presents a layered convergence of blockchain and digital twin technologies specifically designed for smart hospital environments. The model follows a structured multi-layer approach consisting of a physical layer (patients, medical devices, and hospital infrastructure), a data acquisition layer (IoT sensors, EHR systems, and gateways), a blockchain trust layer, a digital twin modeling layer, and an application layer supporting analytics and clinical decision-making. Such layered digital twin architectures have been widely recognized in recent healthcare studies as essential for scalability, modularity, and real-time responsiveness in complex clinical systems (Noeikham et al., 2024).

Figure 1. Blockchain–digital twin integrated architecture for smart hospitals

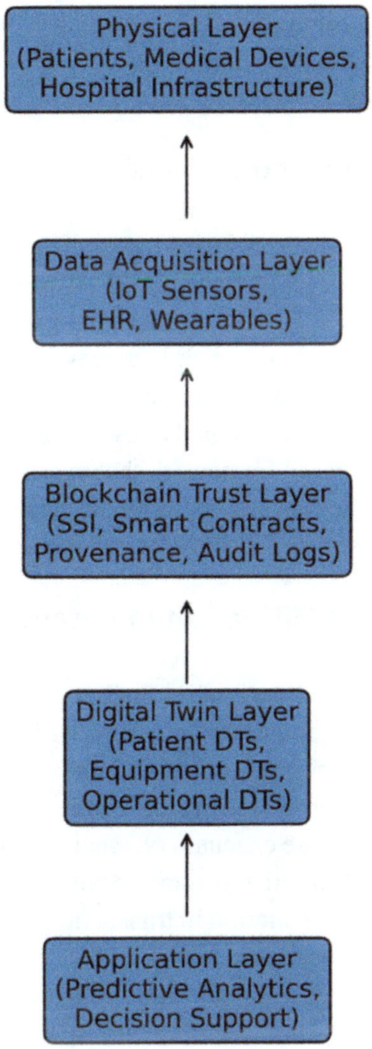

Source: Author (2026)

9.2. Blockchain as Trust and Governance Layer

In this design, blockchain acts as a trust and governance layer and not a high-frequency clinical data repository. Off-chain, patient and device data occurring in high volumes are stored in secure hospital or cloud environments, and cryptographic hashes and timestamps, device identifiers, and decentralized identifiers are immutably recorded on the blockchain. This design guarantees provenance of data, resistance to tampering, and auditing transparency without adding latency to the hospital operations, which are time-sensitive, in accordance with the recent blockchain-enabled healthcare designs (Kasyapa & Vanmathi, 2024).

9.3. Smart Contracts to Update of DT

Smart contracts entrenched within the blockchain layer are what will dictate how digital twin models are accessed, updated and synchronized. Such self-executable contracts implement patient consent using self-sovereign identity solutions and verify that the only verified and authorized sources of data can cause digital twin updates. As an illustration, updates of a patient digital twin are made only in case, sensor data are verified and predetermined consent conditions are met. This model of governance is a contract-based framework that builds trust in a digital twin simulation and prediction outputs, in line with recent healthcare patient digital twin applications that are secured using blockchain technology (Amofa et al., 2024).

9.4. Hybrid Design and Mitigation to Latency

In order to overcome the challenge of scalability and latency in real-time digital twins' synchronization, the proposed architecture will use a hybrid, on-chain and off-chain approach backed by permissioned blockchain networks. Digital twin state-change hashes and access logs are stored in blockchain, and computationally intensive analytics and model execution are executed off-chain in the digital twin layer. It has been demonstrated that such multi-layer and localized blockchain designs can be used to achieve a high level of reduction in transaction latency and at the same time maintain security and consistency of real time IoT-based systems, and are therefore applicable in cyber-physical systems like smart hospitals (Elomda et al., 2025).

9.5. Values to Smart Hospitals

The architecture allows the use of blockchain as a governance backbone of digital twins, which enhances secure predictive analytics, transparent accountability and robust smart hospital operations. Capacity forecasting of ICUs, prediction of equipment failures, and patient modeling with verified and auditable streams of data can be supported by digital twins without harming data integrity and privacy. Recent literature highlights that these highly interconnected blockchain-digital twin systems are essential to the credible and scalable and regulation-conformable intelligent hospital systems (Hemdan & Sayed, 2025).

10.0. BLOCKCHAIN-SECURED DIGITAL TWINS FOR SMART HOSPITAL OPERATIONS

Digital twins (DTs) used in smart hospital settings are dynamic cyber-physical models (similar to simulated artifacts) of patients, hospital units, and hospital infrastructure, instead of non-changing simulated artifacts. These DTs are based on high-frequency data streams on Internet of Medical Things (IoMT) devices, electronic health records, and operational systems of hospitals. Nevertheless, the accuracy and clinical utility of DT-based insights rely crucially on the credibility, provenance, and control of the underlying data. The solution to these issues is offered by blockchain technology, which introduces the concept of a decentralized trust layer that ensures the security of the DT data flows and governance among the stakeholders of the hospital (Fuller et al., 2020; Katsoulakis et al., 2024).

At the patient level, blockchain-secured DTs store an unalterable and verifiable record of physiological data and diagnostic outcomes as well as clinical interventions. The update operation on patient DT is cryptographically associated with its source data, which guarantees provenance and traceability. This feature is specifically useful in high-stress scenarios like intensive care, ED where predictive analytics systems based on DT (early warning systems, or treatment response simulation) need a strong guarantee of the data integrity. As shown by previous researchers, blockchain-supported DTs promote trust in patient-specific models by deterring unauthorized data editing and providing clear auditability (Amofa et al., 2024; Roehrs et al., 2017).

At the operational level, hospital DTs simulate the flow of patients, bed occupancy, employee, and resource availability in each department. With blockchain, the operational data that supply these DTs, including admissions, discharges, and equipment supply, become tamper-resistant and auditable. Indicatively, an ICU capacity DT can be used to simulate surge conditions on blockchain-authenticated inputs by assisting in defensible and transparent decision-making during pandemics or mass-casualty incidents. This type of operational intelligence by DT is in line with previous studies indicating that trusted data infrastructures play a vital part in hospital-scale deployment of DT (Jones et al., 2020)

Naturally, on the infrastructure level, DTs are some of the most important hospital resources, such as imaging systems, surgical equipment, and energy management systems. These DTs can facilitate predictive maintenance and lifecycle management using blockchain-secured sensor reading, maintenance, and compliance check logs. This is because blockchain records are immutable, which means that infrastructure DTs capture reliable system states and minimize downtime and safety risks in mission-critical hospital settings (Fuller et al., 2020; Kherbache et al., 2021).

Notably, blockchain is not an alternative to DT intelligence but controls the DT lifecycle. Smart contracts specify when and who can update particular views of the DT, and under which circumstances, simulations using DT can be used to make a clinical or administrative decision. This design style of governance transforms DTs into decision-support systems that can be trusted and are part of hospital functions. The suggested solution puts blockchain in the role of a governance and accountability layer of DTs, which is a step forward compared to the current implementations of healthcare DTs, which do not have a strong trust and control infrastructure (Agbo et al., 2019; Elomda et al., 2025).

11.0. PRELIMINARY SIMULATION AND DEPLOYMENT SCENARIO

Even though this chapter is conceptual in tone, a prototype deployment scenario is established in advance to illustrate the technical feasibility and operational applicability of the suggested blockchain-digital twin architecture in the smart hospital settings. According to previous studies, healthcare blockchain and digital twin systems Preliminary experiments with simulation, prototype processes, or hypothetical deployments are an established and efficient system to test the complex cyber-physical system before actual implementation (Agbo et al., 2019; Fuller et al., 2020).

11.1. Simulation Design and Assumptions

The simulated situation takes into account a medium sized intelligent hospital that has several clinical units such as an intensive care, emergency, and diagnostic unit. Hospital information systems, patient monitoring devices, and medical equipment produce constant data streams, which are updated on respective digital twins. An authorized blockchain network is presumed that is under use in a hospital consortium, which will be used to verify identities, enforce consent, and record audits using smart contracts. As in the conventional design of healthcare blockchain, the data with a high frequency is processed and saved off-chain, and the cryptographic hash, metadata, and access-control record are written to the blockchain where they cannot be changed. This architectural assumption is slightly similar to previous researches highlighting that hybrid on-chain/ off-chain models would play a critical role in maintaining performance, privacy, and regulatory compliance in healthcare systems (Kuo et al., 2017; Hylock & Zeng, 2019).

Evaluation Metrics: In order to measure the behavior of the system under the actual conditions of a hospital, the simulation is directed to the indicative performance measures utilized most of the time in blockchain-based healthcare and IoT testing. These includes,

Transaction throughput, which is the quantity of blockchain transactions created in order to verify the consent and update the state of the digital twin.

Latency is the duration to authenticate identity and to record a digital twin update.

Rate of data integrity verification, which is the ratio of successful blockchain hash-based data twin verification.

Scalability, which is measured considering the behavior of the system as the number of patients, devices, and digital twins grows.

The metrics are commonly used in the assessment of blockchain-enabled healthcare facilities and offer viable foundation to the feasibility analysis (Agbo et al., 2019; Elomda et al., 2025).

11.2. Observations from the Simulations Scenario

The simulation deployment shows that the suggested architecture is applicable to the near-real-time digital twin synchronization in cases when blockchain is deployed as a governance and verification layer instead of a data transport mechanism. Permissioned consensus systems have low validation times on identity and consent transactions, and off-chain digital twin computing on scalable analytics. The findings are aligned with the existing literature on healthcare digital twin and blockchain that indicate that hybrid structures yield a substantial decrease in latency with ensuring data integrity and auditability (Fuller et al., 2020; Elomda et al., 2025). The findings are that blockchain-based digital twins can be technically implemented in hospitals in terms of ICU monitoring, emergency access control, and predictive equipment maintenance.

11.3. Hospital Deployment Implication

Regarding deployment, the simulation indicates the significance of a gradual process of implementation in real hospital setting. The first use can be non-supreme, like equipment monitoring or administrative process, and then gradually expanded to patient-centric digital twins, when the governance mechanisms and compliance with the current hospital systems are proven. These results support the main idea of the chapter that the convergence of blockchain and digital twins is not only a theoretical concept, but can be implemented in reality given the limitations of hospitals, which is the basis of further pilot studies and empirical validation in clinical environments (Jones et al., 2020; Amofa et al., 2024).

12.0. ETHICAL, REGULATORY, SCALABILITY CONSIDERATIONS IN SMART HOSPITALS

The implementation of blockchain-protected digital twin solutions in intelligent hospitals brings about serious ethical, regulatory, and scaling issues, which need to be settled in order to make it safe, legal, and credible. Since the clinical data is sensitive, and the application of algorithmic decision support is on the rise, the governance mechanisms should be integrated on both technological and organizational levels.

12.1. Patient Autonomy and Ethics

The use of digital twins and blockchain in hospitals means that the use of such technologies is based on ethical governance in which ongoing data gathering, simulation, and pro-gnostication have a direct impact on the clinical decision-making process. The major ethical principles are patient autonomy, informed consent, transparency, and accountability. There is the risk that digital twin systems based on real-time patient data access will strip patients of agency in case there is no clarity in how data access and model decisions are regulated. (Mittelstadt, 2017; Dunphy and Petitcolas, 2018).

12.2. Blockchain-Digital Twin Hospital System Regulatory Compliance

Regulatively, smart hospital systems should be in line with data protection regulations like the General Data Protection Regulation (GDPR) and the Health Insurance Portability and Accountability Act (HIPAA). These standards involve legal data processing, limiting its purpose, minimizing data, and tight access control. Architecture of blockchain architectures should therefore not support identifiable patient data on-chain, but should make use of hashed references and off-chain storage in order to comply (Radanovic and Likic, 2018; Koc, 2024).

12.3. Real-Time Performance Problems and Scalability

Scalability is also a significant technological issue to consider during the implementation of blockchain and real-time digital twins in hospitals. Digital twins need regular data updates at low latency, whereas blockchain networks, especially public chains, may impose a delay on data updates because of overheads on consensus and replication of data. Otherwise, these restrictions can affect real-time monitoring in the critical care units or emergency department. Hybrid architectures are becoming the way to go to contain these challenges. Such designs store high-frequency clinical data and computations of digital twins off-chain, and cryptographic hashes, access logs, and state-change proofs are written to blockchain. (Sadath et al., 2024; Elomda et al., 2025).

12.4. Governance and Risk Mitigation Strategies

Governments of blockchain-digital twin systems at hospitals need to follow co-ordinated technical, ethical, and organizational approaches to achieve good governance. Hospitals should have clear policies that specify who is responsible for the outputs of the digital twins, how to escalate an error created by algorithms, and how to have human controls. Audit trails of blockchain facilitate accountability in recording all data access, model updates and triggers of decisions in a manner that can be verified. In addition, it must be able to interoperate with a large-scale use with legacy hospital systems and regulatory reporting tools. Researchers note that governance-by-design, which entails embedding ethical and regulatory logic into system structures, is more useful than ex post hoc compliance strategies in complex healthcare settings (Agbo et al., 2019; Patel et al., 2024).

13.0. PROPOSED FRAMEWORK: BLOCKCHAIN-BASED PATIENT IDENTITY AND RECORD ECOSYSTEM

A drastic shift in the identity management that gives people control over their private information is Self-Sovereign Identity (SSI). By permitting users to self-sufficiently control their digital identities, this strategy tests traditional unified identity systems. Digital Identity, DID, VC, VP, and Wallet are few of the many essential notions of SSI. A digital identity is an illustration of a person or an object in the digital realm made up of features like name, birthdate, address, and other essential data. Traditional digital identities are more frequently so overseen by corporations or governments. A worldwide unique identifier known as the Decentralized Identifier (DID) allows users and administrations to build their own identifiers without any third-party guidance or assistance. Utilizing cryptographic functions to ensure that all individual users possess the corresponding private key integrated to the DID, these identifiers permit users to offer their proprietorship. Verifiable Credential (VC) is a significantly common data structure used to signify claims about an entity that are tamper-proof and indefinitely cryptographically verifiable. A claim is a declaration about an article that represents a characteristic, like name, address, or date of birth. With verifiable credentials, users can now upload and store numerous claims in a format that is well-matched, cryptographically signed, and completely under their supervision.

If they have verifiable credentials, the user can submit claims to the service provider. An assembly of one or more verifiable credentials from one or more issuers which are shared with the service provider is known as a Verifiable Presentation (VP). As a replacement for using multiple verifiable credentials separately, it is merely a means to represent a collection of distinct credentials selected by the user. The authorship of the set of credentials can be cryptographically confirmed by a digital signature (Gomes et al., 2024).

Figure 2. Self-Sovereign Identity Roles

Source:(Gomes et al., 2024)

(Siyal et al., 2019) the various aspects of smart contracts and blockchain technology were explained to help aid the healthcare industry and transform the entire procedure into a simplified one. As per the research done by them, monitoring and recording medical records plays aa crucial role, and blockchain technology might reduce the data loss and stop data construction, if the data on the ledger is defended.

(Zhang et al., 2017) highlighted the utilization of blockchain and smart contracts and their paramount significance in resolving various healthcare problems. In their most recent works, they recognized various obstacles in the implementation of blockchain technology and used a few of the preliminary steps of the protocol to implement it for diverse healthcare use cases. They have emphasized how building a blockchain-based application can resolve diverse healthcare concerns more effectively. The various uses of blockchain technology for the healthcare system were covered by (Kumar et al., 2018). They have implemented smart contracts for blockchain-based medical systems and sought attention to issues and obstacles in the implementation of blockchain technology.

DT is definitely not just a upfront simulation or a static model; it is an ever-transforming model that tracks its overall lifecycle to keep a check and optimize its functions while always being conscious of the events happening in its physical twin. Real-time data uploading made possible by IoT devices and sensor technology enables synchronization between the DT and its physical counterpart, and big data storage capacities allow the preservation of historical data that may be helpful to the DT.

For example, future states of the physical twin can be predicted by AI algorithms. Additionally, a DT can apply preventive maintenance procedures by simulating new configurations (Kherbache et al., 2021).

Figure 3. Model of Blockchain–Digital Twin Integrated Smart Hospital

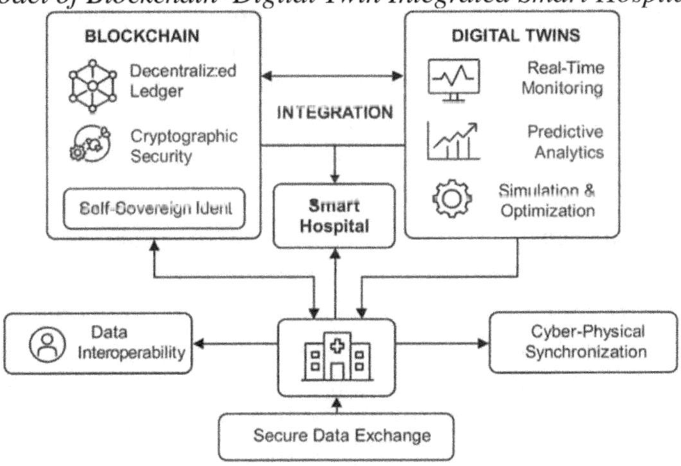

Source: (Author, 2026)

14.0. LIMITATIONS AND FUTURE RESEARCH DIRECTIONS

Although blockchain-guaranteed digital twin systems present a great opportunity in the development of smart hospital systems, certain drawbacks should be taken into consideration to guarantee the attainment of realistic conception of the proposed structure. Such constraints cut across technical, organizational, and regulatory levels and provide valuable research directions in the future.

Limitations Connectivity with the Past Infrastructure: The majority of hospitals have heterogeneous and legacy health information systems, proprietary medical devices and silo databases. Any implementation of blockchain and digital twin architecture in these environments creates challenges regarding interoperability, data harmonization and compatibility of the system. Even though the exchange of data between various entities can be facilitated by standards, including HL7 FHIR, integration with blockchain-based governance and real-time models of a digital twin is highly complicated and resource-consuming (Hylock & Zeng, 2019; Roehrs et al., 2017).

Organizational Readiness and Human Factors: Blockchain-secured digital twins need an organization to change significantly to be implemented. Low technical skills, workflow resistance and distrust of decision support based on algorithms can slow adoption. The lack of explainability and transparency of digital twin insights might lead to the unwillingness of clinicians to trust it without the human-in-the-loop design (Mittelstadt, 2017; Jones et al., 2020).

Scalability and Real-Time Constraints: Even though hybrid on-chain/off-chain architectures address the issues of latency, the problem of scalability remains since the hospital systems have to grow to thousands of patients, devices, and digital twins. Real-time responsiveness in safety critical environments like intensive care units is a challenging task that must be optimized in architecture and must be constantly observed in terms of architectural performance, as well as the choice of suitable permissioned consensus mechanisms (Elomda et al., 2025; Kuo et al., 2017).

Uncertainty in Regulation and Law: The healthcare policies on the protection of data, accountability of algorithms, and clinical decision support remain in development. The use of digital twins in predictive or prescriptive clinical insights can become more regulated. In addition, the immutability of blockchain may be against the regulatory demands of data correction or destruction, which requires specific attention to design options like off-chain storage and cryptographic referencing (Dunphy and Petitcolas, 2018; Agbo et al., 2019).

15.0. FUTURE RESEARCH DIRECTIONS

Hospital-based Empirical Validation: The next research direction of the blockchain-digital twin system needs to be the empirical assessment of the systems by pilot implementations in the actual hospital setting. These studies would be able to compare the performance metrics such as latency, throughput, data integrity, clinical impact, and user acceptance across various departments in a hospital (Amofa et al., 2024; Fuller et al., 2020).

Integration and Standardization Structures: The next step in enhancing the interface that can allow a smooth connection between blockchain systems, digital twin models, and hospital information systems is to conduct further research and create universal interfaces that can work with all three. Interoperability strategies among vendors and standards would be compared in comparative studies, which would help in supporting scalable and vendor-neutral adoption (Hylock & Zeng, 2019).

Trusted-Governance AI Enhanced Digital Twins: Artificial intelligence and machine learning when combined with digital twins have a potential to create more advanced predictive and prescriptive analytics. The next-generation studies must look into the possible application of blockchain-based governance to guarantee transparency, bias reduction, and accountability in AI-driven digital twins applications applied in clinical decision support (Mittelstadt, 2017; Katsoulakis et al., 2024).

Applications in the post-Pandemic/Emergency Preparedness: The COVID-19 pandemic revealed the dismal weakness in hospital capacity planning and coordination. Future studies can focus on how digital twins secured by blockchain can be used to promote emergency preparedness, surge management, and cross-hospital coordination in cases of public health emergencies (Jones et al., 2020; Amofa et al., 2024).

16.0. CONCLUSION

This chapter highlighted the major flaws of the current hospital information systems by introducing a proposal of integrated blockchain-digital twin framework to secure smart, interoperable and intelligent hospitals. The proposed solution allows managing patient identity, proving data immutability, and access control, and use digital twins to model and predict decisions in a variety of clinical, operational, and infrastructural areas by placing blockchain as a layer of governance and trust. The presented governance architecture and maturity structure offers a systematic direction concerning the adoption of the hospital-scale, covering interoperability, scalability, and ethical compliance gaps. All in all, the chapter lays a solid and viable groundwork to the next generation of smart hospital systems, and provides a pathway to the future of empirical validation and actual implementation of the same.

17.0. PRACTICAL IMPLICATIONS

Applicability of the Blockchain-Secured Digital Twins in Hospitals: The combination of blockchain and digital twin technologies are the technology to enable the development of the hospital-specific intelligent applications, and beyond generic digital health systems. Digital twins are used in smart hospitals, which are constantly synchronized cyber-physical models of patients, clinical units, and infrastructure, and blockchain ensures data integrity, provenance, and governance. Such convergence allows reliable real-time analytics, optimization of operations, and decision-making, which comply with regulations in complex hospital settings (Fuller et al., 2020; Jones et al., 2020). Using blockchain technology to build the strong digital asset management tools for the financial operations and systems up to date (Geetha et al., 2024).

Intensive Care Unit Capacity Prediction and Surge Controlling: ICUs are logically under resourced, especially during the emergence of a pandemic. ICU capacity can be simulated using digital twins that are secured by blockchain and combine real-time data of patient monitors, ventilators, admission systems and staffing schedules. Blockchain provides the impossibility to ensure a stream of data serving the ICU digital twin is indestructible and verifiable, which allows for effective predictions of bed occupancy and equipment supply. This type of predictive modeling can facilitate crisis surge planning and clear allocation of resources in advance (Manteghinejad and Javanmard, 2021; Amofa et al., 2024).

Identity Verification and Rapid Onboarding in Emergency Department: Patients who cannot give identity information or medical history are common in the emergency departments. Self-sovereign identity (SSI) facilitated by blockchain enables emergency clinicians to check the identity attribute of patients safely, by means of decentralized identifiers and verifiable credentials. Smart contracts are used to impose contextual and time-constrained access to vital health information whereas blockchain audit trails guarantee accountability. The respective patient digital twin is constantly updated as emergency interventions take place, so the continuity of care between departments in the hospitals is ensured (Dunphy and Petitcolas, 2018; Javed et al., 2021).

Anticipatory repair of Hospital equipments: Hospitals rely on high-value medical devices like imaging devices, surgical robots and life-support devices. The performance degradation of medical equipment and prediction of failures can be designed with digital twins that utilize continuous sensor information. Blockchain makes these data streams secure, authentic, and traceable, and compliance activities and maintenance records are logged in with irreversibility. Such a practice minimizes any unplanned downtimes, promotes patient safety, and facilitates regulatory audits within hospital setups (Fuller et al., 2020; Kherbache et al., 2021). Blockchain technology ensures that secure storage of data prediction while smart contracts facilitate the automated model execution (Kumar et al., 2023).

Safe Interdepartmental Information Exchange and Care Co-ordination: Hospital care needs to be coordinated well to include the departments of radiology, laboratories, pharmacy and the inpatient wards. Digital twins that are secured by blockchains facilitate the ability to share data interoperable with the assurance that any updates to the state of the patient are verified, authenticated, and constantly represented across systems. It can be integrated with the interoperability standard like HL7 FHIR to ensure the compatibility with the legacy hospital information systems that minimizes the errors that happen because of discontinuous streams of data (Hylock et al., 2019; Roehrs et al., 2017).

REFERENCES

Agbo, C. C., Mahmoud, Q. H., & Eklund, J. M. (2019, April). Blockchain technology in healthcare: a systematic review. In *Healthcare* (Vol. 7, No. 2, p. 56). MDPI.
Agbo, C. C., Mahmoud, Q. H., & Eklund, J. M. (2019). *Blockchain technology in healthcare: A systematic review. Health Care*, *7*(2), 56. DOI: 10.3390/healthcare7020056 PMID: 30987333

Amofa, S., Xia, Q., Xia, H., Obiri, I. A., Adjei-Arthur, B., Yang, J., & Gao, J. (2024). Blockchain-secure patient Digital Twin in healthcare using smart contracts. *PLoS One*, *19*(2), e0286120. DOI: 10.1371/journal.pone.0286120 PMID: 38422025

Azaria, A., Ekblaw, A., Vieira, T., & Lippman, A. (2016, August). Medrec: Using blockchain for medical data access and permission management. In *2016 2nd international conference on open and big data (OBD)* (pp. 25-30). IEEE.DOI: 10.1109/OBD.2016.21

Cocco, L., & Tonelli, R. (2024). A Self-Sovereign Identity–Blockchain-Based Model Proposal for Deep Digital Transformation in the Healthcare Sector. *Future Internet*, *16*(12), 473. DOI: 10.3390/fi16120473

Cuff, A. (2023). The evolution of digital health and its continuing challenges. *BMC Digital Health*, *1*(1), 3. DOI: 10.1186/s44247-022-00004-x PMID: 38014367

Dunphy, P., & Petitcolas, F. A. P. (2018). A first look at identity management schemes on the blockchain. *IEEE Security and Privacy*, *16*(4), 20–29. DOI: 10.1109/MSP.2018.3111247

Dwivedi, S. K., Amin, R., & Vollala, S. (2020). Blockchain based secured information sharing protocol in supply chain management system with key distribution mechanism. *Journal of Information Security and Applications*, *54*, 102554. DOI: 10.1016/j.jisa.2020.102554

Elomda, B. M., Abdelaty Abdelbary, T. A., Hassan, H. A., Hamza, K. S., & Kharma, Q. (2025). An enhanced multi-layer blockchain security model for improved latency and scalability. *Information (Basel)*, *16*(3), 241. DOI: 10.3390/info16030241

Elomda, B. M., Ahmed, A. I., El-Sayed, A., & Hassan, M. M. (2025). An enhanced multi-layer blockchain security model for real-time IoT applications. *Information (Basel)*, *16*(3), 241. Advance online publication. DOI: 10.3390/info16030241

Fuller, A., Fan, Z., Day, C., & Barlow, C. (2020). Digital twin: Enabling technologies, challenges, and open research. *IEEE Access : Practical Innovations, Open Solutions*, *8*, 108952–108971. DOI: 10.1109/ACCESS.2020.2998358

Garg, M., Liu, X., Vassilaki, M., Petersen, R. C., Sauver, J. S., & Sohn, S. (2023, December). Navigating Sex-Specific Disease Dynamics in Incident Dementia. In *2023 IEEE International Conference on Bioinformatics and Biomedicine (BIBM)* (pp. 4065-4072). IEEE. DOI: 10.1109/BIBM58861.2023.10385324

Geetha, B. T., Kafila, K., Ram, S. T., Narkhede, A. P., Ahmad, A. Y. B., & Tiwari, M. (2024, March). Creating resilient digital asset management frameworks in financial operations using blockchain technology. In *2024 International Conference on Trends in Quantum Computing and Emerging Business Technologies (pp.* 1-7*).* IEEE. DOI: 10.1109/TQCEBT59414.2024.10545263

Gomes, B., Eisa, S., Matos, D. R., & Pardal, M. L. (2024). Decentralized Storage and Self-Sovereign Identity for Document-Based Claims. *arXiv preprint arXiv:2411.16987.*

Hemdan, E. E. D., & Sayed, A. (2025). Smart and Secure Healthcare with Digital Twins: A Deep Dive into Blockchain, Federated Learning, and Future Innovations. *Algorithms*, *18*(7), 401. DOI: 10.3390/a18070401

Hylock, R. H., & Zeng, X. (2019). A blockchain framework for patient-centered health records and exchange (Health Chain). *Journal of Medical Systems*, *43*(10), 1–9. DOI: 10.1007/s10916-019-1412-5

Javed, I. T., Alharbi, F., Bellaj, B., Margaria, T., Crespi, N., & Qureshi, K. N. (2021). Health-id: A blockchain-based decentralized identity management for remote healthcare. Healthcare. 2021; 9: 712. *Cybersecurity and the Digital Health, 175.* Advance online publication. DOI: 10.3390/healthcare9060712 PMID: 34200778

Jones, D., Snider, C., Nassehi, A., Yon, J., & Hicks, B. J. (2020). Characterizing the digital twin: A systematic literature review. *CIRP Journal of Manufacturing Science and Technology*, *29*, 36–52. DOI: 10.1016/j.cirpj.2020.02.002

Kasyapa, M. S. B., & Vanmathi, C. (2024). Blockchain integration in healthcare: A comprehensive investigation of use cases, performance issues, and mitigation strategies. *Frontiers in Digital Health*, *6*, 1359858. DOI: 10.3389/fdgth.2024.1359858 PMID: 38736708

Katsoulakis, K., Chatzichristofis, S. A., Roussos, G., & Panayiotou, C. (2024). Digital twins in healthcare: A scoping review of current applications, challenges, and future directions. *NPJ Digital Medicine*, *7*(1), 73. Advance online publication. DOI: 10.1038/s41746-024-01073-0 PMID: 38499608

Kherbache, M., Maimour, M., & Rondeau, E. (2021). When digital twin meets network softwarization in the industrial IoT: Real-time requirements case study. *Sensors (Basel), 21*(24), 8194. DOI: 10.3390/s21248194 PMID: 34960288

Koc, S. (2024). Legal Compliance protocols for Blockchain smart contracts: A new era of regulatory compliance. *Authorea Preprints.* DOI: 10.36227/techrxiv.172954185.58874599/v1

Kostkova, P. (2015). Grand challenges in digital health. *Frontiers in Public Health, 3*, 134. DOI: 10.3389/fpubh.2015.00134 PMID: 26000272

Kumar, P. R., Meenakshi, S., Shalini, S., Devi, S. R., & Boopathi, S. (2023). Soil Quality Prediction in Context Learning Approaches Using Deep Learning and Blockchain for Smart Agriculture. In Effective AI, Blockchain, and E-Governance Applications for Knowledge Discovery and Management (pp. 1-26). IGI Global. DOI: 10.4018/978-1-6684-9151-5.ch001

Kumar, T., Ramani, V., Ahmad, I., Braeken, A., Harjula, E., & Ylianttila, M. (2018, September). Blockchain utilization in healthcare: Key requirements and challenges. In *2018 IEEE 20th International conference on e-health networking, applications and services (Healthcom) (pp. 1-7). IEEE.* DOI: 10.1109/HealthCom.2018.8531136

Kuo, T. T., Kim, H. E., & Ohno-Machado, L. (2017). Blockchain distributed ledger technologies for biomedical and health care applications. *Journal of the American Medical Informatics Association : JAMIA, 24*(6), 1211–1220. DOI: 10.1093/jamia/ocx068 PMID: 29016974

Manteghinejad, A., & Javanmard, S. H. (2021). Challenges and opportunities of digital health in a post-COVID19 world. *Journal of Research in Medical Sciences : the Official Journal of Isfahan University of Medical Sciences, 26*(1), 11. DOI: 10.4103/jrms.JRMS_1255_20 PMID: 34084190

Mettler, M. (2016, September). Blockchain technology in healthcare: The revolution starts here. In *2016 IEEE 18th international conference on e-health networking, applications and services (Healthcom)* (pp. 1-3). IEEE.

Mittelstadt, B. (2017). Ethics of the algorithm: Key problems and solutions. *Philosophy & Technology, 30*(4), 1–26. DOI: 10.1007/s13347-016-0229-9

Mohammadi, A., Mehrabi, A., & Yousefi, H. (2024). SCALHEALTH: A scalable blockchain-based framework for secure IoT healthcare systems. *arXiv preprint.* https://arxiv.org/abs/2403.08068

Noeikham, P., Buakum, D., & Sirivongpaisal, N. (2024). Architecture designing of digital twin in a healthcare unit. *Health Informatics Journal*, *30*(4), 14604582241296792. Advance online publication. DOI: 10.1177/14604582241296792 PMID: 39447608

. Patel, N. A., Ingle, P. S., Patsamatla, S. K., Omotunde, H., & Ingole, B. S. (2024). Integration of Blockchain and AI for Enhancing Data Security in Healthcare: A Systematic Review. *Library of Progress-Library Science, Information Technology & Computer, 44(3).*

Radanović, I., & Likić, R. (2018). Opportunities for use of blockchain technology in medicine. *Journal of Medical Systems*, *42*(8), 152. DOI: 10.1016/j.ijpe.2008.03.010 PMID: 29974270

Rao, C. B., Suryakanthi, K., Banappagoudar, S. B., Geetha, B. T., Kaur, S., & Kaur, H. (2023, December). Entrepreneurship and innovation in the age of artificial intelligence: A blockchain approach. In *2023 IEEE International Conference on ICT in Business Industry & Government (ICTBIG)* (pp. 1-6). IEEE. DOI: 10.1109/ICTBIG59752.2023.10456198

Roehrs, A., Da Costa, C. A., da Rosa Righi, R., & De Oliveira, K. S. F. (2017). Personal health records: A systematic literature review. *Journal of Medical Internet Research, 19*(1), e5876. DOI: 10.2196/jmir.5876 PMID: 28062391

Sadath, L., Mehrotra, D., & Kumar, A. (2024). Scalability performance analysis of blockchain using hierarchical model in healthcare. *Blockchain in Healthcare Today*, *7*, 10–30953. DOI: 10.30953/bhty.v7.295 PMID: 38715761

Siyal, A. A., Junejo, A. Z., Zawish, M., Ahmed, K., Khalil, A., & Soursou, G. (2019). Applications of blockchain technology in medicine and healthcare: Challenges and future perspectives. *Cryptography*, *3*(1), 3. DOI: 10.3390/cryptography3010003

. St Clair, J., Ingraham, A., King, D., Marchant, M. B., McCraw, F. C., Metcalf, D., & Squeo, J. (2020). Blockchain, interoperability, and self-sovereign identity: trust me, it's my data. *Blockchain in Healthcare Today, 3*, 10-30953.https://doi.org/ . v3.122DOI: 10.30953/bhty

Tobin, A., & Reed, D. (2017). *The inevitable rise of self-sovereign identity*. Sovrin Foundation.

Zhang, P., White, J., Schmidt, D. C., & Lenz, G. (2017, October). Design of blockchain-based apps using familiar software patterns to address interoperability challenges in healthcare. In Proceedings of the PLoP-24th Conference on Pattern Languages of Programs, Vancouver, BC, Canada (pp. 22-25). https://doi.org/ DOI: 10.5555/3290281.3290304

Zhuang, Y., Shyu, C. R., Hong, S., Li, P., & Zhang, L. (2023). Self-sovereign identity empowered non-fungible patient tokenization for health information exchange using blockchain technology. *Computers in Biology and Medicine*, *157*, 106778. DOI: 10.1016/j.compbiomed.2023.106778 PMID: 36934533

KEY TERMS AND DEFINITIONS

Blockchain: It is a decentralized and distributed ledger that stores transactions in verifiable and immutable way. The blockchain is applied in intelligent hospital to secure the governance of health data, identity control and access, in addition to auditability of health data to many stakeholders.

Digital Twin (DT): This term describes a virtual object (a patient, medical device, hospital unit) that is constantly updated based on real-time data. Digital twins aid in predictive analytics, simulation, and optimization of operations in hospitals.

Self-Sovereign Identity (SSI): A decentralized identity model that enables people to dictate their digital identities and consent preference. SSI in hospital settings allows patients to control the provision of access to their health data with the help of decentralized identifiers and verifiable credentials.

Smart Contracts: Computer scripts that execute automatically and are deployed on blockchain platforms and execute specified rules and conditions. Patient consent, data access permissions, policy of data updating, and policies of smart hospitals are managed by smart contracts.

Smart Hospital: A digitally-enabled hospital that enables cyber-physical systems, real-time data-based analytics, and intelligent technologies to improve clinical-decision making, operational efficiency, and patient safety.

Technology: Technology is the application of the scientific knowledge, tools and techniques in practice with the aim of developing solutions to solve the problems or to better human life.

Chapter 9
Comparative Perspectives on Digital Health Transformation of Blockchain and Digital Twin Integration in Estonia and Saudi Arabia

Anvita Rose
http://orcid.org/0009-0004-0807-3922
Christ (Deemed to be) University, Delhi NCR, India

Khushboo Malik
Christ (Deemed to be) University, Delhi NCR, India

ABSTRACT

This chapter examines the integration of blockchain and digital twin technologies in transforming healthcare systems, focusing on Estonia and Saudi Arabia. Estonia's mature e-governance infrastructure, built on the X-Road interoperability platform and blockchain validation, supports comprehensive electronic health records and secure data exchange. Saudi Arabia's Vision 2030 and National Transformation Program accelerate modernization through AI, IoMT, smart hospitals, and blockchain-based services. The chapter analyzes how blockchain enhances data integrity, privacy, and interoperability, while digital twins enable real-time monitoring, predictive diagnostics, and operational optimization. Comparative insights highlight strengths, challenges, and governance implications, proposing a unified framework for ethics, transparency, and sustainability in digital healthcare ecosystems.

DOI: 10.4018/979-8-3373-8177-0.ch009

INTRODUCTION

Global health systems are undergoing a profound digital transformation driven by rapid advances in data-intensive technologies. What began as a relatively straightforward transition from paper-based records to electronic formats has evolved into a complex ecosystem in which intelligent, interoperable, and predictive infrastructures actively mediate healthcare delivery (Khosrow-Pour, 2015). Within this transformation, two technologies **blockchain** and **digital twins** play complementary and increasingly central roles by enhancing data integrity, operational efficiency, and evidence-based predictive decision-making in ways that conventional health information systems cannot achieve. (Fuller et al., 2020; Khosrow-Pour, 2015)

Blockchain technology introduces a distributed and tamper-resilient ledger that directly addresses the long-standing fragmentation, inconsistency, and security vulnerabilities of health data. In traditional healthcare environments, patient information is typically dispersed across institutional silos comprising hospitals, laboratories, insurers, and public agencies (Kuo et al., 2017). This fragmentation generates inefficiencies, duplication of diagnostics, clinical errors, and heightened exposure to cyber threats. Blockchain mitigates these risks by ensuring that every clinical update, prescription, or diagnostic request is time-stamped, cryptographically linked, and verified through distributed consensus mechanisms. Transparency and accountability are thus embedded directly within system architecture rather than relying solely on policy-based compliance (Agbo et al., 2019; Khosrow-Pour, 2015).

In contrast, **digital twin technology** introduces a forward-looking and predictive dimension to healthcare. Digital twins create dynamic virtual representations of patients, medical devices, and even entire hospital systems by integrating real-time data streams such as biometrics, medical imaging, laboratory results, and environmental indicators (Bruynseels et al., 2018; Fuller et al., 2020). These virtual models enable personalized diagnostics, early risk identification, adaptive therapeutic planning, predictive equipment maintenance, and workflow optimization (Corral-Acero et al., 2020). When deployed alongside blockchain-based data verification, digital twins operate on a trusted data foundation, supporting the development of intelligent, responsible, and patient-centric healthcare systems.

The COVID-19 pandemic significantly accelerated the adoption of these advanced technologies while simultaneously exposing the structural weaknesses of conventional healthcare infrastructures (Ting et al., 2020). Data bottlenecks, limited interoperability, shortages of critical resources, and an absence of predictive capacity constrained effective responses across many health systems (WHO, 2020). Blockchain and digital twins address these vulnerabilities by providing what may be conceptualized as the memory and foresight of resilient healthcare systems: blockchain secures reliable records of past and present clinical events, while digital twins enable real-time simulation and forecasting of future clinical and operational scenarios (Fuller et al., 2020; Kuo et al., 2017).

To illustrate how these technologies are operationalized within differing governance and institutional contexts, this chapter adopts a comparative perspective focusing on **Estonia** and **Saudi Arabia** (Khosrow-Pour, 2015). Estonia, with decades of experience in digital governance, has developed a citizen-centric digital ecosystem anchored in secure national digital identities. Its X-Road data exchange platform connects more than 1,000 institutions, integrating healthcare with broader public services and enabling blockchain-based verification of electronic health records nationwide (Kalvet, 2012; Vassil, 2016). High levels of public trust, robust privacy protections, and extensive interoperability have allowed Estonia to deploy blockchain at scale while advancing research into patient-centered digital twins for chronic disease management and population-level health modeling. (Khosrow-Pour, 2015; Bruynseels et al., 2018)

Saudi Arabia, by contrast, represents a model of rapid, top-down digital modernization. Under Vision 2030 and the National Transformation Program, the Kingdom has invested heavily in digital hospitals, artificial intelligence, telemedicine, and national data governance frameworks to transform healthcare delivery at scale (Kingdom of Saudi Arabia, 2016; Vision 2030, 2016). With the digital health market projected to reach USD 11.07 billion by 2033(Market Research Future, 2023), initiatives such as **Seha Virtual Hospital** the world's largest virtual hospital enable large-scale deployments of advanced care models across vast geographic distances. Saudi Arabia's focus on operational digital twins for intensive care units, emergency departments, and surgical workflows reflects national priorities shaped by population size, geographic dispersion, and systemic efficiency. (Fuller et al., 2020)

A comparison of these two models underscores how contextual factors shape digital health strategies. Estonia emphasizes trust-based governance, identity infrastructure, and incremental innovation, whereas Saudi Arabia relies on centralized coordination, strategic investment, and rapid scaling (Vassil, 2016; Kingdom of Saudi Arabia, 2016). Together, these cases demonstrate that digital health transformation is as much a governance and institutional challenge as it is a technological one, requiring societal readiness, aligned incentives, and adaptive regulatory frameworks (WHO, 2021; Khosrow-Pour, 2015). In conclusion, blockchain and digital twins represent a paradigm shift toward secure, predictive, and patient-centric healthcare systems. While they reshape clinical workflows, operational management, and data governance, they also raise important ethical, legal, and interoperability considerations. Lessons drawn from Estonia and Saudi Arabia provide a valuable framework for policymakers, healthcare leaders, and researchers seeking to design intelligent, transparent, and resilient health ecosystems for the twenty-first century.

1: GLOBAL SHIFT TOWARD SMART HEALTHCARE

1.1 From Digitization to Intelligent Health Ecosystems

The global healthcare sector is witnessing a transition from basic digitization to fully integrated smart healthcare ecosystems. Early digitization efforts focused primarily on converting analog records into digital formats, thereby improving storage efficiency and accessibility (Khosrow-Pour, 2015). While this shift represented a necessary first step, it did little to resolve deeper structural challenges such as interoperability, data governance, predictive capacity, and system-wide coordination (WHO, 2021). Contemporary smart healthcare systems move beyond static digitization toward adaptive, data-driven environments capable of learning from continuous streams of clinical and operational data.

Smart healthcare ecosystems are defined by their ability to integrate heterogeneous data sources including electronic health records, medical imaging, Internet of Medical Things (IoMT) devices, genomic databases, and public health surveillance systems into a unified analytical framework. Artificial intelligence and advanced analytics transform these data into actionable insights, while cloud and edge computing infrastructures ensure scalability and real-time responsiveness. Within this ecosystem, blockchain and digital twin technologies perform complementary roles: blockchain establishes trust, integrity, and accountability, while digital twins enable simulation, prediction, and optimization.

1.2 Blockchain as the Trust Layer of Digital Health

Blockchain technology introduces a structural solution to long-standing issues of trust and data integrity in healthcare. Unlike centralized databases, which rely on institutional authority and perimeter-based security, blockchain operates as a distributed ledger maintained collectively by authorized participants (Agbo et al., 2019). Each transaction is cryptographically linked to the previous one, creating an immutable chain of records that can be independently verified.

In healthcare contexts, blockchain does not typically store raw clinical data directly on-chain. Instead, it stores cryptographic hashes or metadata that verify the authenticity and integrity of data stored off-chain in institutional repositories (Azaria et al., 2016). This hybrid approach ensures compliance with data protection regulations while preserving the core benefits of immutability and auditability. By embedding verification mechanisms directly into the data exchange process, blockchain transforms trust from a policy-based construct into a technical guarantee.

Key advantages of blockchain in healthcare include:

- **Reduction of data fragmentation** through verifiable cross-institutional exchange;
- **Enhanced cybersecurity** via tamper-evident recordkeeping;
- **Transparent audit trails** for regulatory compliance and patient oversight; and
- **Automated governance** through smart contracts that enforce access rules and consent conditions.

1.3 Digital Twins as Engines of Prediction and Personalization

While blockchain secures the past and present of healthcare data, digital twins extend healthcare capabilities into the future. Digital twins enable the creation of continuously updated virtual models that mirror the real-time state of patients, medical devices, or healthcare facilities. These models support predictive analytics by simulating how systems are likely to respond under different conditions.

In clinical settings, patient-specific digital twins allow healthcare professionals to simulate disease progression, test alternative treatment strategies, and identify early warning signals before adverse events occur. At the operational level, hospital digital twins enable administrators to optimize bed utilization, staffing levels, operating room schedules, and equipment maintenance. These capabilities are particularly valuable in high-pressure environments such as intensive care units and emergency departments.

Digital twins derive their power from the convergence of multiple technologies, including AI, high-performance computing, IoMT sensors, and interoperable data standards (Fuller et al., 2020; Islam et al., 2015). Their effectiveness, however, is contingent on the quality, integrity, and timeliness of underlying data an area where blockchain-based verification provides critical support.

1.4 Acceleration Through Crisis: Lessons from the COVID-19 Pandemic

The COVID-19 pandemic highlighted the limitations of conventional healthcare infrastructures and underscored the necessity of intelligent, predictive systems. Many countries struggled with fragmented data systems, delayed reporting, and limited capacity to anticipate surges in demand. In contrast, systems equipped with interoperable digital platforms, real-time analytics, and predictive modeling demonstrated greater resilience.

Blockchain and digital twin technologies gained renewed attention during this period as tools capable of enhancing transparency

2: ESTONIA'S DIGITAL HEALTH AND BLOCKCHAIN ECOSYSTEM

2.1 Overview of Estonia's e-Health Journey

Estonia is widely regarded as a global frontrunner in digital governance, and its healthcare system is a direct beneficiary of this long-standing digital legacy. Since the early 2000s, the country has pursued a deliberate and coordinated strategy to develop a nationwide e-governance infrastructure that today underpins nearly all public services, including healthcare (Khosrow-Pour, 2015; Vassil, 2016). Rather than digitizing healthcare as a standalone sector, Estonia embedded health services within a broader digital state architecture, thereby ensuring institutional coherence, interoperability, and long-term sustainability.

At the core of this transformation lies Estonia's national digital identity (e-ID) system, which provides every resident with a secure and universally recognized means of authentication. This digital identity enables citizens to access a wide range of public and private services healthcare (Khosrow-Pour, 2015; Vassil, 2016), taxation, social security, and administrative services through a single trusted interface. Within healthcare, the e-ID framework allows citizens to view and manage their electronic health records (EHRs), access e-prescriptions, authorize data sharing, and interact seamlessly with clinics, pharmacies, laboratories, and insurers within an integrated digital ecosystem. (European Commission, 2023)

By 2024, Estonia achieved a perfect score of 100% in the European Union's e-Health maturity assessment, placing it among a very small group of countries offering citizens complete digital access to their health records (European Commission, 2023). This milestone reflects not only advanced technological implementation but also strong institutional coordination and high levels of public trust. Further reinforcing its leadership, Estonia ranked first in interoperability in a 2025 global industry assessment, reporting a 99.1% national health data-sharing rate among healthcare providers (OECD, 2025). Together, these indicators demonstrate Estonia's ability to operationalize digital health infrastructure at a national scale with near-universal coverage.

2.2 Comparative Table: Estonia vs. EU-27 (2024)

Table 1 situates Estonia's e-health performance within the broader EU-27 context and provides a comparative baseline for evaluating global healthcare digitization. The data illustrate Estonia's transition from partial digital adoption to full systemic maturity, particularly in interoperability, universal access, and comprehensive data integration. (European Commission, 2023), (OECD, 2025; Khosrow-Pour, 2015)

Table 1. Comparative Assessment of Estonia's e-Health Performance Against the EU-27 Average (2024)

Indicator	Estonia	EU-27 Average (2024)	Interpretation
EHR Access Maturity Score (composite)	100% (European Commission, 2023; OECD, 2025)	≈ 83%(European Commission, 2023)	Estonia has achieved full maturity; the EU average remains uneven and transitional.
Population technically able to access EHRs	100%(European Commission, 2023)	~85–90% (varies by country) (European Commission, 2023)	Estonia ensures universal access, while several EU states still face systemic gaps.
Availability of all data categories (prescriptions, lab results, medical imaging, device data)	100% across categories (European Commission, 2023)	Medical imaging ≈ 26%; device data ≈ 55%	Estonia provides comprehensive data availability; EU averages reveal fragmentation.
Provider connectivity and data supply (public & private)	All relevant provider categories connected(European Commission, 2023; Vassil, 2016)	Public ≈ 79%; Private ≈ 59%(European Commission, 2023; Vassil, 2016)	Estonia's integrated model significantly outperforms EU norms.
Interoperability / data-sharing rate among providers	≈ 99.1% (global top rank, 2025) (OECD, 2025; Khosrow-Pour, 2015)	No unified metric; generally lower (OECD, 2025; Khosrow-Pour, 2015)	Estonia sets a global benchmark for interoperable health data exchange.

2.3 Core Architectural Elements: e-ID, X-Road, and Decentralized Records

The effectiveness of Estonia's digital health ecosystem rests on three tightly integrated architectural components: the national e-ID system, the X-Road data exchange platform, and a decentralized data storage model.

The e-ID system functions as the trust anchor of the ecosystem. All residents and authorized healthcare institutions authenticate themselves using secure digital credentials, enabling verified access to health data and digital signatures. Patients can monitor access logs showing when and by whom their records are accessed, reinforcing transparency, accountability, and confidence in digital healthcare services.

Complementing this identity framework is X-Road, a decentralized interoperability platform rather than a centralized database (Kalvet, 2012). Hospitals, laboratories, pharmacies, and insurers retain custody of their own data while enabling encrypted, logged, and time-stamped data exchanges under standardized protocols (European Commission, 2023). This federated architecture ensures institutional autonomy while allowing seamless nationwide interoperability.

Although not all medical records are stored directly on a blockchain, the system reflects core blockchain principles through cryptographic verification, immutable audit trails, and distributed trust. Estonia employs cryptographic hashing mechanisms to verify the integrity of health records, ensuring that any unauthorized modification is immediately detectable without exposing sensitive patient data (Agbo et al., 2019).

2.4 Outcomes: Clinical, Administrative, and Societal Benefits

Estonia's mature digital health ecosystem produces benefits across multiple levels of the healthcare system.

For patients, citizens enjoy real-time access to their complete medical histories, including prescriptions, laboratory results, imaging, and device-related data. Patients retain control over data-sharing decisions, determining when and with whom their information is accessed. This transparency restores agency, strengthens trust, and minimizes inappropriate data access.

For healthcare providers, interoperable EHRs reduce administrative delays, prevent redundant diagnostics, and enhance clinical decision-making (European Commission, 2023). Clinicians benefit from holistic patient histories regardless of where care is delivered. Electronic prescriptions and shared diagnostic data simplify coordination across primary, secondary, and specialized care.

For public health and research, nationwide health data captured under unified standards support evidence-based epidemiological modeling, resource allocation, and outcome tracking. The decentralized yet interoperable architecture enables large-scale analytics while minimizing privacy risks.

For system resilience, the federated design minimizes single points of failure. Distributed data repositories, cryptographic verification, and identity-based authentication ensure that localized disruptions do not compromise national healthcare operations.

Empirical evaluations reinforce these outcomes. In the 2025 global interoperability rankings, Estonia ranked first among 18 high-income countries, with evaluators citing seamless clinical coordination, real-time access to comprehensive patient records, and high provider satisfaction with system usability and reliability (OECD, 2025).

2.6 Key Lessons from Estonia for Global Health Systems

Estonia's experience offers several transferable lessons for countries seeking to build or reform digital health systems:

1. **Begin with a universal digital identity infrastructure** to establish trust and accountability.

2. **Adopt a federated rather than monolithic data architecture** to avoid single points of failure.
3. **Align regulatory and governance frameworks** with technical architecture.
4. **Prioritize transparency and patient agency** to build trust and adoption.
5. **Design for extensibility** to accommodate future technologies such as IoMT devices and digital twins.

Collectively, these lessons demonstrate that achieving a mature and trustworthy digital health ecosystem depends less on technology alone and more on governance design, civic trust, and architectural foresight

3: SAUDI ARABIA'S VISION 2030 AND THE SMART HOSPITAL REVOLUTION

3.1 Introduction: Digital Transformation as a National Strategy

Saudi Arabia's healthcare modernization under **Vision 2030** represents one of the most ambitious and centrally coordinated digital health transformations currently underway worldwide (Vision 2030, 2016). In contrast to countries such as Estonia where digital health evolved incrementally over decades Saudi Arabia's approach is strategic, investment-driven, and explicitly designed to re-engineer healthcare into a fully technology-enabled, integrated ecosystem within a compressed timeframe (Kingdom of Saudi Arabia, 2016). Health sector reform is positioned as a cornerstone of the Kingdom's broader agenda for economic diversification, innovation, and long-term sustainability.

Vision 2030 places healthcare at the intersection of public welfare and national competitiveness, recognizing that advanced health systems are essential to productivity, demographic resilience, and social stability (WHO, 2021). Emerging technologies artificial intelligence (AI), blockchain, the Internet of Medical Things (IoMT), telemedicine, and digital twins are deployed not as isolated innovations but as mutually reinforcing components of a future-ready health infrastructure (Fuller et al., 2020; Kuo et al., 2017). These technologies aim to enhance clinical quality, improve hospital efficiency, reduce geographic disparities, and enable data-driven decision-making across the continuum of care.

The scale of this transformation is reflected in market projections. Saudi Arabia's digital health market is expected to reach USD 11.07 billion by 2033, growing at a compound annual growth rate (CAGR) of 18.79%, one of the highest globally (Market Research Future, 2023). This growth is driven by rising healthcare demand, demographic pressures, and sustained government investment in smart healthcare infrastructure. The Kingdom's health sector reform, operationalized through the National Transformation Program (NTP), focuses on four strategic pillars:

1. Comprehensive digitalization of healthcare facilities;
2. Privatization and restructuring of service delivery through health clusters;
3. Strengthening public–private partnerships; and
4. Nationwide adoption of interoperable digital platforms to enhance patient safety and continuity of care.

This section examines how Saudi Arabia is constructing a digital-first healthcare ecosystem, situating its progress within global benchmarks and highlighting the growing role of blockchain and digital twin technologies in shaping future smart hospital architectures (Kingdom of Saudi Arabia, 2016).

3.2 Saudi Arabia's Smart Hospital Revolution

Smart hospitals constitute the operational backbone of Saudi Arabia's digital health transformation. Unlike conventional hospitals that merely digitize records, smart hospitals integrate automated systems, advanced analytics, IoMT-enabled medical devices, and remote clinical oversight into a unified, intelligent infrastructure. Together, these components function as a "digital nervous system" capable of sensing, analyzing, and responding to clinical and operational conditions in real time.

In 2024, the Saudi smart hospital market was valued at approximately USD 674.9 million and is projected to exceed USD 1.7 billion by 2033, reflecting strong institutional adoption of advanced healthcare technologies (Market Research Future, 2023). This rapid growth is underpinned by three structural drivers. First, consolidated political and financial support has enabled rapid modernization across public healthcare institutions. Second, the organization of healthcare delivery into large-scale hospital clusters allows targeted and standardized digital upgrades across regions. Third, sustained investment in workforce development has produced a growing cadre of clinicians trained in telemedicine, digital diagnostics, and AI-assisted decision support (WHO, 2021).

Concrete implementations of smart hospital technologies across the Kingdom include:

1. AI-assisted radiology and pathology workflows;
2. Automated medication dispensing systems and pharmacy robotics;
3. IoMT-enabled continuous patient monitoring;
4. Real-time location systems (RTLS) for asset and patient flow management;
5. Predictive analytics dashboards for emergency demand forecasting; and

6. Centralized command centers linking tertiary, secondary, and community hospitals.

These developments illustrate that Saudi Arabia is not merely aligning with global digital health standards but actively redefining them through top-down policy direction, strategic investment, and coordinated implementation (Kingdom of Saudi Arabia Vision 2030, 2016)

3.3 The Rise of Virtual Healthcare: Seha Virtual Hospital

One of the most internationally visible outcomes of Saudi Arabia's digital health agenda is the establishment of Seha Virtual Hospital, widely recognized as the world's largest fully integrated virtual hospital (Ministry of Health Saudi Arabia, 2022). Unlike conventional telemedicine platforms that facilitate isolated clinician–patient interactions, Seha Virtual Hospital operates as a centralized, technology-enabled hub providing continuous access to multidisciplinary expertise, advanced diagnostics, and specialized care regardless of patient location (WHO, 2021).

Seha Virtual Hospital currently supports more than 130 peripheral hospitals across the Kingdom (Ministry of Health Saudi Arabia, 2022) and enables a range of advanced services that would otherwise require access to tertiary care centers, including:

- Remote stroke diagnosis and intervention support;
- Virtual intensive care unit (vICU) surveillance;
- Remote cardiac monitoring;
- Teleradiology and telepathology services;
- Virtual rehabilitation and post-acute care; and
- AI-assisted triage and diagnostic decision support.

The platform integrates digital twin–like simulation dashboards within centralized command-and-control centers, allowing clinicians to anticipate patient deterioration, optimize bed utilization, and manage clinical workflows proactively. By extending specialist expertise to remote and underserved regions, Seha Virtual Hospital significantly reduces geographic inequities in access to high-quality care and advances the Kingdom's objective of universal healthcare coverage.

3.4 Growth of Healthcare Workforce and Digital Capacity

Saudi Arabia's digital transformation is reinforced by sustained expansion of its healthcare workforce alongside targeted investments in digital capacity building (Kingdom of Saudi Arabia, 2016). By 2024, the Kingdom employed approximately:

- **129,772 physicians**,
- **243,336 nurses**, and
- Thousands of allied health professionals across diverse clinical disciplines.

Workforce expansion has been accompanied by structured investments in clinical informatics and digital health training (WHO, 2021), ensuring that healthcare professionals are equipped to operate within technology-intensive environments. Unlike many healthcare systems where digital transformation is slowed by legacy infrastructure and workforce resistance, Saudi Arabia's reform strategy embeds digital competencies directly into institutional restructuring (Kingdom of Saudi Arabia, 2016). As a result, digital adoption is framed not as an add-on but as an integral component of professional practice.

3.5 Comparative Table: Saudi Arabia's Digital Health Capacity (2024)

Table 2 highlights a health system undergoing rapid transition toward digital maturity, supported by both supply-side capacity (infrastructure, workforce, capital) and demand-side drivers (patient adoption, remote care needs).

Table 2. Saudi Arabia's Digital Health Capacity Indicators (2024)

Indicator	Value (2024)	Relevance to Digital Transformation
Total Hospitals	516 (Ministry of Health Saudi Arabia, 2024)	Broad physical infrastructure supporting digital integration
Physicians	129,772(Ministry of Health Saudi Arabia, 2024)	Expanding workforce capable of adopting health IT systems
Nurses	243,336 (Ministry of Health Saudi Arabia, 2024)	Enables scalability of digital inpatient and outpatient workflows
Digital Health Market Size	USD 674.9 million (Market Research Future, 2023)	Reflects strong investment in smart hospital and IoMT technologies
Telemedicine Adoption	High (Ministry of Health Saudi Arabia, 2022; Vision 2030, 2016)	Driven by Seha Virtual Hospital and national platforms
CAGR (2023–2033)	18.79%(Market Research Future, 2023)	Among the highest projected growth rates globally

3.6 Privatization and Health Sector Restructuring

A further defining feature of Saudi Arabia's health transformation is the strategic move toward privatization, with a target of 65% private sector participation under Vision 2030 (Vision 2030, 2016). This restructuring includes plans for the privatization of approximately 290 government hospitals, reorganization of nearly 2,300 primary health centers, establishment of decentralized health clusters, and adoption of value-based healthcare financing models (Kingdom of Saudi Arabia, 2016).

Privatization functions not merely as an economic reform but as a catalyst for digital innovation. Competitive pressures, performance incentives, and accountability mechanisms encourage private providers to adopt digital solutions more rapidly, accelerating the diffusion of innovation across the health sector. At the same time, the growing number of independent actors increases the need for secure, transparent, and interoperable data-sharing mechanisms conditions under which blockchain-based architectures become particularly valuable.

3.7 National Digital Platforms and Interoperability Goals

Saudi Arabia's National e-Health Strategy prioritizes the development of integrated digital platforms that enable secure, standardized data exchange across public and private healthcare institutions (Ministry of Health Saudi Arabia, 2023).

Key national platforms include: (Ministry of Health Saudi Arabia, 2023; Vision 2030, 2016)

- **NABIDH** (Unified EHR platform for Riyadh),
- **NPHIES** (National Platform for Health Insurance and E-Claims),
- **Wasfaty** (Digital prescription platform),
- **Mawid** (National appointment booking system), and
- **Seha** (Central telemedicine platform).

Together, these platforms represent a structural shift toward nationwide interoperability, enabling horizontal data flows across institutional boundaries. As the ecosystem grows in complexity, blockchain emerges as a governance enabler by providing verifiable audit trails, safeguarding data integrity, and simplifying compliance across a multi-provider landscape.

3.8 Why Saudi Arabia Is Poised for Blockchain Adoption

Several structural characteristics make Saudi Arabia's healthcare ecosystem particularly conducive to blockchain adoption:

- High-volume data flows generated by smart hospitals and national platforms; (Ministry of Health Saudi Arabia, 2023)
- Complex multi-actor interactions involving insurers, regulators, and private providers; (Kingdom of Saudi Arabia, 2016)
- Rapid innovation requiring scalable and trustworthy governance frameworks; (WHO, 2021) and
- Strong political commitment ensuring long-term sustainability. (Vision 2030, 2016)

Where traditional EHR systems struggle with transparency and cross-institutional trust, blockchain offers verifiable data integrity. Where centralized databases face security and governance challenges, distributed ledgers provide tamper-resistant architectures. In an increasingly privatized and interoperable healthcare landscape, blockchain thus functions not merely as a technological enhancement but as a foundational governance layer supporting Saudi Arabia's emerging smart hospital ecosystem

4: BLOCKCHAIN APPLICATIONS IN DATA INTEGRITY, CONSENT, AND SECURITY

As healthcare systems evolve toward fully digital and interoperable ecosystems, ensuring data integrity, security, transparency, and patient trust become a foundational requirement rather than a secondary concern. Conventional centralized health databases, while efficient in early digitization phases, are increasingly inadequate for modern healthcare environments characterized by high data volumes, multi-provider interactions, cross-border data flows, and rising cybersecurity threats. Centralized architectures remain vulnerable to single points of failure, unauthorized manipulation, and systemic breaches.

Blockchain technology offers a fundamentally different paradigm. By introducing a distributed, cryptographically secured ledger, blockchain enables tamper-evident, auditable, and verifiable transactions without relying on institutional trust alone. In Estonia, blockchain underpins national e-Health data verification through the Keyless Signature Infrastructure (KSI), ensuring record integrity at a nationwide scale (Vassil, 2016). In Saudi Arabia, rapid digital expansion, privatization, and the emergence of multi-provider ecosystems create a compelling case for blockchain-enabled interoperability, consent management, and governance (Kingdom of Saudi Arabia, 2016; Kuo et al., 2017). Together, these contexts illustrate how blockchain can provide a resilient foundation for scalable, trustworthy, and future-ready healthcare infrastructures across diverse national settings.

4.1 Ensuring Data Integrity Through Immutable Ledger Mechanisms

Data integrity is central to patient safety and clinical effectiveness. Inaccurate or manipulated records can lead to misdiagnosis, delayed treatment, inappropriate medication, and systemic inefficiencies. Traditional healthcare information systems store patient data within institution-specific servers or centralized repositories, exposing them to cyberattacks, accidental overwrites, insider manipulation, and inconsistent versioning.

Blockchain addresses these vulnerabilities through multiple structural mechanisms:

1. Creation of Time-Stamped, Immutable Records

Every healthcare transaction whether a diagnostic update, laboratory report, prescription entry, or imaging request is recorded on the blockchain with a cryptographic signature and time stamp (Azaria et al., 2016). Once validated and added to the ledger, the record becomes immutable. Any attempt to alter the data retroactively is immediately detectable, ensuring accountability and preserving clinical accuracy (Kuo et al., 2017).

2. Cryptographic Linking Through Hash Chains

Each block in the blockchain contains a cryptographic hash of the preceding block. This sequential linking ensures that even minor alterations to historical records disrupt the entire chain and are instantly flagged. Such architecture guarantees end-to-end integrity across all participating healthcare institutions (Kuo et al., 2017).

3. Comprehensive Auditability and Traceability

Blockchain generates an immutable audit trail for every data access request, modification attempt, or clinical transaction. This enables real-time and retrospective oversight by administrators, regulators, and patients, fostering unprecedented transparency in health data governance.

4. Interoperability Without Centralization

Rather than acting as a centralized data repository, blockchain functions as a verification and coordination layer across distributed systems. For example:

- In **Estonia**, blockchain verifies data consistency across hospitals, laboratories, insurers, and primary care units. (Vassil, 2016)
- In **Saudi Arabia**, blockchain supports validation of data authenticity across public and private providers operating within health clusters. (Vision 2030, 2016)

In both cases, blockchain enhances interoperability while preserving institutional autonomy.

4.2 Blockchain for Advanced Consent Management

Dynamic, patient-centric consent management remains one of the most complex challenges in digital healthcare. Traditional consent mechanisms paper-based forms or static digital agreements are difficult to update, enforce, and audit (Khosrow-Pour, 2015). They often fail to reflect the evolving preferences of patients in data-intensive environments.

Blockchain reconceptualizes consent as a living digital asset, governed automatically through smart contracts and recorded immutably on a distributed ledger. (Szabo, 1997; Azaria et al., 2016).

Key Enhancements Enabled by Blockchain:

1. **Granular Consent Control**

Patients can specify exactly which provider, specialist, insurer, or research entity may access their data, for what purpose, and for what duration.

2. **Real-Time Consent Modification**

Consent can be modified or revoked instantly. Access rights are updated across all integrated systems without administrative delay.

3. **Immutable Authorization History**

Every consent action granting, modifying, or revoking access is permanently recorded, creating a tamper-evident audit trail.

4. **Reduced Administrative Burden**

Smart contracts automatically enforce consent conditions, eliminating the need for manual verification by institutional authorities.

5. **Cross-Border and Multi-Provider Compliance**

In European contexts such as Estonia, blockchain supports GDPR principles of transparency, accountability, and reversibility. (European Parliament & Council of the European Union, 2016). In Saudi Arabia, it enables secure consent governance across increasingly complex public–private provider networks.

4.3 Blockchain-Based Consent and Data Access in Healthcare

Figure 1 illustrates the complete lifecycle of consent and data access within a blockchain-enabled healthcare system (Azaria et al., 2016). The workflow demonstrates how patient identity verification, smart contract execution, secure data access, and audit logging are coordinated across a distributed ledger. This architecture ensures transparency, real-time control, and patient-centric governance while maintaining data integrity and security.

Figure 1. Blockchain-Based Consent and Data Access Workflow in Healthcare

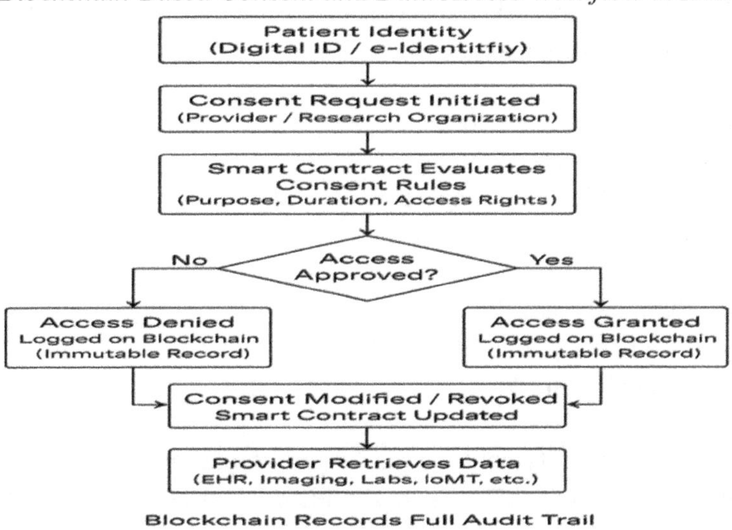

(Adapted from Azaria et al., 2016; Kuo et al., 2017; Agbo et al., 2019).

4.4 Enhancing Security Through Cryptographic Algorithms and Distributed Validation

Blockchain security is grounded in a combination of cryptographic algorithms, decentralized validation, and permissioned consensus mechanisms optimized for healthcare environments.

Core Security Features Include:

Public–Private Key Encryption

Each patient and provider is assigned a unique cryptographic key pair (Nakamoto, 2008). Data access requires authorization through the private key, ensuring confidentiality even across distributed networks (Agbo et al., 2019).

Permissioned Consensus Protocols

Healthcare blockchains typically employ enterprise-grade consensus mechanisms such as:

- Practical Byzantine Fault Tolerance (PBFT), (Castro & Liskov, 1999)
- Delegated Proof of Authority (DPoA),
- Raft-based or permissioned consensus frameworks (e.g., Hyperledger Fabric). (Androulaki et al., 2018)

These protocols balance performance, scalability, and regulatory compliance.

Resilience Against Cyber Threats

Blockchain architectures are inherently resistant to: (Agbo et al., 2019)

- Data tampering,
- Man-in-the-middle attacks,
- Unauthorized overwriting of records,
- Insider manipulation.

Because no single entity controls the ledger, compromising the system would require simultaneous breaches across multiple nodes an exceedingly difficult task. (Nakamoto, 2008)

4.5 Applications Across Healthcare Domains

Blockchain applications extend across multiple healthcare domains:

1. **Electronic Health Records (EHRs):** Unified, verifiable patient records across institutions (Azaria et al., 2016).

2. **Pharmaceutical Supply Chains:** End-to-end traceability from manufacturer to patient, reducing counterfeit risks. (Tseng et al., 2018)
3. **Insurance and Claims Processing:** Smart contracts automate claims adjudication, minimizing fraud and delays. (Kuo et al., 2017)
4. **Clinical Research:** Immutable research logs ensure reproducibility and data integrity. (Agbo et al., 2019)
5. **IoMT Device Security:** Blockchain-based identity verification prevents spoofing and unauthorized data injection from medical devices. (Reyna et al., 2018)

4.6 Estonia and Saudi Arabia: Complementary Blockchain Pathways

Estonia represents a trust-centric blockchain model, where citizen participation, transparency, and digital literacy underpin adoption (Vassil, 2016). Saudi Arabia exemplifies a scale-driven and investment-led model, where blockchain supports interoperability, governance, and data integrity in a rapidly expanding multi-provider ecosystem. (Vision 2030, 2016)

Together, these approaches demonstrate that blockchain adoption in healthcare is not monolithic. Instead, it adapts to national governance structures, institutional capacity, and strategic priorities offering multiple pathways toward secure, interoperable, and patient-centered digital health systems

5: DIGITAL TWIN TECHNOLOGIES IN PREDICTIVE AND PERSONALIZED HEALTHCARE

Digital twin technology, originally developed in aerospace engineering and advanced manufacturing, is rapidly emerging as one of the most transformative innovations in contemporary healthcare (Fuller et al., 2020). This accelerated translation into the health sector is driven by the convergence of real-time clinical data, advanced simulation environments, artificial intelligence (AI), and the proliferation of Internet of Medical Things (IoMT) devices. (Reyna et al., 2018) In healthcare, a digital twin refers to a dynamic, continuously updated virtual representation of a physical entity, which may include an individual patient, a specific organ system, a medical device, a clinical workflow, or even an entire hospital ecosystem.

Unlike static health records or conventional decision-support tools, digital twins evolve in real time by ingesting continuous data streams from sensors, imaging systems, electronic health records, and wearable devices. This enables clinicians and administrators to simulate scenarios, predict outcomes, and optimize both clinical and operational decisions before interventions are implemented in the physical world.

Global market projections underscore the rapid acceleration of digital twin adoption in healthcare. In 2024, the global healthcare digital twin market was valued at approximately USD 1.2 billion, and it is projected to reach USD 9.5 billion by 2030, reflecting a compound annual growth rate (CAGR) of nearly 40%. (MarketsandMarkets, 2023) This growth is propelled by advances in AI-driven analytics, high-performance computing, cloud infrastructures, and the increasing availability of real-time patient data.

Digital twins are increasingly deployed across multiple healthcare domains, including:

- Predictive diagnostics,
- Personalized treatment planning,
- Hospital and clinical operations optimization,
- Surgical simulation and planning,
- Drug development and clinical trials, and
- Long-term monitoring of chronic diseases.

This section examines the architectural foundations, applications, and future potential of digital twin technologies, drawing comparative insights from Estonia's digitally mature healthcare ecosystem and Saudi Arabia's rapidly expanding smart hospital infrastructure.

5.2 Architectural Foundations of Digital Twin Systems

A healthcare digital twin system is built upon a multi-layered architecture that enables seamless synchronization between physical and virtual environments (Fuller et al., 2020). These systems typically consist of five interconnected layers:

1. Physical Layer

This layer includes the real-world entities being modeled, such as patients, organs, medical devices, hospital infrastructure, equipment, and clinical workflows. (Bruynseels et al., 2018).

2. Data Acquisition Layer

Real-time data is collected through IoMT devices, wearable sensors, imaging systems, laboratory information systems, and hospital information systems (Reyna et al., 2018).. Continuous data inflow is essential for maintaining an accurate and dynamic digital representation.

3. Integration and Interoperability Layer

This layer enables secure data exchange across heterogeneous systems using application programming interfaces (APIs), healthcare interoperability standards such as **HL7-FHIR**, and blockchain-based validation mechanisms to ensure data integrity and authenticity. (Kuo et al., 2017; Khosrow-Pour, 2015).

4. Simulation and Analytics Layer

Advanced AI models, predictive algorithms, physics-based simulations, and real-time analytics engines operate within this layer (Tao et al., 2019). These tools allow the digital twin to generate forecasts, identify anomalies, and simulate alternative intervention scenarios.

5. Digital Twin Interface Layer

The interface layer translates complex analytics into actionable insights through clinical dashboards, risk prediction scores, operational alerts, and personalized treatment recommendations for clinicians and administrators. (Bruynseels et al., 2018).

Together, these layers enable continuous feedback loops between real and virtual systems, supporting data-driven clinical decision-making and large-scale health system optimization.

Figure 2 illustrates the multi-layered architecture of a digital twin within a smart hospital environment, highlighting data acquisition sources, interoperability frameworks, AI-based simulation engines, and front-end clinical decision-support interfaces.

Figure 2. Digital Twin Architecture in a Smart Hospital

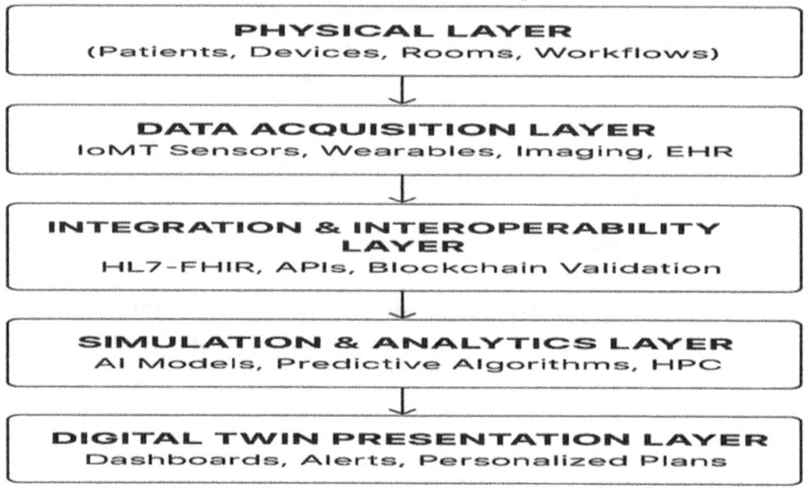

Sources: Fuller et al. (2020), Tao et al. (2019), Bruynseels et al. (2018)

5.4 Applications of Digital Twins in Predictive Healthcare

5.4.1 Patient-Specific Digital Twins

Patient-specific digital twins represent one of the most clinically transformative applications of this technology. These twins model an individual's physiological and behavioural state in real time by integrating:

- Vital signs,
- Diagnostic imaging data,
- Laboratory test results,
- Genomic and molecular information, and
- Behavioural and lifestyle indicators.

Predicting Disease Progression

Digital twins enable clinicians to simulate disease trajectories and anticipate complications before they manifest clinically (Fuller et al., 2020). Examples include:

- Cardiovascular risk prediction using hemodynamic simulations, (Tao et al., 2019);
- Modeling tumor growth and treatment response in oncology, (Bruynseels et al., 2018)

- Forecasting diabetic complications based on glucose trends and metabolic patterns. (Reyna et al., 2018).

Personalizing Therapeutic Strategies

Treatment plans can be tested virtually before implementation (Bruynseels et al., 2018). Clinicians may simulate:

- Insulin dosage adjustments,
- Chemotherapy regimens,
- Rehabilitation strategies following injury or surgery.

This reduces trial-and-error approaches and enhances patient safety. (Fuller et al., 2020).

Enhancing Early-Warning Systems

By continuously processing real-time biosensor data, digital twins detect subtle physiological deviations earlier than conventional monitoring systems, enabling timely clinical intervention.

5.5 Digital Twins in Smart Hospitals and Clinical Operations

Beyond individual patients, digital twins are increasingly applied at the hospital and system level, modeling entire clinical ecosystems. These operational digital twins capture patient flows, bed occupancy, staffing patterns, and equipment utilization, supporting optimized resource allocation in large healthcare networks.

Key operational capabilities include:

1. **Emergency Department Demand Forecasting:** AI-driven digital twins predict patient inflows, allowing dynamic reallocation of staff, beds, and diagnostic resources. (Tao et al., 2019).
2. **Operating Room Scheduling Optimization:** Digital twins identify workflow bottlenecks in surgical pathways, reducing cancellations, idle time, and procedural delays. (Fuller et al., 2020)
3. **Intensive Care Unit (ICU) Resource Management:** Simulation of ICU capacity, nurse-to-patient ratios, and ventilator availability enhances resilience during crises such as pandemics or mass-casualty events. (WHO, 2021).
4. **Equipment Lifecycle and Predictive Maintenance:** High-value assets such as MRI scanners, ventilators, and laboratory analyzers are monitored in real time to anticipate failures and optimize maintenance schedules. Saudi Arabia's Seha Virtual Hospital exemplifies operational digital twin adoption, using centralized

monitoring dashboards to oversee patient care and resource utilization across more than 130 connected healthcare facilities. (Vision 2030, 2016).

5.6 Digital Twins for Chronic Disease Management

Chronic diseases account for over 74% of global mortality, according to the World Health Organization. Digital twins offer transformative potential for long-term disease management by enabling continuous monitoring and individualized interventions. (Bruynseels et al., 2018).

A. Cardiovascular Diseases
    - Simulation of cardiac stress responses,
    - Prediction of arrhythmias using ECG trend analysis,
    - Modeling patient-specific blood flow dynamics.

B. Diabetes
    - Virtual insulin dosage optimization,
    - Continuous glucose pattern monitoring,
    - Prediction of dietary and lifestyle impacts on glycemic control.

C. Respiratory Diseases
    - Lung digital twins model oxygen exchange efficiency,
    - Predict pulmonary deterioration,
    - Optimize inhaler and ventilation therapies.

Estonia's advanced digital infrastructure enables seamless integration of such models, while Saudi Arabia's rapidly expanding IoMT ecosystem accelerates deployment in large-scale chronic disease programs. (Vision 2030, 2016).

5.7 Digital Doubles for Precision Surgery and Medical Training

1. Preoperative Planning

Surgeons increasingly rely on 3D digital replicas of organs to simulate complex procedures (Tao et al., 2019; Fuller et al., 2020) such as:

- Cardiac bypass grafting,
- Tumor resection,
- Orthopedic reconstructive surgery. (Bruynseels et al., 2018).

This enhances surgical precision and reduces intraoperative risks.

2. Intraoperative Navigation

Digital twins integrated with real-time imaging systems support augmented surgical guidance, improving accuracy during procedures.

3. Medical Education and Training

Medical students and residents train in immersive virtual environments that accurately replicate anatomical structures and clinical scenarios (Tao et al., 2019). Saudi tertiary hospitals are increasingly adopting 3D anatomical modeling, while Estonian research institutions are advancing predictive surgical simulation platforms. (Vision 2030, 2016; Vassil, 2016).

5.8 Integration of Digital Twins with Predictive Analytics and Artificial Intelligence

Digital twins are intrinsically dependent on AI-driven analytics for prediction, anomaly detection, and scenario simulation. When integrated with high-performance computing, these systems can process:

- Millions of physiological data points,
- Thousands of concurrent clinical interactions,
- Large-scale hospital operational datasets.

This makes digital twin platforms indispensable for:

- Epidemic forecasting,
- Hospital capacity planning,
- Real-time patient risk scoring,
- Personalized treatment recommendations.

5.9 Blockchain as a Supportive Governance Layer for Digital Twins

Digital twins generate massive volumes of real-time and high-sensitivity health data, necessitating robust mechanisms for security, validation, and controlled sharing. Blockchain technology provides a complementary governance layer by ensuring:

- **Data Integrity:** Simulation inputs remain accurate and tamper-resistant.
- **Transparency:** All access and modifications to digital twins are traceable.

- **Access Control:** Patient-centric permission management across institutions.
- **Auditability:** Regulatory compliance in high-risk settings such as ICUs, oncology units, and surgical theaters.

Saudi Arabia's multi-provider healthcare ecosystem benefits significantly from blockchain-enabled governance (Vision 2030, 2016), while Estonia's existing blockchain-based data verification systems are inherently compatible with digital twin platforms (Vassil, 2016).

6: COMPARATIVE ANALYSIS OF SMART HEALTHCARE TRANSFORMATION IN ESTONIA AND SAUDI ARABIA

The evolution of smart healthcare ecosystems in Estonia and Saudi Arabia illustrates two structurally distinct yet complementary pathways toward digital health transformation. While both countries leverage advanced technologies such as blockchain, artificial intelligence, and digital twins, their trajectories differ significantly in governance philosophy, population scale, institutional maturity, and implementation strategy. A comparative examination of these models provides valuable insights into how national context shapes the design, pace, and outcomes of digital healthcare innovation.

Estonia, with a population of approximately 1.3 million, represents one of the most digitally mature healthcare systems globally (OECD, 2020). Nearly 99% of prescriptions and approximately 95% of patient health records are fully digitized (European Commission, 2019). The country's X-Road interoperability platform enables seamless, secure data exchange across public and private institutions, while the deployment of Keyless Signature Infrastructure (KSI) blockchain ensures data integrity, auditability, and transparency across the national e-Health system (Kuo et al., 2017). Within this trusted digital foundation, Estonia has begun the incremental integration of digital twin technologies, particularly in chronic disease management, preventive care, and population-level public health modeling.

Saudi Arabia, by contrast, operates at a vastly different scale, serving a population exceeding 32 million (World Bank, 2022). Under Vision 2030 and the National Transformation Program, the Kingdom has pursued rapid and centralized digital modernization across its healthcare sector (Vision 2030, 2016). Significant investments have been made in electronic health records, artificial intelligence, telemedicine, and operational digital twins (WHO, 2021), exemplified by initiatives such as Seha Virtual Hospital, currently the world's largest virtual hospital network (Ministry of Health Saudi Arabia, 2022).Whereas Estonia emphasizes trust-based governance and gradual innovation, Saudi Arabia prioritizes speed, scale, efficiency, and systemic modernization, reflecting its demographic size, geographic breadth, and strategic national planning objectives.

6.1 Governance Models and Digital Health Strategy

A key differentiator between the two countries lies in their governance models. Estonia adopts a citizen-centric, bottom-up approach, where digital healthcare initiatives are embedded within a broader national digital identity and e-governance ecosystem. Citizens actively participate in data governance through transparent access logs, consent mechanisms, and strong legal protections. Trust in public digital systems is reinforced by long-standing digital literacy programs and institutional transparency.

Saudi Arabia follows a government-led, top-down investment model, where large-scale reforms are coordinated centrally through ministries and national digital authorities (Vision 2030, 2016). This approach enables rapid deployment of infrastructure and advanced technologies but also introduces challenges related to workforce readiness, interoperability alignment, and uniform adoption across public and private providers.

6.2 Comparative Readiness for Blockchain–Digital Twin Integration

Table 3 provides a structured comparison of Estonia and Saudi Arabia across governance, digital identity, health-record digitization, blockchain adoption, strategic focus, population scale, strengths, and implementation challenges. The table highlights how Estonia's maturity lies in interoperability and trust, while Saudi Arabia's comparative advantage lies in financial capacity, technological ambition, and large-scale deployment potential.

Table 3. Comparison of Estonia and Saudi Arabia in Blockchain–Digital Twin Readiness

Attribute / Factor	Estonia	Saudi Arabia
Governance Style	Citizen-centric, bottom up (Vassil, 2016)	Government-led, top-down investment (Vision 2030, 2016)
Identity / Digital ID	Universal e-ID card used broadly (European Commission, 2019)	National ID + biometrics / national e-services (Vision 2030, 2016)
Health-Record Digitization	Nearly universal EHR coverage (OECD, 2020)	Partial and uneven nationwide coverage (WHO, 2021)

continued on following page

Table 3. Continued

Attribute / Factor	Estonia	Saudi Arabia
Data Integrity / Blockchain Use	KSI blockchain used nationally (Kuo et al., 2017)	Pilot initiatives; non-uniform adoption (Agbo et al., 2019)
Digital Health Focus	Interoperability, unified records, public health (OECD, 2020)	Hospital systems, telemedicine, remote care (WHO, 2021)
Scale (Population)	Small population enables rapid integration (World Bank, 2022)	Large population enables scale but adds complexity (World Bank, 2022)
Strengths	Trust, interoperability, transparency (Vassil, 2016; Khosrow-Pour, 2015)	Investment capacity, modernization speed (Vision 2030, 2016)
Challenges	Limited data scale for AI-driven care (Fuller et al., 2020)	Integration gaps, privacy governance, workforce readiness (WHO, 2021; Khosrow-Pour, 2015)

6.3 Digital Maturity Profiles: Visual Comparative Analysis

Figure 3 visually illustrates the contrasting digital maturity profiles of Estonia and Saudi Arabia. Estonia demonstrates exceptional strength in governance, interoperability, and blockchain-enabled trust, while Saudi Arabia shows rapid advancement in AI maturity, operational digital twins, and hospital-scale innovation.

Figure 3. Comparative Digital Health Maturity Profiles

Estonia – Mature Digital Health Ecosystem

Indicator	Maturity	Visual Scale
Interoperability	Very High	■ ■ ■ ■ ■ ■ ■
Blockchain	High	■ ■ ■ ■ ■ ■ ■
AI Maturity	High	■ ■ ■ ■ ■ ■ ■
Digital Twins	Moderate	■ ■ ■ ■ ■
Governance	Very High	■ ■ ■ ■ ■ ■ ■
Cybersecurity	High	■ ■ ■ ■ ■ ■ ■

Saudi Arabia – Rapidly Advancing Digital Health Ecosystem

Indicator	Maturity	Visual Scale
Interoperability	High	■ ■ ■ ■ ■ ■ ■
Blockchain	Moderate	■ ■ ■ ■ ■
AI Maturity	Very High	■ ■ ■ ■ ■ ■ ■
Digital Twins	High	■ ■ ■ ■ ■ ■ ■
Governance	High	■ ■ ■ ■ ■ ■
Cybersecurity	High	■ ■ ■ ■ ■ ■ ■

6.4 Synthesis: Complementary Pathways to Smart Healthcare

Ultimately, Estonia and Saudi Arabia represent two successful but structurally distinct models of digital health transformation (OECD, 2020). Estonia exemplifies the ideal of a trust-based, interoperable, and citizen-empowered healthcare ecosystem, (Vassil, 2016) where blockchain serves as a foundational verification layer and digital twins evolve incrementally within a stable governance framework. Saudi Arabia, conversely, demonstrates how ambitious national vision, centralized coordination, and sustained investment can rapidly modernize healthcare infrastructure at scale, even in complex and geographically diverse environments.

Rather than competing paradigms, these models are complementary. Estonia offers lessons in governance design, transparency, and interoperability, while Saudi Arabia provides insights into scaling innovation, mobilizing resources, and accelerating systemic change. Together, they illustrate that the successful deployment of blockchain- and digital twin-enabled smart healthcare systems depends not on a single universal blueprint, but on context-sensitive alignment between technology, governance, and societal readiness

7: ETHICAL, LEGAL, AND INTEROPERABILITY CHALLENGES IN BLOCKCHAIN- AND DIGITAL TWIN–ENABLED HEALTHCARE

7.1 Introduction

As healthcare systems evolve toward intelligent, predictive, and data-driven ecosystems, blockchain and digital twin technologies are increasingly positioned as foundational infrastructures. Blockchain introduces immutable, auditable data architectures, while digital twins enable dynamic simulations of patients, clinical workflows, and entire hospital systems. Together, these technologies promise unprecedented improvements in efficiency, transparency, personalization, and anticipatory care.

However, the same characteristics that make these technologies transformative also generate complex ethical, legal, and interoperability challenges. Issues surrounding patient privacy, data ownership, consent, algorithmic transparency, accountability, and cross-institutional compatibility pose significant barriers to responsible and scalable adoption. Despite global momentum, fewer than 40% of OECD countries currently operate fully interoperable electronic health record (EHR) systems, and only 28% have implemented structured AI-based clinical governance frameworks

(OECD, 2020), underscoring the gap between technological potential and institutional readiness.

This section critically examines these challenges through the comparative experiences of Estonia and Saudi Arabia, two nations at different stages of digital health maturity. By synthesizing ethical theory, legal frameworks, and technical constraints, the section develops a multi-layered understanding of the risks and trade-offs confronting policymakers, healthcare providers, technologists, and regulators in the deployment of blockchain- and digital twin–enabled healthcare systems.

7.2 Ethical Issues: Privacy, Autonomy, and Algorithmic Transparency

7.2.1 Patient Privacy and Data Autonomy

Patient privacy and autonomy remain the most prominent ethical concerns in advanced digital healthcare systems. Blockchain's immutability ensures data integrity and trust but introduces tension with established medical ethics principles, particularly the right of patients to amend, restrict, or erase personal information. Healthcare data including genetic, behavioral, psychological, and biometric data are among the most sensitive forms of personal information.

Digital twins further intensify these concerns by generating predictive insights that extend beyond observable clinical facts. A digital twin may forecast disease progression, organ failure risk, or behavioral susceptibility, effectively creating future-oriented personal data. Ethical questions arise regarding who controls these predictions, how they are communicated, and whether patients can opt out of their generation or use.

7.2.2 Tension Between Immutability and the "Right to Be Forgotten"

A fundamental ethical and legal contradiction exists between blockchain's immutable design and regulatory rights such as the European Union's GDPR Article 17, which grants individuals the "right to be forgotten." (European Parliament & Council of the European Union, 2016). Permanent storage of personal data on-chain may violate such provisions.

Estonia addresses this challenge through a hybrid blockchain architecture, storing only cryptographic hashes or digital signatures on-chain while retaining raw medical data in off-chain repositories under institutional control. This approach preserves verifiability without compromising erasure rights. Saudi Arabia's Personal Data Protection Law (PDPL) similarly emphasizes data minimization, retention limits, and purpose limitation, (Saudi Data & AI Authority, 2021) encouraging comparable hybrid architectures to balance integrity with privacy compliance.

7.2.3 Ethical Risks of Predictive Digital Twin Simulations

Digital twins, by design, are predictive and probabilistic. While this enhances preventive care, it introduces significant ethical risks. Predictive insights related to heart failure, cancer susceptibility, neurodegenerative conditions, or mental health disorders may:

- Influence insurance eligibility or premium calculations,
- Affect employability or workplace accommodations,
- Generate psychological distress or health anxiety,
- Lead to stigmatization or self-fulfilling behavioral outcomes.

Ethically responsible deployment requires strict governance over prediction disclosure, purpose limitation, and interpretability, ensuring that predictive outputs support care without undermining patient dignity or autonomy.

7.2.4 Algorithmic Transparency and Bias

Digital twins rely heavily on machine learning and AI models trained on large clinical datasets. If these datasets lack demographic diversity, predictions may embed systemic bias. A 2023 *Lancet Digital Health* review found significant overrepresentation of populations from the United States and Western Europe in medical AI training datasets, with underrepresentation of Middle Eastern, African, and South Asian populations. (The Lancet Digital Health, 2023).

For Saudi Arabia characterized by demographic diversity and multinational populations this presents substantial risks of miscalibration and inequitable outcomes (WHO, 2021). Estonia, while digitally mature, faces limitations related to population homogeneity, potentially restricting the generalizability of predictive models. (OECD, 2020).

Ethically robust digital twin systems must therefore incorporate: (WHO, 2021; Khosrow-Pour, 2015)

- Explainable AI mechanisms,
- Regular bias audits,
- Population-specific recalibration,
- Transparent documentation of model limitations.

7.3 Legal and Regulatory Challenges

Healthcare is among the most heavily regulated sectors globally, and emerging technologies such as blockchain and digital twins strain existing legal frameworks. No comprehensive global legal regime currently governs blockchain use in healthcare, and even fewer jurisdictions explicitly regulate digital twin simulations.

7.3.1 Data Ownership and Jurisdictional Complexity

Health data ownership varies across jurisdictions:

- **Estonia:** Patients retain ownership; institutions act as custodians. (Vassil, 2016).
- **Saudi Arabia:** Mixed custodial ownership under PDPL with expanding patient rights. (Saudi Data & AI Authority, 2021).
- **European Union:** GDPR centers ownership and consent with the data subject. (European Parliament & Council of the European Union, 2016).
- **United States:** Institutional ownership predominates under HIPAA. (U.S. Department of Health & Human Services, 2013).

Blockchain complicates these distinctions because data verification occurs across distributed nodes that may span multiple jurisdictions, (Finck, 2019) raising unresolved questions regarding data residency, applicable law, and regulatory authority. (Kuo et al., 2017).

7.3.2 Liability for Digital Twin–Assisted Decisions

A major unresolved legal issue concerns liability when digital twin predictions influence clinical outcomes. If a simulation inaccurately predicts stability and delays intervention, responsibility may be contested among:

- Software vendors,
- Clinicians applying the model,
- Hospitals deploying the system,
- Regulatory bodies approving its use.

No jurisdiction has fully resolved these questions. Emerging legal scholarship proposes shared liability models, similar to those used in autonomous vehicle regulation, combining vendor accountability, clinical oversight, and institutional governance.

7.3.3 Regulatory Alignment and Certification Standards

Global regulators have begun addressing these gaps:

- The **European Medicines Agency (EMA)** is exploring digital twins in drug modeling. (European Medicines Agency, 2022).
- The **U.S. FDA** has issued preliminary guidance on virtual clinical trials. (U.S. Food & Drug Administration, 2023).
- The **World Health Organization (WHO)** 2023 Digital Health Strategy calls for AI governance frameworks. (WHO, 2021).
- Saudi Arabia's **SFDA** is developing certification pathways for digital health products and telemedicine platforms. (Saudi Food & Drug Authority, 2022).

Despite these efforts, regulatory fragmentation persists. (OECD, 2020) Large-scale adoption requires clarity on (Finck, 2019; WHO, 2021):

- Legal recognition of blockchain records,
- Enforceability of smart contracts,
- Accuracy thresholds for digital twin outputs,
- Rules governing cross-system and cross-border data exchange.

7.4 Interoperability Challenges: Technical, Semantic, and Institutional Dimensions

Interoperability is a foundational requirement for both blockchain and digital twin systems. Digital twins depend on continuous, high-quality data flows from EHRs, IoMT devices, imaging systems, and laboratory platforms, while blockchain relies on standardized inputs to maintain verifiable audit trails. Yet in 2024, only 13 OECD countries report high national interoperability readiness. (OECD, 2020).

7.4.1 Technical Interoperability Barriers

Many healthcare providers operate proprietary EHR systems lacking standardized APIs or FHIR-compatible outputs. (Health Level Seven International [HL7], 2019). Blockchain cannot validate inconsistent or unstructured data efficiently. Saudi Arabia addresses this through national mandates such as NPHIES and NABIDH (Saudi Ministry of Health, 2022) while Estonia's X-Road demonstrates how a unified interoperability backbone accelerates integration.

7.4.2 Semantic Interoperability Challenges

Semantic interoperability ensures that data have consistent meaning across systems. Digital twins require standardized terminologies such as SNOMED CT, ICD-11, LOINC, and DICOM to accurately simulate physiological processes (World Health Organization, 2019; SNOMED International, 2022). Estonia aligns with EU-wide standards, while Saudi Arabia continues national efforts to unify terminologies across public and private providers.

7.4.3 Institutional and Cultural Interoperability

Beyond technology, interoperability requires cultural alignment. Blockchain's transparency may face resistance in organizations accustomed to siloed data control. Digital twins demand cross-departmental collaboration, challenging traditional clinical hierarchies. Estonia benefits from high digital trust and literacy, whereas Saudi Arabia must invest in clinician training and public engagement across culturally diverse populations.

Ethical Risk Spectrum for Digital Twins

- **Low Risk:** Operational twins, workflow optimization, vital-sign simulations
- **Medium Risk:** Organ models, ICU digital twins
- **High Risk:** Genomic prediction, behavioral modeling, mental health simulations

Table 4. Key Ethical, Legal, and Technical Risks with Mitigation Strategies

Risk Category	Why It Matters	Mitigation Strategies
Consent & Autonomy	Continuous monitoring requires informed, ongoing consent	Dynamic consent platforms; smart contracts; re-consent workflows
Privacy / Re-identification	High re-identification risk from merged datasets	Off-chain storage; tokenization; differential privacy
Algorithmic Bias	Risk of inequitable care outcomes	Bias audits; representative datasets; explainability
Legal Non-compliance	GDPR, PDPL violations carry penalties(European Parliament & Council of the European Union, 2016; Saudi Data & AI Authority, 2021)	DPIAs; regulatory pre-submissions; local data strategies
Interoperability Failures	Semantic mismatches undermine safety	FHIR/DICOM/OMOP standards; canonical models. (HL7, 2019; SNOMED International, 2022)

continued on following page

Table 4. Continued

Risk Category	Why It Matters	Mitigation Strategies
Security & Key Management	Key compromise risks impersonation	HSMs; PKI rotation; multi-signature governance
Accountability & Liability	Blurred responsibility in AI-assisted care	Human-in-the-loop controls; governance boards

7.5 Concluding Reflections

Ethical, legal, and interoperability challenges are not peripheral obstacles but central determinants of success for blockchain- and digital twin–enabled healthcare systems. Estonia and Saudi Arabia demonstrate that while technological capability is essential, sustainable adoption depends on governance design, regulatory clarity, cultural readiness, and ethical foresight. Addressing these challenges proactively is critical to ensuring that intelligent healthcare systems enhance trust, equity, and patient well-being rather than amplifying existing risks

8: FRAMEWORK FOR BLOCKCHAIN–DIGITAL TWIN INTEGRATION IN SMART HEALTHCARE SYSTEMS

8.0 Introduction to the Integration Framework

The preceding sections of this chapter examined blockchain and digital twin technologies as distinct yet complementary innovations, analyzed their implementation within the healthcare ecosystems of Estonia and Saudi Arabia, and critically evaluated the ethical, legal, and interoperability challenges associated with their deployment. Building upon these insights, Section 8 synthesizes the analytical findings into a unified, implementable framework for the integration of blockchain and digital twin technologies within real-world smart hospital infrastructures.

This integration framework is designed to serve as a strategic reference model for national governments, ministries of health, hospital networks, regulators, and digital health architects seeking to transition toward secure, predictive, and interoperable healthcare systems. Importantly, the framework is technology-agnostic and context-adaptive, allowing it to be applied through phased customization in low-, middle-, and high-income healthcare systems.

The framework draws inspiration from multiple sources:

- Estonia's trust-by-design and interoperability-first digital governance model (Vassil, 2016);
- Saudi Arabia's rapid, investment-driven smart hospital modernization under Vision 2030 (Vision 2030, 2016);
- International standards, including WHO Digital Health Guidelines and HL7-FHIR interoperability frameworks; (WHO, 2021; HL7, 2019) and
- Recent interdisciplinary research on the convergence of blockchain, artificial intelligence (AI), and the Internet of Medical Things (IoMT) in healthcare. (Kuo et al., 2017; Fuller et al., 2020).

At its core, the framework is guided by four foundational design principles: (Khosrow-Pour, 2015)

- **Security-by-design:** Blockchain ensures tamper-proof, auditable medical data flows;
- **Prediction-by-design:** Digital twins enable simulation and forecasting of clinical and operational events;
- **Interoperability-by-design:** FHIR-driven architectures enable cross-institutional data exchange;
- **Ethics-by-design:** Privacy, consent, fairness, and accountability are embedded within system architecture rather than treated as external compliance requirements.

8.1 Architectural Framework for Blockchain–Digital Twin Integration

The proposed architectural framework conceptualizes blockchain and digital twins as mutually reinforcing layers within a unified smart healthcare ecosystem rather than as standalone technologies.

Figure 4 illustrates an integrated architecture in which blockchain governs and validates data flows, while digital twins interpret, simulate, and predict clinical and operational scenarios. The architecture incorporates:

- IoMT-enabled data acquisition from patients, devices, and hospital systems; (WHO, 2021)
- Interoperable data pipelines compliant with HL7-FHIR standards; (HL7, 2019)
- Blockchain-based consent management, identity verification, and audit logging; (Finck, 2019)

- AI-powered simulation engines for patient-level and hospital-level digital twins; (Fuller et al., 2020); and
- Real-time clinical and administrative decision-support dashboards. (OECD, 2020).

Figure 4.

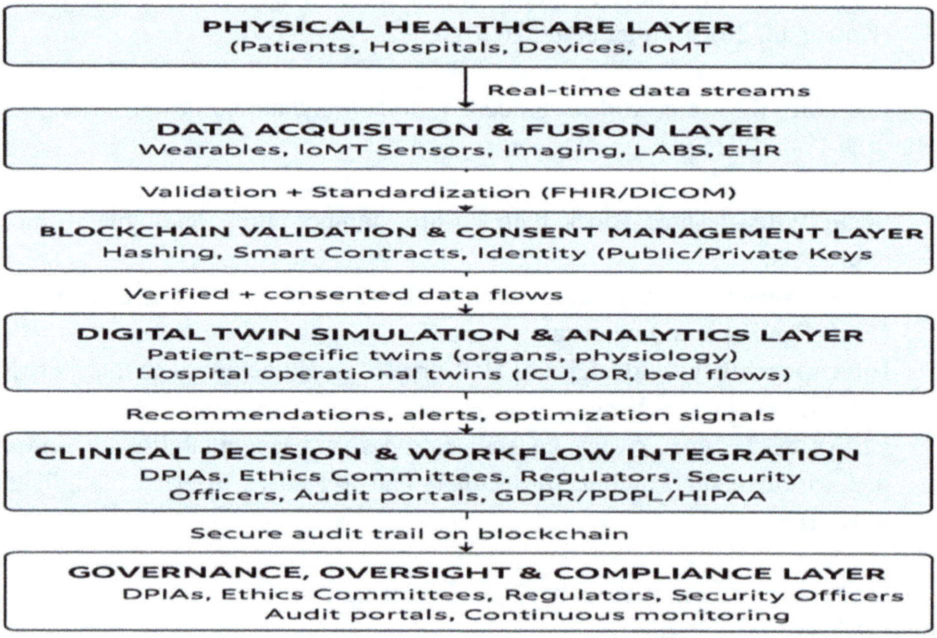

PHYSICAL HEALTHCARE LAYER
(Patients, Hospitals, Devices, IoMT
Real-time data streams
DATA ACQUISITION & FUSION LAYER
Wearables, IoMT Sensors, Imaging, LABS, EHR
Validation + Standardization (FHIR/DICOM)
BLOCKCHAIN VALIDATION & CONSENT MANAGEMENT LAYER
Hashing, Smart Contracts, Identity (Public/Private Keys
Verified + consented data flows
DIGITAL TWIN SIMULATION & ANALYTICS LAYER
Patient-specific twins (organs, physiology)
Hospital operational twins (ICU, OR, bed flows)
Recommendations, alerts, optimization signals
CLINICAL DECISION & WORKFLOW INTEGRATION
DPIAs, Ethics Committees, Regulators, Security
Officers, Audit portals, GDPR/PDPL/HIPAA
Secure audit trail on blockchain
GOVERNANCE, OVERSIGHT & COMPLIANCE LAYER
DPIAs, Ethics Committees, Regulators, Security Officers
Audit portals, Continuous monitoring

Within this architecture, blockchain functions as a trust and governance layer, ensuring that data inputs to digital twins are authentic, complete, and traceable. Digital twins, in turn, transform validated data into predictive intelligence, enabling proactive care delivery, operational optimization, and strategic planning.

8.3 Phased National Roadmap for Blockchain–Digital Twin Integration

To operationalize the framework, a four-phase national implementation roadmap is proposed (WHO, 2021). This phased approach reduces institutional risk, supports incremental learning, and aligns technological deployment with regulatory readiness.

PHASE 1 — Foundation: Digital Infrastructure and Interoperability

Objectives:

- Establish a national digital identity (e-ID) framework;
- Deploy a FHIR-based health data exchange platform;
- Implement baseline cybersecurity and data protection controls;
- Develop IoMT device certification and onboarding standards;
- Initiate blockchain pilots focused on data integrity verification.

Illustrative Examples:

- *Estonia:* X-Road interoperability infrastructure combined with universal e-ID. (Vassil, 2016)
- *Saudi Arabia:* NABIDH and NPHIES platforms enabling regional and national data exchange. (Saudi Ministry of Health, 2022).

This phase establishes the technical and institutional prerequisites for scalable digital health transformation.

PHASE 2 — Blockchain Rollout for Data Integrity and Consent Governance

Objectives:

- Deploy a nationwide blockchain ledger for health data verification;
- Implement smart contracts for dynamic, patient-controlled consent;
- Integrate blockchain audit trails into EHR systems;
- Train clinicians and administrators on access governance and data stewardship.

Key Outputs:

- A national trust layer for healthcare data;
- Transparent, immutable access logs;
- Secure cross-hospital authentication and data validation mechanisms.

This phase institutionalizes trust, accountability, and transparency across the healthcare ecosystem.

PHASE 3 — Digital Twin Development (Pilot and Scale)

Objectives:

- Launch patient-level digital twin pilots (e.g., cardiology, diabetes, oncology);
- Develop operational digital twins for ICUs, operating rooms, and emergency departments;
- Integrate IoMT-based predictive analytics;
- Establish high-performance computing (HPC) and AI infrastructure.

Key Outputs:

- Predictive early-warning systems;
- Scenario-based clinical and operational simulations;
- Measurable reductions in adverse events and resource inefficiencies.

Saudi Arabia is already advancing through this phase via smart hospitals and Seha Virtual Hospital, demonstrating the feasibility of large-scale operational twins. (Saudi Ministry of Health, 2022).

PHASE 4 — Fully Integrated Smart Healthcare Ecosystem

Objectives:

- Enable bidirectional integration between blockchain and digital twin systems;
- Establish AI governance boards for oversight and accountability;
- Implement real-time national digital hospital operations;
- Introduce public transparency and performance reporting mechanisms;
- Continuously retrain AI and simulation models using validated data.

Key Outputs:

- National smart health command centers;
- Fully digital, predictive hospital networks;
- Trust-driven, patient-centered data ecosystems.

In comparative terms, Estonia is currently closest to achieving this level of integration at a national scale.

8.4 Comparative Implementation Models: Estonia and Saudi Arabia

Table 5 highlights how Estonia and Saudi Arabia operationalize similar technologies through fundamentally different governance and implementation strategies. Together, they demonstrate that no single pathway exists, but successful integration depends on alignment between technology, governance, and societal context.

Table 5. Comparative Blockchain–Digital Twin Integration Approaches

Framework Component	Estonia Approach	Saudi Arabia Approach
Foundational Identity	Universal digital e-ID	National ID + digital health platforms (Vision 2030, 2016; Saudi Ministry of Health, 2022)
Data Exchange System	X-Road (high maturity)	NABIDH + NPHIES (rapidly scaling) (Saudi Ministry of Health, 2022)
Blockchain Role	Data integrity verification	Inter-hospital data governance and insurance
Digital Twin Focus	Patient-level twins, national analytics	Hospital operational twins, remote monitoring
Governance Style	Citizen-trust, bottom-up	State-driven, top-down
Technical Strength	Interoperability and public trust	Scale and rapid innovation (Saudi Ministry of Health, 2022)
Key Challenges	Scaling advanced AI models	Workforce digital readiness

8.5 Synthesis: Why Blockchain–Digital Twin Integration Requires Joint Architecture

Blockchain and digital twin technologies, when deployed independently, deliver only partial value:

- **Blockchain alone** cannot generate predictive insights;
- **Digital twins alone** cannot guarantee data trust, provenance, or accountability.

When integrated within a unified architecture:

- **Blockchain** ensures data reliability, integrity, and auditability;
- **Digital twins** transform reliable data into predictive intelligence;
- **IoMT** supplies continuous real-time signals;
- **FHIR interoperability** ensures semantic consistency across systems;

- **Governance layers** enforce ethical, legal, and clinical safeguards.

The resulting healthcare system is:

- **Transparent** in data usage and access;
- **Predictive** in clinical and operational decision-making;
- **Interoperable** across institutional and national boundaries;
- **Patient-centered** through consent-driven data governance;
- **Legally and ethically compliant** by design.

9: POLICY RECOMMENDATIONS AND FUTURE RESEARCH DIRECTIONS

9.1 Introduction: The Imperative for Governance, Standards, and Scientific Foresight

The integration of blockchain and digital twin technologies into healthcare represents a paradigm shift from reactive, episodic care toward predictive, data-driven, and patient-centered health systems. Blockchain ensures the integrity, security, and auditability of medical records, while digital twins enable real-time simulation of patient physiology, disease progression, and treatment outcomes. Combined, these technologies promise enhanced personalization, simulation-driven decision-making, and operational transparency.

However, technological potential alone is insufficient. Without coherent policy frameworks, adoption can be fragmented, ethically problematic, and legally ambiguous. Today, only 23% of countries have a national AI governance strategy, and even fewer incorporate explicit guidelines for blockchain or digital twin adoption in healthcare. Hospitals lacking secure and interoperable systems are projected to face quadrupled cybersecurity threats by 2030, underscoring the urgency for governance interventions.

Countries such as Estonia, Singapore, South Korea, and Saudi Arabia demonstrate the advantages of coordinated digital healthcare strategies (OECD, 2023). Yet, most nations remain trapped in fragmented digital silos, limiting data sharing, cross-institutional collaboration, and predictive modeling. Against this backdrop, this chapter offers an integrated policy and research agenda, identifying mechanisms for ethical, legal, operational, and technical alignment of next-generation healthcare technologies.

Key objectives include:

- Establishing robust national governance structures.
- Embedding ethics, transparency, and privacy in predictive healthcare systems.
- Ensuring interoperability and standardization for cross-institutional and cross-border collaboration.
- Developing digital literacy and workforce capabilities.
- Guiding future research to expand the scientific, technological, and policy frontier.

9.2 Policy Recommendations for National Healthcare Transformation

The transformation toward predictive, simulation-driven healthcare requires coordinated policy interventions across multiple domains, including governance, ethics, interoperability, infrastructure, and workforce development. Fragmented strategies risk inefficiencies, technology misalignment, and potential harm to patients. Based on global best practices, we outline a comprehensive policy framework for national-level adoption.

9.2.1 Establishing National Governance Authorities

Countries should create National Digital Health Authorities (NDHAs) (WHO, 2021). or equivalent regulatory bodies responsible for oversight of blockchain systems, digital twin accuracy, and AI safety. Dedicated authorities ensure legal enforceability, standardization, and accountability across both public and private healthcare sectors.

Global examples include:

- **Estonia** – Information System Authority (RIA) centralizes health data oversight, ensuring interoperability and secure system certification. (Vassil, 2016).
- **Saudi Arabia** – Saudi Data & AI Authority (SDAIA) consolidates predictive health governance under a centralized, well-funded institution, enabling nationwide digital health initiatives. (Vision 2030, 2016; SDAIA, 2021).

Core functions of an NDHA include:

- Certification of blockchain node operators.
- Legal oversight of smart contracts in healthcare.
- Audit trail compliance for clinical data and transactions.
- Verification of digital twin simulation safety and accuracy.

- Coordination of national cyber-defense for healthcare institutions.

By instituting NDHAs, nations can preempt regulatory gaps, reduce technological fragmentation, and maintain public trust.

9.2.2 Enhancing Ethical and Privacy Protections

Predictive healthcare systems raise new ethical, legal, and social concerns (Bruynseels et al., 2018). Digital twins produce detailed simulations that may generate algorithmically derived risk scores, potentially inducing patient anxiety or enabling misuse in employment and insurance. Blockchain's immutability conflicts with privacy rights such as GDPR's Article 17 (Finck, 2019). ("right to be forgotten"), necessitating new approaches to ethical system design.

Recommended ethical measures include:

- **Explainability mandates:** Digital twin predictions must be interpretable and clinically justifiable.
- **Annual algorithmic bias audits:** To prevent disparities in simulation outcomes for diverse populations.
- **Privacy-preserving computation:** Leveraging zero-knowledge proofs, homomorphic encryption, or secure multi-party computation.
- **Patient-controlled consent dashboards:** Allowing granular permissions for data use, sharing, and deletion.
- **Cultural competency protocols:** Ensuring models are sensitive to demographic, regional, and socio-economic diversity.

Estonia's transparent access logs build trust (Vassil, 2016) by allowing patients to see who accessed their data, while Saudi Arabia's Personal Data Protection Law (PDPL) enforces purpose-limited usage of sensitive health data. (SDAIA, 2021)

9.2.3 Mandating Interoperability and Standards Compliance

Interoperability is the cornerstone of a scalable, predictive healthcare system. National mandates on data standards, APIs, and semantic harmonization prevent fragmented, siloed digital ecosystems.

Global evidence highlights success factors:

- **OECD (2023) Health Data Governance Report**: Countries with national interoperability mandates adopt advanced technologies 40–60% faster than those without. (OECD, 2023).

- **Estonia** – X-Road architecture enables seamless data exchange across healthcare institutions. (Vassil, 2016).
- **Saudi Arabia** – Harmonization via NPHIES and NABIDH standards ensures consistent, computable data for digital twins. (Saudi Ministry of Health, 2022)

Key interoperability mandates:

- FHIR-based national EHR architecture. (HL7, 2019)
- Adoption of SNOMED CT, ICD-11, LOINC terminologies.
- DICOM compliance for imaging and radiology data.
- Universal Internet of Medical Things (IoMT) certification standards.
- Mandatory secure API integration for hospital systems.

These policies ensure reliable digital twin simulations, consistent clinical events, and auditable blockchain logs.

9.2.4 Investing in Digital Talent and Healthcare Workforce Transformation

Human capital is critical for operationalizing predictive healthcare systems. Digital literacy for clinicians, data scientists, and hospital administrators ensures accurate interpretation, ethical application, and secure management of emerging technologies. (OECD, 2020; Khosrow-Pour, 2015).

Core training domains include:

- AI ethics and predictive modeling interpretation.
- Digital twin simulation literacy and validation.
- Blockchain auditing and trust framework assessment.
- Telemedicine and remote monitoring operations.
- Continuous professional education on regulatory updates and cybersecurity best practices.

Global example:

- **Saudi Arabia Vision 2030:** Nationwide digital upskilling program targeting healthcare professionals. (Vision 2030, 2016).

Estonia: Early digital literacy programs integrated into public education, enabling long-term societal readiness for AI and blockchain adoption. (Vassil, 2016).

Table 6. Policy Priorities for Blockchain–Digital Twin Integration

Policy Domain	Key Actions	International Examples
Governance	Establish NDHA, certify blockchain nodes, enforce audit trails	Estonia (RIA), Saudi Arabia (SDAIA)
Ethics & Privacy	Explainable predictions, bias audits, consent dashboards	GDPR, PDPL
Interoperability	FHIR EHRs, SNOMED CT, secure API integration	Estonia (X-Road), Saudi Arabia (NPHIES)
Workforce	AI & digital twin training, telemedicine skill-building	Saudi Vision 2030, Estonia digital literacy

9.3 Future Research Directions in Predictive and Trusted Healthcare

Blockchain–digital twin ecosystems open **multidisciplinary research opportunities**, (Fuller et al., 2020; Kuo et al., 2017). spanning medicine, computer science, data governance, ethics, and public policy. Addressing these research priorities is essential for the next decade of intelligent healthcare.

9.3.1 Explainable Digital Twins and Model Transparency

Digital twins currently function as "black boxes" (Bruynseels et al., 2018), limiting clinicians' ability to justify decisions. Research must focus on:

- Visual explanation frameworks for predictive models.
- Human-understandable physiological modeling.
- Uncertainty quantification methods to improve clinical trust.
- Personalized calibration to reflect individual patient variability.

Europe's Horizon Research Programs emphasize explainable AI; (European Commission, 2020). similar efforts are required to standardize explainable digital twin models.

9.3.2 Scalable and Sustainable Blockchain Architectures

Healthcare blockchains must scale efficiently to support nationwide or international deployments without excessive energy or computational costs. Key research areas include:

- Lightweight consensus algorithms.
- Off-chain privacy-preserving storage solutions.
- Energy-efficient validation mechanisms.
- Distributed clinical analytics integrated with blockchain.

Example: Singapore's 2024 blockchain pilot demonstrates successful multi-clinic, scalable data exchange for clinical research and patient care. (OECD, 2023).

9.3.3 Ethical Simulation Frameworks and Patient-Centered Predictive Rights

Digital twins introduce questions about predictive rights: patients' control over risk predictions, how forecasts are communicated, and potential impacts on insurance or employment. Research must address:

- Defining ethical prediction thresholds.
- Assessing psychological effects of risk forecasting.
- Promoting social equity in predictive healthcare.
- Establishing rights to limit or oppose predictive simulations.

The U.S. AI Bill of Rights serves as an early model for integrating patient-centered safeguards in predictive systems. (White House Office of Science and Technology Policy, 2022).

9.3.4 Global Interoperability and Cross-Border Digital Twin Mobility

For medical tourism and migrant populations, digital twins must be portable internationally while preserving privacy and data sovereignty. Key research directions:

- Cross-border data governance frameworks.
- International registry of validated digital twin models.
- Global FHIR-based reference architectures.
- Regional blockchain health networks for secure data exchange.

Case study: Estonia-Finland cross-border prescription system provides proof of concept for secure international digital health interoperability. (Vassil, 2016).

9.3.5 Research Roadmap for the Next Decade

Table 7. Research Roadmap Flow

Timeframe	Focus Areas
2025–2027	Interoperability foundations, explainable digital twin models
2027–2030	Scalable blockchain infrastructures, clinical twin validation
2030–2034	Ethical predictive rights, cross-border twin mobility
2034–2035	Fully integrated, predictive, patient-centered smart health ecosystems

9.4 Conclusion: A Pathway to Predictive, Trusted, and Globally Interoperable Healthcare

Blockchain and digital twin technologies can transform healthcare systems (Fuller et al., 2020). into predictive, transparent, and equitable environments. Estonia and Saudi Arabia illustrate two complementary strategies: (Vassil, 2016; Vision 2030, 2016). incremental, trust-driven innovation versus rapid, nationally coordinated transformation.

Successful adoption requires more than technology:

- Strong governance and legal frameworks.
- Ethical foresight embedded in digital twins and blockchain.
- Interoperable standards for national and international data exchange.
- Digital literacy and workforce readiness.

By implementing the policy recommendations and pursuing the research directions outlined here, countries can develop healthcare systems that are not only technologically advanced but resilient, equitable, and aligned with human values. (WHO, 2021).

REFERENCES

Agbo, C. C., Mahmoud, Q. H., & Eklund, J. M. (2019). Blockchain technology in healthcare: A systematic review. *Health Care*, *7*(2), 56. DOI: 10.3390/healthcare7020056 PMID: 30987333

Androulaki, E., Barger, A., & Bortnikov, V.. (2018). Hyperledger Fabric: A distributed operating system for permissioned blockchains. *Proceedings of the Thirteenth EuroSys Conference*. DOI: 10.1145/3190508.3190538

Azaria, A., Ekblaw, A., Vieira, T., & Lippman, A. (2016). MedRec: Using blockchain for medical data access and permission management. *Proceedings of IEEE Open & Big Data Conference*. DOI: 10.1109/OBD.2016.11

Bruynseels, K., Santoni de Sio, F., & van den Hoven, J. (2018). Digital twins in health care: Ethical implications of an emerging engineering paradigm. *Frontiers in Genetics*, *9*, 31. DOI: 10.3389/fgene.2018.00031 PMID: 29487613

Corral-Acero, J., Margara, F., Marciniak, M., Rodero, C., Loncaric, F., Feng, Y., Gilbert, A., Fernandes, J. F., Bukhari, H. A., Wajdan, A., Martinez, M. V., Santos, M. S., Shamohammdi, M., Luo, H., Westphal, P., Leeson, P., DiAchille, P., Gurev, V., Mayr, M., & Lamata, P. (2020). The 'digital twin' to enable the vision of precision cardiology. *European Heart Journal*, *41*(48), 4556–4564. DOI: 10.1093/eurheartj/ehaa159 PMID: 32128588

European Commission. (2019). Digital economy and society index (DESI) report: Estonia.

European Commission. (2023). eHealth digital maturity assessment of EU member states 2024 report. Publications Office of the European Union.

European Medicines Agency. (2022). Digital transformation of medicines regulation: Strategic reflection.

European Parliament & Council of the European Union. (2016). *Regulation (EU) 2016/679*. General Data Protection Regulation.

Finck, M. (2019). Blockchain and the General Data Protection Regulation. *European Data Protection Law Review*, *5*(1), 17–37. DOI: 10.21552/edpl/2018/1/6

U.S. Food & Drug Administration. (2023). Artificial intelligence/machine learning (AI/ML)-based software as a medical device action plan.

Fuller, A., Fan, Z., Day, C., & Barlow, C. (2020). Digital twin: Enabling technologies, challenges and open research. *IEEE Access : Practical Innovations, Open Solutions*, *8*, 108952–108971. DOI: 10.1109/ACCESS.2020.2998358

Health Level Seven International (HL7). (2019). FHIR release 4 (R4) specification.

Islam, S. M. R., Kwak, D., Kabir, M. H., Hossain, M., & Kwak, K. S. (2015). The Internet of Things for health care: A comprehensive survey. *IEEE Access : Practical Innovations, Open Solutions*, *3*, 678–708. DOI: 10.1109/ACCESS.2015.2437951

Kalvet, T. (2012). Innovation: A factor explaining e-government success in Estonia. Electronic Government, an International Journal, 9(2), 142–157.

Khosrow-Pour, M. (Ed.). (2015). *Encyclopedia of information science and technology* (3rd ed.). IGI Global.

Kingdom of Saudi Arabia. (2016). *National Transformation Program 2020*. Government of Saudi Arabia.

Kuo, T. T., Kim, H. E., & Ohno-Machado, L. (2017). Blockchain distributed ledger technologies for biomedical and health care applications. *Journal of the American Medical Informatics Association : JAMIA*, *24*(6), 1211–1220. DOI: 10.1093/jamia/ocx068 PMID: 29016974

Market Research Future. (2023). Saudi Arabia digital health and smart hospital market forecast to 2033.

Market Research Future. (2023). Saudi Arabia digital health market forecast to 2033.

Ministry of Health Saudi Arabia. (2022). Seha Virtual Hospital initiative report.

Ministry of Health Saudi Arabia. (2022). Seha Virtual Hospital official report.

Ministry of Health Saudi Arabia. (2023). National e-Health platform overview.

Ministry of Health Saudi Arabia. (2023). National e-Health strategy and digital platforms overview.

Ministry of Health Saudi Arabia. (2024). Health statistical yearbook 2024.

Nakamoto, S. (2008). Bitcoin: A peer-to-peer electronic cash system.

OECD. (2020). Health in the digital age: OECD health policy studies. https://doi.org/DOI: 10.1787/0a5e3f3a-en

OECD. (2023). Health data governance for the digital age.

Organisation for Economic Co-operation and Development (OECD). (2025). *Digital government and health data interoperability benchmarking report*. OECD Publishing.

Organisation for Economic Co-operation and Development (OECD). (2025). *Digital health interoperability benchmarking report*. OECD Publishing.

Reyna, A., Martín, C., Chen, J., Soler, E., & Díaz, M. (2018). On blockchain and its integration with IoT. *Future Generation Computer Systems*, *88*, 173–190. DOI: 10.1016/j.future.2018.05.046

Saudi Data & AI Authority. (2021). *Personal Data Protection Law*. PDPL.

Saudi Data & AI Authority (SDAIA). (2021). *Personal Data Protection Law*. PDPL.

Saudi Food & Drug Authority. (2022). Digital health and telemedicine regulatory framework.

Saudi Ministry of Health. (2022). National Platform for Health Information Exchange Services (NPHIES) framework.

Saudi Ministry of Health. (2022). National Health Information Exchange (NPHIES) framework.

Saudi Ministry of Health. (2022). NPHIES and national digital health transformation framework.

SNOMED International. (2022). SNOMED CT global clinical terminology standards.

Tao, F., Zhang, H., Liu, A., & Nee, A. Y. C. (2019). Digital twin in industry: State-of-the-art. *IEEE Transactions on Industrial Informatics*, *15*(4), 2405–2415. DOI: 10.1109/TII.2018.2873186

The Lancet Digital Health. (2023). Representation and fairness in medical AI datasets. The Lancet Digital Health.

Ting, D. S. W., Carin, L., Dzau, V., & Wong, T. Y. (2020). Digital technology and COVID-19. *Nature Medicine*, *26*(4), 459–461. DOI: 10.1038/s41591-020-0824-5 PMID: 32284618

Tseng, J. H., Liao, Y. C., Chong, B., & Liao, S. W. (2018). Governance on the drug supply chain via blockchain technology. *International Journal of Environmental Research and Public Health*, *15*(6), 1055. DOI: 10.3390/ijerph15061055 PMID: 29882861

U.S. Department of Health & Human Services. (2013). Summary of the HIPAA privacy rule.

Vassil, K. (2016). Estonian e-government ecosystem: Foundation, applications, outcomes.

Vision 2030. (2016). Kingdom of Saudi Arabia Vision 2030.

White House Office of Science and Technology Policy. (2022). Blueprint for an AI Bill of Rights.

World Bank. (2022). World development indicators: Population data.

World Health Organization. (2019). *International classification of diseases* (11th ed.).

World Health Organization. (2021). *Global strategy on digital health 2020–2025*. WHO.

World Health Organization (WHO). (2020). *Strengthening the health systems response to COVID-19*. WHO Regional Office for Europe.

Chapter 10
Revolutionizing Research:
Blockchain Technology in Healthcare

Urmila Pilania
http://orcid.org/0000-0002-9251-8514
Manav Rachna University, Faridabad, India

Manoj Kumar
http://orcid.org/0000-0002-9841-8207
Manav Rachna University, Faridabad, India

ABSTRACT

The healthcare research field is struggling with several ongoing problems like ensuring data is accurate, being open and clear, connecting different systems, keeping information safe, and building trust. Things such as broken health records, studies that can't be repeated, people changing data without permission, and patients not having control over their medical information are making it harder to move forward with scientific research and new ideas. In this situation, blockchain technology has come up as a big change that can really improve healthcare research by offering ways to manage data that are spread out, can't be changed, and are transparent. This paper looks at how blockchain can change the way healthcare research is done, help people work together securely, and build trust between those involved. Blockchain uses a system where data is stored across a network of computers, making it almost impossible to change or fake. This helps keep research data honest and makes it easier to check and track throughout the research process.

DOI: 10.4018/979-8-3373-8177-0.ch010

1 INTRODUCTION

In an epoch increasingly characterized by digital alteration and data-driven decision-making, blockchain is a disruptive force that cuts through several industries, including healthcare. Initially conceived as the basis for cryptocurrencies like Bitcoin, blockchain has since gone beyond its financial roots to pledge to change how sensitive information is handled, exchanged, and secured in the healthcare industry. Various issues confront healthcare systems globally, with criticality among them being the secure and efficient management of patient health records. In the past, healthcare data has been confined within fragmented systems, which have led to inefficiencies in information exchange, interoperability problems, and increased chances of data breaches. These issues disrupt patients' privacy and hinder medical research, clinical trials, and quality care (Yaqoob et al., 2020).

Blockchain technology offers new solutions to these long-standing problems by changing how data is stored, accessed, and validated. Blockchain is a decentralized, undying ledger recording communications across a network of computers. The digital ledger process cannot be changed, and it records transactions across numerous computers to ensure privacy and transparency (Pilania et al., 2023). In it, data is divided into "blocks" and connected in time to design a "chain". Every block in the chain comprises many transactions linked by cryptography to the preceding one, making it hard to alter any data in one block without changing all others following it. Unlike traditional databases, which depend on a central authority for validation and maintenance purposes, blockchain works through a consensus mechanism whereby there must be an agreement from all concerned parties before any alteration is completed. Basic blockchain architecture is represented in Figure 1 (Khezr et al., 2019).

It keeps records, which makes it difficult for hackers to hack the system, and the information is kept on the blockchain, thus making it safe and incontrovertible. It is a Distributed Ledger Technology (DLT), which uses a digital format to record transactions and related data in multiple locations simultaneously (Pilania et al., 2024). Every computer in the blockchain network preserves a duplicate of the ledger where communications are logged to avoid a single failure. Additionally, all images are modified and validated concurrently. Blockchain is also reflected as a dataset type, but it varies from traditional datasets in many ways in how it records and manages data. Instead of storing data in rows, columns, tables, and files as traditional databases do, blockchain stores data in chunks connected by digital chains (Alqahtani et al., 2023).

Figure 1. Blockchain Architecture

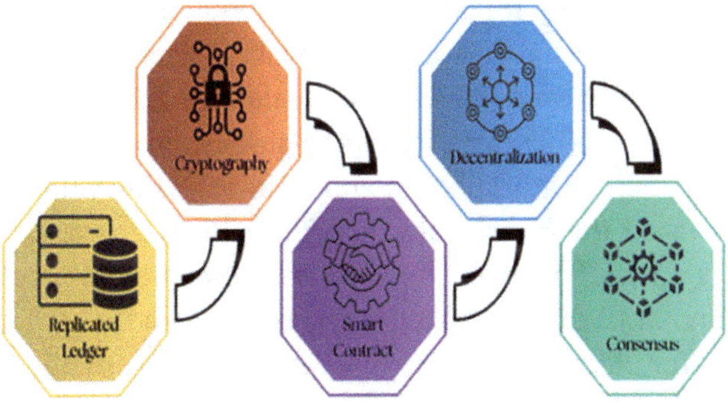

It is a decentralized dataset succeeded by computers in a point-to-point network in place of a central server, as in a traditional dataset. Founded on the Bitcoin blockchain in 2009, Bitcoin and cryptocurrency were popular applications of blockchain (Baygin et al., 2019). Because of that, blockchain and bitcoin are used mostly with substitutes like Bitcoin Cash, which uses public ledgers. However, since Bitcoin's launch, the useful private ledger blockchain has stretched to include other requests. Logistics companies use blockchain to track and trace products during production (Justinia, 2019).

The coming together of blockchain, digital twinning, DID, and smart contracts is creating a strong new way to build safe, independent, and trustworthy digital systems. Digital twins help with real-time tracking, testing, and predicting outcomes in areas like healthcare, manufacturing, smart cities, and supply chains. However, the usual centralized setup of these systems brings up issues like data reliability, compatibility between systems, managing identities, and ensuring trust (Habib et al., 2022).

Blockchain helps solve these problems by offering a shared, unchangeable record that keeps track of events and changes in digital twins. By linking encrypted versions of twin data to the blockchain, we can verify where the data came from and make sure it's genuine, without sharing private details. This makes it easier to trust each other in situations where many different groups are involved. The DID adds another layer by giving control over digital identities to individuals and things, like assets, devices, twins, and users (Xu et al., 2019).

This ensures that access is secure, permissions are well-managed, and rules about data use are followed. Smart contracts act as the automation part, running rules and making payments automatically based on what's happening in the digital twin, such as when a service is delivered or a performance level is met. Together, these technologies create a secure, compatible, and independent digital environment that makes it possible to verify digital twins, control identities in a decentralized way, and exchange value smoothly for advanced smart systems (Pilania et al., 2023).

Blockchain can serve as a trust and provenance layer across different organizations for Health Level Seven (HL7) Fast Healthcare Interoperability Resources (FHIR) by permanently storing cryptographic hashes, timestamps, and digital signatures of FHIR resources at important stages in their lifecycle, without keeping actual clinical data on the blockchain. FHIR's built-in Provenance, AuditEvent, and Meta features track who created the data and its version history. These features create hashed summaries that are linked to the blockchain through smart contracts. This setup allows for clear and tamper-proof auditing. The method works without changing current HL7/FHIR processes and ensures data integrity, prevents denial of actions, and meets regulatory standards during audits and when data is reused (Kassab et al., 2019).

1.1 Centralized, Decentralized, and Distributed Blockchain

Blockchain is classified into centralized, decentralized, and distributed. A single entity handles a centralized blockchain. Only one person is responsible for handling and validating all the transactions. That person is also accountable for the maintenance of the ledger. As a single person handles it, it provides fast transactions, is simple to implement and manage, and provides accountability. Because of a single point of contact, it goes down when the central server fails. It is not very transparent, and an unauthorized person can hack data. A private company blockchain is an example of a centralized blockchain (Habib et al., 2022).

In a decentralized blockchain, control is given to all participating nodes. Proof of Work (PoW) and Proof of Stake (PoS) are utilized to authenticate communications, as they are controlled by all the nodes present in the blockchain, which are transparent and more secure. It is also resistant to censorship. It has a slow transaction speed compared to the centralized blockchain. Its monitoring can be more complex compared to the centralized blockchain. Its examples include Bitcoin and Ethereum (Xu et al., 2019).

Figure 2. Blockchain Categories: Centralized

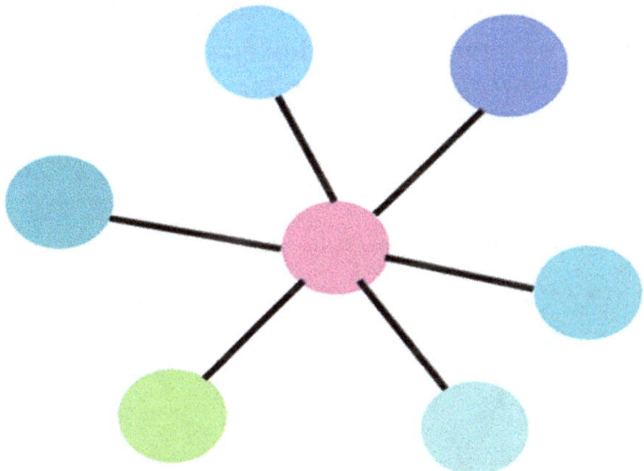

Figure 3. Blockchain Categories: Decentralized

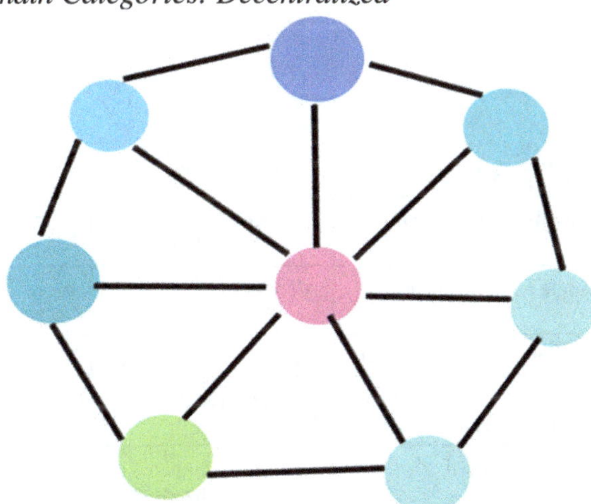

In a distributed blockchain ledger, it is replicated and is in shared mode with all the blocks in the network. All the nodes may not have identical power. The network can be centralized or decentralized, but data is always distributed. The distribution follows the redundancy rule in this type of blockchain. In it, data is backed up in multiple nodes. The network will be functional if some of the nodes fail to participate. The data is scalable. The synchronization problem is widespread in nodes (Pilania et al., 2023).

One example of a distributed blockchain is Google Drive. Figures 2, 3, and 4 represent all three blockchains: Centralized Decentralized, and Distributed, respectively. The figure shows how the nodes are linked to each other for data sharing and controlling the participants' activities. Table 1 represents the more concise differences among all three types of blockchains.

Figure 4. Blockchain Categories: Distributed

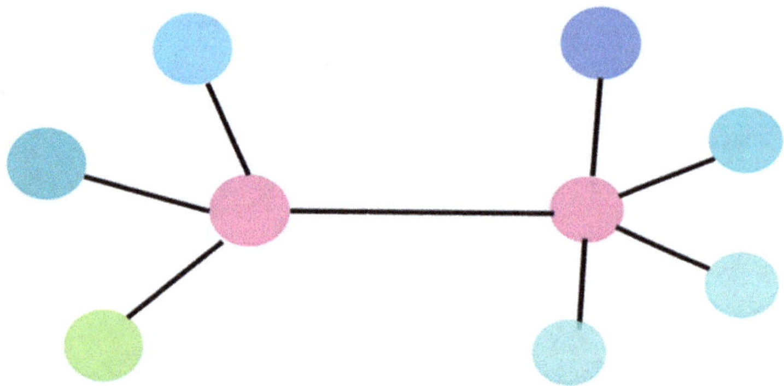

Table 1. Blockchain Types (Kassab et al., 2019)

Characterstic	Centralized Blockchain	Decentralized Blockchain	Distributed Blockchain
Control	Single point of contact	All nodes have controls	It can follow both centralized and decentralized
Data Storage	Single central point of contact	All participating nodes	It is replicated between nodes
Failure Risk	If the central point of contact fails, then the network fails	Fault tolerance is low	The risk of failure is low because of redundancy
Speed	High speed	IT is slow compared to centralized	Its speed depends on many factors
Examples	Private banks	Bitcoin, Ethereum	Ripple, Hyperledger Fabric

1.2 Layered Blockchain Architecture

Figure 5 represents the layered architecture of the blockchain. Table 2 describes the role of each layer with distinct parameters and applications. The functions and responsibilities of each layer are explained step by step. Hardware acts as the foundation of blockchain. It has different components like nodes, servers, devices, and connections, which help operate the blockchain. It provides computing resources, enables point-to-point communication in different nodes present in the blockchain, and stores and replicates blockchain data (Bell et al., 2018).

Table 2. Role of Layers (Abd Elaziz et al., 2024)

Blockchain Layer	Function of Layer	Real-World Example
Infrastructure	It includes hardware, nodes, and a network	Its examples are computers and servers
Information	In it, information is stored in a ledger, blocks, and hashing	Its example is blockchain data
Network Protocol	It includes communication and peer-to-peer sharing	In it, the Gossip protocol is functional
Consensus	Consensus is the agreement mechanism in it	It is dependent on PoW and PoS
Incentive	Economic model	BTC rewards, ETH staking
Smart Contract	It includes logic & smart contracts	Its examples are EVM and chaincode
Application	End-users are aware of the application layer, and it acts as an interface	Its examples are Wallets, dApps, and NFTs

Its example includes nodes that validate Bitcoin transactions. The combination of data and network layers is the second layer of blockchain, which acts as a ledger. It contains blocks, transactions, and hash functions. It is responsible for how data is to be stored in blocks. It is responsible for hashing and confirms immutability, synchronization, and transparency in blockchain (Ismail et al., 2019). One example of a data layer function is transaction data stored in Bitcoin blocks. The consensus layer is basically the agreement in blockchain. Its basic components include PoW and PoS. It confirms the agreement of all the nodes in the ledger. It is responsible for making trust between nodes and securing data without the intervention of the central authorities (Fusco et al., 2020).

The incentive layer is responsible for the payments in blockchain. It motivates users to make payments and aligns individual incentives with data safety. Its components are transaction fees, rewards, and staking. At the contract layer, logics and rules are defined for the blockchain. It includes smart contracts, scripts, and virtual machines. It is responsible for the automation of agreements between nodes. It is also responsible for the execution of decentralized applications. It defines governance rules and regulations. It's an example that includes Ethereum smart contracts and Hyperledger. At this layer, users are active and participate in the blockchain. It has DApps, wallets, and DeFi as main components. It is responsible for providing services to the users. It can handle real-world problems. An example is the MetaMask wallet (Katuwal et al., 2018).

Figure 5. Layers in Blockchain (Yaqoob et al., 2019)

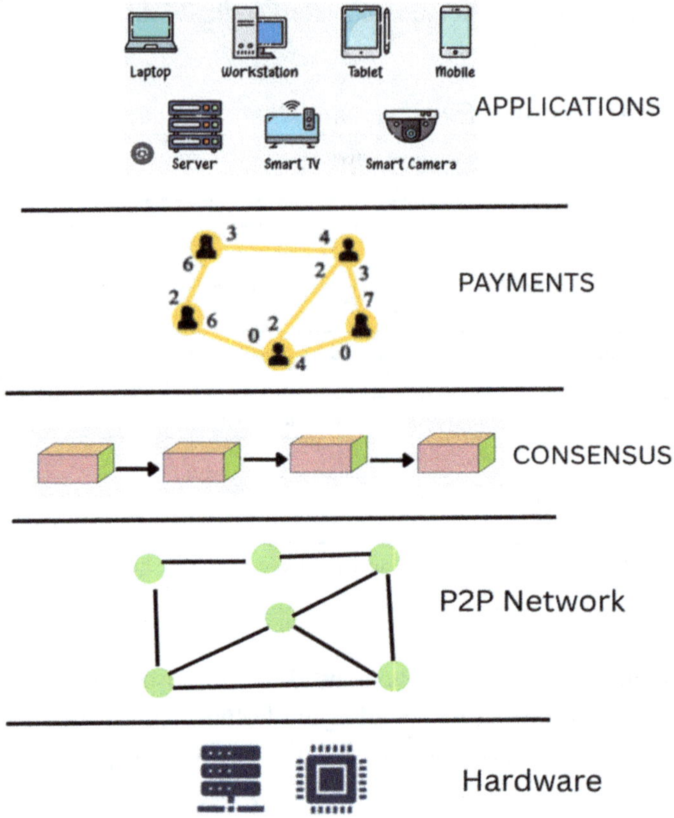

2 LITERATURE REVIEW

Table 3 analyzes the literature summary with blockchain technology in the healthcare sector. A few papers are studied and summarised below:

Table 3. Literature Summary

Title	Author	Date	Literature Survey
Blockchain for Digital Twins: Recent Advances and Future Research Challenges (Yaqoob et al., 2020)	Ibrar Yaqoob, Khaled Salah, Mueen Uddin, Raja Jayaraman, Mohammed Omar, and Muhammad Imran		Blockchain-integrated digital twins, which are virtual models that represent real-world systems using multiple physics-based simulations, allow for secure, decentralized, and unchangeable sharing of data in Industry 4.0. These digital twins support activities like designing, testing, monitoring, diagnosing, and predicting the future performance of systems. They also help ensure that data is traceable, meets regulations, is genuine, maintains quality, and ensures safety. This approach highlights important uses, how different technologies work together, and the areas where more research is needed.
Blockchain Technology in Healthcare Industry (Ghayvat et al., 2023)	Ketan Gupta; Nasmin Jiwani; Md Haris Uddin Sharif; Nirmal Adhikari; Neda Afreen	2022	Blockchain technology in healthcare provides improved security and obstruction for patient data. It could reshape the industry toward patient-centered care and transform electronic health record management.
Blockchain technology in Healthcare (Khosla et al., 2022)	Anita Khosla, Shruti Vashist, Geeta Nijhawan	2022	Blockchain is used to store and share electronic patient health data. The authors discuss the many challenges and benefits of using blockchain in health.
Blockchain Technology in Healthcare Industry (Rakic, 2018)	Dean Rakic	2019	Blockchain in the health industry enhances communication, real-time predictive analytics, trend analysis, and evidence-based medicine. It accelerates the efficiency of health care, the accuracy of diagnosis, and the quality of outcomes.
Enabling Blockchain with IoMT Devices for Healthcare (Almalki et al., 2022)	Jameel Almalki, Waleed Al Shehri, Rashid Mehmood, Khalid Alsaif, Saeed M. lshahrani, Najlaa Jannah and Nayyar Ahmed Khan	2024	This study introduces a healthcare prototype that combines blockchain and artificial intelligence with the Internet of Medical Things. It uses an edge–cloud architecture along with smart contracts to securely collect, analyze, and make decisions about patient data while protecting privacy. The system was tested using a COVID-19 dataset on a peer-to-peer network based on Hyperledger.
Innovating Healthcare With Blockchain Technology: A Comprehensive Review (John Shiny, 2024)	John Shiny J.	2024	Blockchain technology ensures that healthcare data is secure, transparent, and immutable. Challenges in health information management include patient records and information sharing. Enhance reliable and safe health information.

3 BLOCKCHAIN IN HEALTHCARE

Blockchain technology assists the health care sector by improving information management, enhancing interoperability, and streamlining medical supply chains and payments. Some ways blockchain is utilized in healthcare are given in Figure 6 and each of the point is discussed in detail in subsections.

3.1 Patient Information Management

An important application of blockchain in health care is the organization of patient data. Whether it's storing medical data, social privacy numbers, or financial details, blockchain encryption systems provide a method for data storage. The utilization of DLT confirms that patient medical data is securely transferred, preventing access to information. Additionally, blockchain guarantees the immutability of data. Once data is chronicled on the blockchain network, it cannot be transformed without all parties' consent. This feature maintains the accuracy and genuineness of information over time. It facilitates seamless data sharing among medical professionals while ensuring the integrity of the information (Chen et al., 2019).

3.2 Recording Clinical Trial Data

In research settings like trials for medications or disease studies, vast amounts of data must be recorded accurately. Blockchain's immutability characteristic safeguards the reliability of trial data by preventing alterations. It also plays a role in documenting every modification made during trials and tracking these changes effectively (Agbo & Mahmoud, 2020). This data is accessed by the medical professionals for giving online treatment to the patients. The online monitoring of the patient helps them to avoid physical moments and in that time they can take care of themselves.

3.3 Pharmaceutical Supply Chain Management

Fake pills are a significant problem in the healthcare system; however, these could be unsafe for patients. Fake capsules may also include poisonous materials that might adversely affect an affected person's health. Generally, illegal pills are repackaged using faux labels after their expiry, inflicting excessive fitness challenges. As per the National Crime Prevention Council, more than 10% of medications in the global supply chain are fake. Using blockchain, the supply chain issue could be resolved (Islayem et al., 2025).

3.4 Telemedicine and far-flung Tracking

Telemedicine could deliver smooth entry to first-class healthcare for people living in remote regions. It depends on the communication between patients and the healthcare professionals. The wearable sensors could be used to collect data from the patients. Then, based on the collected data, the patient can make suggestions for taking the medicine. All this communication could happen remotely, promoting telemedicine using blockchain and IoT wearables (Pirtle & Ehrenfeld, 2018).

Figure 6. Blockchain in Healthcare

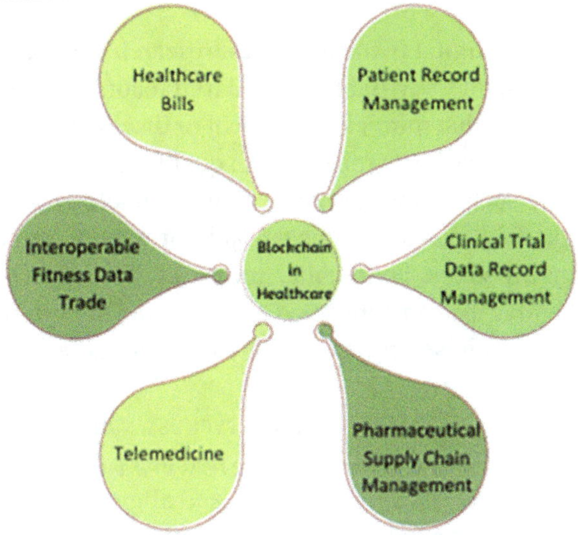

3.5 Interoperable Fitness Data Trade

Sometimes, sufferers need to seek expert advice and complete statistics on their health history for the best results. Patient data could be collected using IoT devices, collected data is stored using cloud computing, and then, using computational techniques, data analysis is done, and based on that analysis, medical professionals suggest medicine to the patient (Taherdoost, 2023).

3.6 Healthcare Bills

Hospitals generate many transactions daily for claims. This procedure includes sharing credit card and financial institution account data. The developing quantity of records, opening incidents, and safeguarding reimbursement details have become more vital than ever. Blockchain utilizes hashing to guard information from unauthorized users. These transactions form a chain, and that chain is immune to unauthorized users. It additionally facilitates rationalized healthcare payments by eliminating intermediaries, resulting in quicker payments and decreased charges (Singh et al., 2020).

3.7 Blockchain-Enabled Digital Twins for Clinical Research

Blockchain-powered digital twins in clinical research connect virtual patient or disease models with reliable, verifiable clinical trial records. A digital twin is a living computational model that mimics real patient or disease behavior using clinical data and simulations. Its accuracy relies on the quality, origin, and trustworthiness of the data, which are secured through blockchain technology. Blockchain keeps a permanent, time-stamped record of clinical trial information like protocol versions, data timelines, consent status, and quality measures. Sensitive patient data stays off the blockchain and is instead connected using unique digital fingerprints called cryptographic hashes. This setup provides a clear, traceable record of the entire clinical trial process.

The unchangeable data on the blockchain serves as a validation system for digital twins. When real-world clinical data is used to update or run simulations on a digital twin, the system checks the data's integrity and alignment with the trial's rules using blockchain records. Any changes to the digital twin, like model updates or simulation results, can be tied back to the blockchain, making the process repeatable and trackable. Together, blockchain and digital twins create a safe and dependable system that boosts data accuracy, helps meet regulatory standards, and increases trust in research and decisions made by AI in clinical settings (Kerrison et al., 2023).

3.8 Secure Operational Data Flow

The section shows how blockchain not only protects research data but also secures the flow of operational data in smart hospitals. These hospitals use many systems that constantly generate data from electronic health records, medical devices, clinical platforms, and administrative tools. Blockchain can serve as a tamper-proof layer that records metadata and transactions across all these systems, ensuring transparency, data accuracy, and responsibility in everyday hospital activities.

In managing medical devices and assets, blockchain creates unchangeable records of how devices are used, maintained, calibrated, and their real-time status, which helps with compliance and patient safety. It also helps control who has access to clinical systems and patient information, making it easier to track who did what and hold them accountable based on their roles. Furthermore, blockchain enhances supply chain management by offering full visibility into the movement of medicines and equipment, helping to prevent fake products and errors in inventory. Covering these operational uses gives a clearer picture of how blockchain supports the creation of secure and connected smart hospital systems (Girardi et al., 2020).

3.9 Blockchain with IoMT

Blockchain can play an important role in keeping track of and confirming high-frequency data from IoMT devices used in everyday medical care and research studies like pragmatic clinical trials. These devices constantly send streams of data, such as vital signs, activity levels, and how well they're working. By storing encrypted hashes and details about these data streams on a blockchain, each piece of data gets a secure timestamp and is connected to its source. This ensures the data hasn't been changed after it was collected.

Instead of keeping all the raw data directly on the blockchain, it's used as a way to verify off-chain data by linking it to an unchangeable record. This helps doctors and researchers check if the data is accurate, confirm when it was collected, and ensure that research procedures were followed, either in real time or later. In trials that take place within regular medical settings, blockchain timestamps help tell the difference between normal care data and data collected for research, while keeping a single, clear record. This builds trust in the data from IoMT devices, helps meet legal requirements, and improves the accuracy of both medical decisions and research results (Almalki et al., 2022).

3.10 Smart Contract Architecture

A smart contract setup for a unified smart hospital can be built as a layered system that connects electronic health records, research databases, and ethics boards using a permissioned blockchain network. The blockchain holds smart contracts that set up rules for governance, access control, consent handling, and audit needs. However, all sensitive clinical and research information stays safely stored off-chain in the existing hospital and research systems.

Secure middleware and APIs connect EHRs and research databases to the blockchain. These connections activate smart contracts whenever data is accessed, updated, or reused. The contracts log time-stamped metadata and cryptographic hashes to form unchangeable audit trails and check if protocols are followed, all without revealing patient information. Separate smart contracts for ethics and consent store approvals, consent status, and changes. These contracts automatically check if someone is eligible before their data is used for research. This whole setup allows for clear governance, safe data sharing, and ongoing compliance with regulations in both patient care and clinical research (Amofa et al., 2024).

3.11 Decentralized Identity System

A decentralized identity (DID) system for smart hospitals can work with current hospital single sign-on (SSO) systems and national eHealth IDs, while also allowing patients to have control over their data through dynamic consent. Each person involved—like patients, doctors, researchers, and hospitals—is given a DID based on blockchain. This DID is like a digital identity that connects to trusted sources, such as hospitals or government eHealth services, instead of replacing the existing ways people identify themselves.

Hospitals and eHealth organizations give out verified digital credentials to these DIDs after someone logs in using standard SSO or eHealth methods. These credentials are given based on the person's role or specific attributes, such as being a patient or a researcher. Dynamic consent is handled using smart contracts linked to the patient's DID, letting individuals easily choose who can access their data, for how long, and for what purpose. Every time someone tries to access data, the system checks if they have the right credentials and if their consent is still active. All these activities are recorded permanently on the blockchain. This setup supports secure authentication, smooth integration between care and research, and safe sharing of data across the smart hospital network (Zhang et al., 2024).

4 BENEFITS OF BLOCKCHAIN TECHNOLOGY

Blockchain benefits many industries worldwide, including banking, education, business, and many more. The significant applications of blockchain are in health care. Blockchain can save costs, provide transparency, ensure data security, seamless data sharing with medical professionals and patients, telemedicine, healthcare bills, health data recording, patient information management, and many more. Its application in the healthcare system is shown in Figure 7, and details of each are also provided.

4.1 Cost Saving

The technology can decrease secretarial tasks' costs, increase productivity, and provide high-speed information exchange. Using it, healthcare professionals do not require hand and paper. The less utilization of paper saves the environment as well. More systems in healthcare are used for sharing medical records, dispensing medications, and processing care and claims, thus reducing costs (El-Gazzar & Stendal, 2020). As health data is available online, which can be utilized by medical professionals, and patients can contact doctors online, this lowers patients' physical visits.

4.2 Transparency

Blockchain in health care could increase transparency by providing a dedicated and dispersed ledger structure that does not permit transactions or information to be altered once recorded. It brings greater transparency to collecting and sharing patient information, medical data, and prescribing information. Every activity is recorded in the blockchain with a timestamp. The authorized members, such as the patient, doctor, labs, insurance company, and hospital, can alter and access the data. Any transaction or alteration done by any stakeholder will be visible to all. All the mentioned stakeholders are accountable for any changes. It also reduces the chances of fraud (Taherdoost, 2023).

Figure 7. Blockchain Benefits

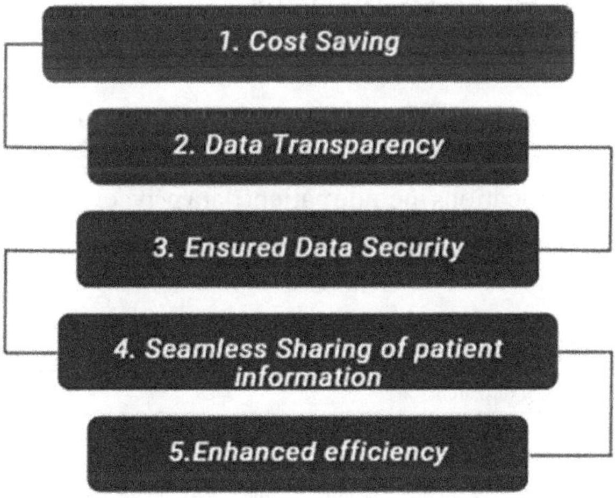

4.3 Ensured Data Security

Health information breaches are the main worry worldwide, disturbing so many people. More than 38 million people will be affected by a health data breach in the first 6 months of 2023 alone, as per a healthcare IT security report. This report highlights the requirement for more secure healthcare. It adds more security to patient data due to its cryptography feature. Because the blockchain transactions are transparent, any alteration made by any stakeholder is visible to all, reducing the chance of data breach. It uses cryptography and hashing for the safety of the patient data. The data is not stored at any single device; it is distributed in the network, reducing the chances of data hacking (Le Nguyen, 2018).

4.4 Seamless sharing of Patient Information

The cryptography characteristics of blockchain confirm the safety of data during communication. Blockchain networks store patient information in a decentralized manner, avoiding the requirement of the central government to control and manage access. This gives patients and authorized participants direct control of their data and facilitates easy portability (Khezr et al., 2019). The interoperable feature of the blockchain allows healthcare stakeholders to access and modify the data without duplication. It also avoids mismatches in information and ensures data transparency. It reduces the paperwork and administrative load of the administrator (Atadoga et al., 2024).

5 APPLICATIONS OF BLOCKCHAIN TECHNOLOGY IN HEALTHCARE

Table 4 represents some examples of blockchain techniques used for real-life applications. Some of the case studies in the table show the applications of blockchain in healthcare. These applications include patient data privacy, electronic data storage, supply chain management, telemedicine, and remote patient health monitoring.

Table 4. Real-Life Applications of Blockchain in Healthcare

1. Blockchain to keep the privacy of patient data		
BurstIQ (https://www.burstiq.com/wp-content/uploads/2018/12/BurstIQ-Cover-Story-Revised-Final12.pdf)	2015, USA	BurstIQ is a platform for securing patient data using blockchain techniques. Due to its decentralized feature, it stores, manages, and shares health data using blockchain. BurstIQ confirms the integrity of patient data due to the immutable nature of blockchain. Patients who are using BurstIQ also confirm complete control over their personal data.
MedicalChain (https://medicalchain.com/Medicalchain-Whitepaper-EN.pdf)	2016, England	MedicalChain is leading the way in bringing blockchain to the health industry. In 2016, many professionals were aware of the power of blockchain, so Medicalchain was proposed to transform the healthcare industry. Patients have complete control over their health data. They give rights to the hospital, doctor, and lab professional; only these persons can access the required data. The decentralized and cryptographic features in blockchain add more security. In 2018, the medical chain launched telemedicine services with the launch of MyClinic.com. The platform allows patients to consult with doctors via video call and settle their payments using "MedToken," a blockchain-based native token for MedicalChain.

continued on following page

Table 4. Continued

Guardtime (https://guardtime.com/about)	2007, Estonia	GuardTime helps healthcare businesses and governments store data with blockchain-based solutions. Health data is sometimes distributed among providers and systems, which causes fragmentation of patient records. GuardTime uses blockchain to create tamper-proof online health data that can only be accessed by authorized users, confirming the accuracy and security of health information. The company operates this data in the US, UK, Switzerland, Estonia, and Singapore.
2. Blockchain for storing medical data		
Avaneer Health (https://avaneerhealth.com/press/avaneer-health-launches-its-decentralized-network-and-platform-to-transform-healthcare-administration/)	2020, USA	Avaneer Health is at the leading edge of utilizing blockchain technology to enhance healthcare facilities. It provides revolutionary and secure methods for improving healthcare transport. It could also manage health data efficiently and adequately. Avaneer Health uses a public ledger to communicate patients' health data, proper claims, and healthcare issuer directories.
Patientory (https://www.f6s.com/company/patientory#about)	2015, USA	The patient uses blockchain to provide solutions to manage health data, enhance transparency, and ensure the security of sensitive medical data. Finally, end-to-end encryption assures that healthcare employees can share health data securely. The company provides a tamper-proof ledger to help healthcare professionals store and transfer all information using a blockchain network.
Medibloc (https://www.biospectator.com/news/view/6509)	2017, USA	MediBloc utilized blockchain for easy access and the safety of secure health data. The decentralized feature helps improve the security of health data. Patients could alter their personal health data and be given the right to access it.
3. Pharmaceutical supply chain management		
Chronicled (https://www.chronicled.com/about-us)	2014, USA	Chronicled is a platform that revolutionizes medication supply chain management by overcoming challenges like fake medications, quality of medicine, data security, and more. The network enables end-to-end transparency of drugs, from manufacturing facilities to end users, thereby curbing malicious activities such as drug smuggling
Blockpharma (https://www.crunchbase.com/organization/blockpharma)	2016, France	Another good example of using blockchain for the health industry is blockchain. The company transforms drug delivery systems for greater transparency, traceability, and security.
4. Blockchain used for telemedicine and remote monitoring		
Robomed Network (https://medium.com/robomed/application-of-blockchain-technology-in-medicine-aa9242628624)	2016, USA	RoboMed is harnessing AI and blockchain to revolutionize telemedicine and remote management in the health industry. The platform enables the delivery of smart wearable devices that collect and transmit real-time data on heart rate, blood pressure, blood sugar levels, and other wearable diagnostic tools. Healthcare providers who securely use blockchain technology can manage patient health data. This helps in the early prediction of health challenges and early action. Telemedicine conferences also provide a platform for patients to consult with doctors remotely.

Real-world hospital projects show that blockchain works best as a tool for governance and auditing, not as a full replacement for existing health IT systems. In Estonia, their e-Health system works with Guardtime to use blockchain-based Keyless Signature Infrastructure (KSI) technology. This helps create secure, unchangeable proof of data integrity and who accessed it, but the actual patient data stays in regular electronic health records. This setup lets doctors keep using their usual systems without changing how they work, while still being able to track any changes. At the Mayo Clinic, similar projects use blockchain to track clinical trial information and patient consent. They store only the unchangeable audit records on the blockchain, while the actual data stays off-chain. These examples show that blockchain can help build trust between different organizations, improve data tracking and security, and make sure systems are ready for regulations, all while keeping the standard ways of sharing health information (Hariharan et al., 2022).

6 CHALLENGES OF BLOCKCHAIN IN THE HEALTHCARE SECTOR

Some of the challenges associated with blockchain in the healthcare industry are given as follows (Attaran, 2022; Angraal et al., 2017; Capece & Lorenzi, 2020; Satamraju & B, 2020; Saranya & Murugan, 2023) in Figure 8:

Figure 8. Challenges Blockchain

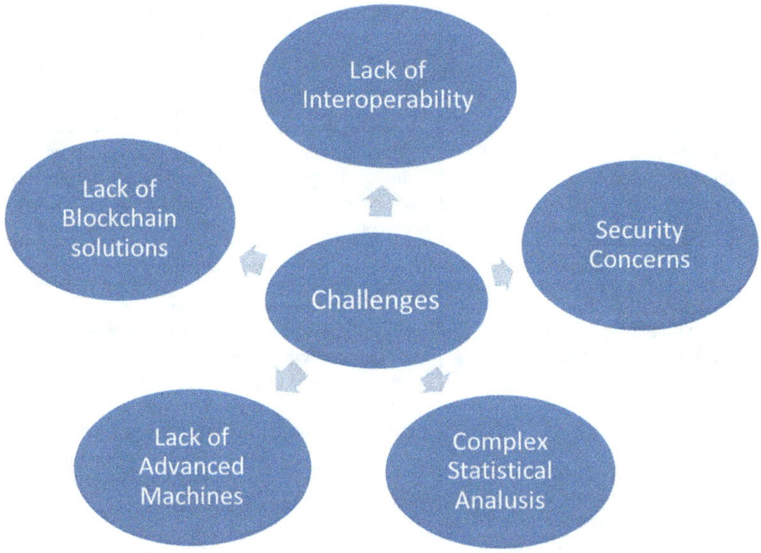

- Lack of studies on blockchain and healthcare
- Potential outcomes and difficulties encountered in a healthcare enterprise
- Patient security concerns
- Potential compromise of the stakeholder community
- Internal machine weaknesses in the healthcare region
- There is a need for a comprehensive evaluation earlier than enforcing blockchain solutions
- Lack of interoperability in healthcare records ecosystems
- Complex and lengthy statistical analyses in healthcare trend evaluation
- Accelerating scientific and biomedical studies, fitness data registry

7 CONCLUSION

In the work, authors have analysed the growing role of blockchain technology in the healthcare industry. The authors started with a discussion of what blockchain is, highlighting its decentralized, transparent, DID, IoMT, digital twinning and secure nature, which makes it an essential tool to address a few ongoing challenges in healthcare. Blockchain is important in terms of healthcare's ability to improve the security of patient data, ensure the integrity of medical records, and facilitate secure information sharing between healthcare providers. The authors also examined blockchain applications in several healthcare domains, including patient data management, EHR, smart healthcare contracts, medication tracking capabilities, clinical trials, and telemedicine. These applications demonstrate the flexibility of blockchain aspects of the healthcare system by improving data transparency, ensuring compliance, and reducing administrative burdens.

Additionally, the authors highlight blockchain's various benefits, like enhanced data security, reduced administrative costs, improved data utilization, and better patient outcomes. The potential of blockchain to provide consistent, searchable, and measurable data is particularly valuable for ensuring the accuracy and reliability of vital health information. Authors have explored top organizations currently leading the way in implementing blockchain solutions in the healthcare industry. These organizations are driving innovation by leveraging the potential of blockchain to address critical issues like fake medications, patient privacy, and access to healthcare.

REFERENCES

Abd Elaziz, M., Al-qaness, M. A., Dahou, A., Al-Betar, M. A., Mohamed, M. M., El-Shinawi, M., Ali, A., & Ewees, A. A. (2024). Digital twins in healthcare: Applications, technologies, simulations, and future trends. *Wiley Interdisciplinary Reviews. Data Mining and Knowledge Discovery*, *14*(6), e1559. DOI: 10.1002/widm.1559

Agbo, C. C., & Mahmoud, Q. H. (2020). Blockchain in healthcare: Opportunities, challenges, and possible solutions. [IJHISI]. *International Journal of Healthcare Information Systems and Informatics*, *15*(3), 82–97. DOI: 10.4018/IJHISI.2020070105

Almalki, J., Al Shehri, W., Mehmood, R., Alsaif, K., Alshahrani, S. M., Jannah, N., & Khan, N. A. (2022). Enabling blockchain with IoMT devices for healthcare. *Information (Basel)*, *13*(10), 448. DOI: 10.3390/info13100448

Almalki, J., Al Shehri, W., Mehmood, R., Alsaif, K., Alshahrani, S. M., Jannah, N., & Khan, N. A. (2022). Enabling blockchain with IoMT devices for healthcare. *Information (Basel)*, *13*(10), 448. DOI: 10.3390/info13100448

Alqahtani, A., Alsubai, S., & Bhatia, M. (2023). Digital-twin-assisted healthcare framework for adult. *IEEE Internet of Things Journal*, *11*(8), 14963–14970. DOI: 10.1109/JIOT.2023.3345331

Amofa, S., Xia, Q., Xia, H., Obiri, I. A., Adjei-Arthur, B., Yang, J., & Gao, J. (2024). Blockchain-secure patient Digital Twin in healthcare using smart contracts. *PLoS One*, *19*(2), e0286120. DOI: 10.1371/journal.pone.0286120 PMID: 38422025

Angraal, S., Krumholz, H. M., & Schulz, W. L. (2017). Blockchain technology: Applications in health care. *Circulation: Cardiovascular Quality and Outcomes*, *10*(9), e003800. DOI: 10.1161/CIRCOUTCOMES.117.003800 PMID: 28912202

Atadoga, A., Elufioye, O. A., Omaghomi, T. T., Akomolafe, O., Odilibe, I. P., & Owolabi, O. R. (2024). Blockchain in healthcare: A comprehensive review of applications and security concerns. *International Journal of Science and Research Archive*, *11*(1), 1605–1613. DOI: 10.30574/ijsra.2024.11.1.0244

Attaran, M. (2022). Blockchain technology in healthcare: Challenges and opportunities. *International Journal of Healthcare Management*, *15*(1), 70–83. DOI: 10.1080/20479700.2020.1843887

Baygin, N., Baygin, M., & Karakose, M. (2019, November). Blockchain technology: applications, benefits and challenges. In *2019 1st International Informatics and Software Engineering Conference (UBMYK)* (pp. 1-5). IEEE. DOI: 10.1109/UBMYK48245.2019.8965565

Bell, L., Buchanan, W. J., Cameron, J., & Lo, O. (2018). Applications of blockchain within healthcare. *Blockchain in Healthcare Today, 1*. Advance online publication. DOI: 10.30953/bhty.v1.8

Capece, G., & Lorenzi, F. (2020). Blockchain and Healthcare: Opportunities and Prospects for the EHR. *Sustainability (Basel), 12*(22), 9693. DOI: 10.3390/su12229693

Chen, H. S., Jarrell, J. T., Carpenter, K. A., Cohen, D. S., & Huang, X. (2019). Blockchain in healthcare: A patient-centered model. *Biomedical Journal of Scientific & Technical Research, 20*(3), 15017. PMID: 31565696

El-Gazzar, R., & Stendal, K. (2020). Blockchain in health care: Hope or hype? *Journal of Medical Internet Research, 22*(7), e17199. DOI: 10.2196/17199 PMID: 32673219

Fusco, A., Dicuonzo, G., Dell'Atti, V., & Tatullo, M. (2020). Blockchain in healthcare: Insights on COVID-19. *International Journal of Environmental Research and Public Health, 17*(19), 7167. DOI: 10.3390/ijerph17197167 PMID: 33007951

Ghayvat, H., Zuhair, M., Shukla, N., & Kumar, N. (2023). Healthcare-CT: Solid PoD and Blockchain-Enabled Cyber Twin Approach for Healthcare 5.0 Ecosystems. *IEEE Internet of Things Journal, 11*(4), 6119–6130. DOI: 10.1109/JIOT.2023.3312448

Girardi, F., De Gennaro, G., Colizzi, L., & Convertini, N. (2020). Improving the healthcare effectiveness: The possible role of EHR, IoMT and blockchain. *Electronics (Basel), 9*(6), 884. DOI: 10.3390/electronics9060884

Habib, G., Sharma, S., Ibrahim, S., Ahmad, I., Qureshi, S., & Ishfaq, M. (2022). Blockchain technology: Benefits, challenges, applications, and integration of blockchain technology with cloud computing. *Future Internet, 14*(11), 341. DOI: 10.3390/fi14110341

Hariharan, U., Dhanakoti, V., Rajkumar, K., & Jeyavel, J. (2022, March). Safeguarding e-healthcare documents utilizing an infrastructure for advanced keyless signature infrastructure blockchain within the cloud. In *2022 International Conference on Emerging Smart Computing and Informatics (ESCI)* (pp. 1-6). IEEE. DOI: 10.1109/ESCI53509.2022.9758266

Islayem, R., Musamih, A., Salah, K., Jayaraman, R., & Yaqoob, I. (2025). Enhancing medical digital twins within metaverse using blockchain, NFTs and LLMs. *Internet of Things : Engineering Cyber Physical Human Systems, 32*, 101648. DOI: 10.1016/j.iot.2025.101648

Ismail, L., Materwala, H., & Zeadally, S. (2019). Lightweight blockchain for healthcare. *IEEE Access : Practical Innovations, Open Solutions*, *7*, 149935–149951. DOI: 10.1109/ACCESS.2019.2947613

John Shiny, J. (2024). Innovating Healthcare with Blockchain Technology. *Cybersecurity and Data Management Innovations for Revolutionizing Healthcare*, 240.

Justinia, T. (2019). Blockchain technologies: Opportunities for solving real-world problems in healthcare and biomedical sciences. *Acta Informatica Medica*, *27*(4), 284. DOI: 10.5455/aim.2019.27.284-291 PMID: 32055097

Kassab, M., DeFranco, J., Malas, T., Laplante, P., Destefanis, G., & Neto, V. V. G. (2019). Exploring research in blockchain for healthcare and a roadmap for the future. *IEEE Transactions on Emerging Topics in Computing*, *9*(4), 1835–1852. DOI: 10.1109/TETC.2019.2936881

Katuwal, G. J., Pandey, S., Hennessey, M., & Lamichhane, B. (2018). Applications of blockchain in healthcare: current landscape & challenges. *arXiv preprint arXiv:1812.02776*.

Kerrison, S., Jusak, J., & Huang, T. (2023). Blockchain-enabled IoT for rural healthcare: Hybrid-channel communication with digital twinning. *Electronics (Basel)*, *12*(9), 2128. DOI: 10.3390/electronics12092128

Khezr, S., Moniruzzaman, M., Yassine, A., & Benlamri, R. (2019). Blockchain technology in healthcare: A comprehensive review and directions for future research. *Applied Sciences (Basel, Switzerland)*, *9*(9), 1736. DOI: 10.3390/app9091736

. Khosla, A., Vashist, S., & Nijhawan, G. (2022). Blockchain Technology in Healthcare. *Blockchain, Artificial Intelligence, and the Internet of Things: Possibilities and Opportunities*, 163-185.

Le Nguyen, T. (2018, August). Blockchain in healthcare: A new technology benefit for both patients and doctors. In *2018 Portland International Conference on Management of Engineering and Technology (PICMET)* (pp. 1-6). IEEE. DOI: 10.23919/PICMET.2018.8481969

Pilania, U., Kumar, M., Singh, S., Adhalkha, P., & Satija, T. (2023, December). Securing Confidential Information on WhatsApp with Blockchain Technology. In *International Conference on Advancements in Smart Computing and Information Security* (pp. 53-61). Cham: Springer Nature Switzerland.

Pilania, U., Kumar, M., Tanwar, R., Upadhyay, P., & Narayan, P. (2024). Music DApp on the Solana Blockchain Platform: Design, Development, and Analysis. In *Quantum and Blockchain-based Next Generation Sustainable Computing* (pp. 121–134). Springer Nature Switzerland. DOI: 10.1007/978-3-031-58068-0_6

Pilania, U., Upadhyay, P., Tanwar, R., & Kumar, M. (2023). A creative domain of blockchain application: NFTs. In *Mobile Radio Communications and 5G Networks: Proceedings of Third MRCN 2022* (pp. 397-406). Singapore: Springer Nature Singapore.

Pirtle, C., & Ehrenfeld, J. (2018). Blockchain for healthcare: The next generation of medical records? *Journal of Medical Systems*, *42*(9), 172. DOI: 10.1007/s10916-018-1025-3 PMID: 30097733

Rakic, D. (2018, March). Blockchain Technology in Healthcare. In *ICT4AWE* (pp. 13-20). DOI: 10.5220/0006531600130020

Saranya, R., & Murugan, A. (2023). A systematic review of enabling blockchain in healthcare system: Analysis, current status, challenges and future direction. *Materials Today: Proceedings*, *80*, 3010–3015. DOI: 10.1016/j.matpr.2021.07.105

Satamraju, K. P., & B, M. (2020). Proof of concept of scalable integration of internet of things and blockchain in healthcare. *Sensors (Basel)*, *20*(5), 1389. DOI: 10.3390/s20051389 PMID: 32138380

Singh, A. P., Pradhan, N. R., Luhach, A. K., Agnihotri, S., Jhanjhi, N. Z., Verma, S., Kavita, , Ghosh, U., & Roy, D. S. (2020). A novel patient-centric architectural framework for blockchain-enabled healthcare applications. *IEEE Transactions on Industrial Informatics*, *17*(8), 5779–5789. DOI: 10.1109/TII.2020.3037889

Taherdoost, H. (2023). Privacy and security of blockchain in healthcare: Applications, challenges, and future perspectives. *Sci*, *5*(4), 41. DOI: 10.3390/sci5040041

Taherdoost, H. (2023). Blockchain and healthcare: A critical analysis of progress and challenges in the last five years. *Blockchains*, *1*(2), 73–89. DOI: 10.3390/blockchains1020006

Xu, M., Chen, X., & Kou, G. (2019). A systematic review of blockchain. *Financial Innovation*, *5*(1), 1–14. DOI: 10.1186/s40854-019-0147-z

Yaqoob, I., Salah, K., Uddin, M., Jayaraman, R., Omar, M., & Imran, M. (2020). Blockchain for digital twins: Recent advances and future research challenges. *IEEE Network*, *34*(5), 290–298. DOI: 10.1109/MNET.001.1900661

Yaqoob, S., Khan, M. M., Talib, R., Butt, A. D., Saleem, S., Arif, F., & Nadeem, A. (2019). Use of blockchain in healthcare: A systematic literature review. *International Journal of Advanced Computer Science and Applications*, *10*(5). Advance online publication. DOI: 10.14569/IJACSA.2019.0100581

Zhang, K., Zhou, H. Y., Baptista-Hon, D. T., Gao, Y., Liu, X., Oermann, E., Xu, S., Jin, S., Zhang, J., Sun, Z., Yin, Y., Razmi, R. M., Loupy, A., Beck, S., Qu, J., & Wu, J. (2024). Concepts and applications of digital twins in healthcare and medicine. *Patterns (New York, N.Y.)*, *5*(8), 101028. DOI: 10.1016/j.patter.2024.101028 PMID: 39233690

Chapter 11
Blockchain and Digital Twins for Smart Hospital Infrastructures:
New Roles for Academic, Clinical, and Medical Libraries

Jogen Sharma
http://orcid.org/0000-0001-7151-0137
KIIT (Deemed to be) University, India

ABSTRACT

The digital twin (DT) and blockchain are accelerating the digital transformation in healthcare. DTs provide the ability to develop real-time virtual models of patients, devices and hospital systems for simulation and optimization, while blockchain provides data security and provenance. However, libraries are still the underrepresented subject in such debates in spite of their knowledge in data stewardship, metadata control and digital preservation. This chapter suggests the Blockchain-Digital Twin-Library Integration Model (BDT-LIM), which describes the way libraries can become smart healthcare ecosystem partners. Libraries are able to store documentation under digital twins, metadata provenance, and long-term preservation and adhere to data practices that are in compliance with FAIR and GDPR. This framework transforms about the libraries as a center of ethical governance, through the fusion of library science, health informatics, and emerging technologies, libraries are re-imagined as places where safe, fair, and sustainable healthcare innovation is assured.

DOI: 10.4018/979-8-3373-8177-0.ch011

1. INTRODUCTION

1.1. Context and Significance

The world has never witnessed such pressure on healthcare systems to achieve operational efficiency, greater accuracy in diagnosis and safety, as the volume of complex clinical data continues to swell exponentially. I"nternet of Medical Things (IoMT) as a set of networked medical equipment, biosensors"(Agua & Correia, 2023) and facility management systems produces operating streams of real-time data that the traditional information management techniques can hardly handle. At the same time, new standards of clinical interoperability and regulatory frameworks such as the General Data Protection Regulation (GDPR), the Health Insurance Portability and Accountability Act (HIPAA) and new standards of transparency, auditability and rigor in data governance require unprecedented transparency, auditability and rigor in data governance.

Digital Twin technology can solve the former issue by developing digital simulations of real-life healthcare entities. A "digital twin is an artificial representation that is aligned with the real one in time, allowing for predictive analysis and optimisation of the process"("AI Technologies for Enhancing Recycling Processes," 2025), as well as safe simulation of clinical situations without the intervention of real patients and surgical practice. The healthcare sector of global digital twins market is estimated to grow significantly until 2030, with applications varying in terms of patient-specific treatment planning to predictive maintenance of medical equipment and optimization of hospital workflow processes.

Blockchain technology can support governance and auditing requirements by offering permanently written and cryptographically verified data on the provenance of information, ensuring that each operation or change in healthcare information systems is permanently recorded and verifiable. Contrary to traditional centralised databases, which can be easily tampered with or modified by an unauthorised entity, the distributed consensus mechanisms in blockchain form a network of systems that cannot easily fail or be altered by a third party.

Nevertheless, both technologies are not entirely the solution to the complex issues of healthcare information management. "Digital twins bring with them unheard-of amounts of data that necessitate discovery systems, memory policies and control systems"(Bhattacharya et al., 2024). Although blockchain provides certain immutability, it generates some new challenges in terms of how data can be organized, meaningfully searched and retrieved and long-term kept. Such combinations of technologies form an information ecosystem that demands the advanced data management, metadata standardization, ethical governance and institutional stewardship systems-exactly the capabilities that libraries have honed over centuries.

1.2. Research Motivation and Problem Statement

Although there is a growing pace in the adoption of digital twins and blockchain technology in healthcare contexts, libraries have been marginally involved in the strategic discourse of their adoption, governance and long-term information stewardship. This peripheralization is an indication of technological specialisation in the healthcare IT departments and a broader sense that the traditional library's functions are no longer relevant in the new areas of technology. As a consequence, the value of libraries as neutral and trusted data intermediaries that can be leveraged to ensure compliance with FAIR (Findable, Accessible, Interoperable, Reusable) data principles, build consistent metadata standards, create adequate digital preservation infrastructure and enable reproducible healthcare research is often ignored during the introduction of the smart hospital.

There are unique gaps in existing innovative hospital models:

(1) Lack of specified roles in information professionals to handle digital twins artifacts and blockchain-based datasets;
(2) The siloing of healthcare data across institutional boundaries, impairs both discoverability and interoperability;
(3) Inadequate metadata and provenance documentation models to digital twins records and blockchain transactions;
(4) Poor long-term preservation policies to support dynamic simulation environments, machine learning models and continuously changing clinical data; and
(5) Poorly defined governance frameworks to provide ethical accountability and compliance responsibility in data steward.

The solution to those gaps requires Library and Information science (LIS) practitioners to develop combination of technical, ethical and organizational skills that will allow libraries to become active strategic participants of smart hospital infrastructure, as opposed to service providers at the margins.

2. LITERATURE REVIEW

2.1. Blockchain and Digital Twins in Health Transformation

Recent entries in Elsevier's Encyclopedia of Operations and Supply Chain Management (Petropoulos et al., 2025) provide such an overview on the trajectory transformation of operations and supply chain management in data-rich environments, adopting artificial intelligence (AI), blockchain and digital twins. These together lend towards organisational resilience, traceability and efficiency in several business verticals including healthcare. The review draws attention to predictive digital modeling and secure data provenance as key pillars of next-generation healthcare systems (Petropoulos et al., 2025).

Monlezun (2025) expands upon this discourse in his ground-breaking work Quantum Health **AI:** The Revolution of Medicine,Public Healthl and Global Health by Elsevier. He explains that the convergence of quantum computing, blockchain and AI will revolutionize healthcare governance and ethics. The book provides a human-focused perspective to the use of technology, with emphasis on the trade-off between privacy, data sovereignty and equal access to healthcare. Underpinning Monlezun's vision of "Quantum AI" is blockchain as an ethical guard rail in digital environments that guarantees traceability, visibility and consent validation with the use of patient data.

Similarly, Oke et al. (2025) Smart Materials and Energy in the Fourth Industrial Revolution (CRC Press), authors position blockchain and smart materials as enablers of sustainable innovation, where smart materials and blockchain are predicted to act as the primary disruptive technology. While the book's emphasis is on material science and energy, it highlights how distributed digital systems[i] such as blockchain are central to maintaining data integrity, lifecycle tracking and responsible automation for smart infrastructure — including healthcare facilities. Collectively, these studies confirm their interdisciplinary implications of blockchain and digital twin in the shaping of smart and sustainable healthcare infrastructures.

2.2. Digital Twins (Simulation, Optimization and Predictive Analytics)

Digital twin (DT) technology matured from the field of industrial usage toward healthcare realm and has been already put into practice for real-time simulation, prediction of patients, medical devices, hospitals. In the Blockchain and Digital Twins for Smart Hospital Infrastructures chapter (Sharma, 2025), DTs allow health institutions to duplicate patient physiology and treatment pathways so as to improve clinical decision making and operational efficiency. These models are further updated with data collected from the Internet of Medical Things (IoMT), electronic health records (EHRs) and biosensors.

Kordi and Weissense (25), for example, propose that the DT framework, through convergence with sustainable AI, can facilitate "synchronous models of digital objects" of healthcare actors- enabling operational foresight and decreased costs. Physicians can simulate patient reactions to treatments or surgeries, which minimizes risks and improves treatment efficiency. Hariyani (2025) and Mehra & Kumar (2025) emphasise that these virtual simulations environments are personalising the onset of personalised medicine, enabling clinicians to pre-test treatment options on patient specific digital twins.

The healthcare digital twin market[mdash]detailing in the recent literature, predicts that by 2030 it will grow tremendously because of its predictive maintenance, workflow management and ongoing clinical monitoring applications (Liu et al., 2025). AI, along with data visualization tools, accelerate this growth as they provide health practitioners with easy to understand patient modelling and outcome prediction dashboards.

2.3. Blockchain (Provenance, Governance and Ethical Consideration of Data)

Thanks to cryptographic consensus, blockchain technology guarantees medical data transactions cannot be tampered with or hidden, ensuring their immutable, transparent and originating nature (Ortiz-Rod et al., 2025). Sharma (2025) elaborates that blockchain can protect health information systems by logging all alterations to patient records, treatment authorizations, and digital twin updates in tamper-evident ledgers. This enduring record increases accountability and follows international data protection practices, including GDPR and HIPAA.

Resilient against unauthorized data modifications and cyber-attacks; Mim (2025) and Singh et al. (2025) highlights that the decentralized nature of blockchai provides resistance to unauthorized data alterations while offering security from digital health challenges. In permissioned blockchains (e.g., Hyperledger Fabric), institutional participants maintain control over access rights, that is, they protect sensitive patient data and goods can still be auditable shared among stakeholders.

In addition, smart contracts based on blockchain technology have proved very valuable in consent management for clinical research. As demonstrated by Sharma (2025) such self-enforcing agreements can program data access, and guarantee that patient consent directives are adhered to exactly. This is especially at play in the context of multi-institution precision medicine research, where Stacks serves as an interface between data from digital twins, genomic records and clinical trials.

2.4. Blockchain and Digital Twins

The blockchain-digital twin-library integration model (BDT-LIM) proposed by Sharma (2025), its six layers covers the digital twin data along with the provenance potential of Block chain which is managed by academic and medical libraries. The model is comprised of (1) a data source layer, (2) a digital twin layer, (3) a blockchain layer, (4) the library repository layers as illustrated above and also further where required, libraries for identitifiers or trees on which models can be estimated), (5) an access and visualization layer by one or more users in need of the model derived information provided at run time and 6. A governance layer.

As the trusted information steward, libraries are expected to oversee digital twin metadata, housing model parameters and long-term digital preservation according to FAIR (Findable, Accessible, Interoperable and Reusable) principles. This entanglement establishes libraries as hub nodes of smart hospital infrastructures serving the purposes of data integrity, reproducibility and ethical governance. The model's novel method of combining established information science with new clinical informatics is concurrent with the areas for future work proposed by Petropoulos et al. (2025) and Monlezun (2025).

With the application of this model, secure interworking between IoMT devices and access to blockchain records, as well as digital twins simulating their behaviour in the context of healthcare will be enabled. It also provides a strong footing for compliance auditing, predictive analytics and AI-driven decision support.

2.5. Library Science and Medical Data Guardianship

The re-purposing of academic, clinical and medical libraries as data governance centres is consistent with the FAIR Principles and the Open Archival Information System (OAIS Reference Model) (Sharma, 2025). Libraries have a historical knowledge of metadata management and a history of preservation and ethical data treatment – all essential competencies for digital health stewardship. Metadata standards for digital twin artifacts and blockchain transactions such as Dublin Core, PREMIS and FHIR can allow libraries to provide extensive documentation about these (and resources derived from them), including chain of custody information.

Sharma (2025) prescribe, that libraries are responsible for version control and provenance tracking of continuously updated healthcare datasets and archival storage. These—including classical library functions—extend librarian activities into health informatics and information technology ethics. Furthermore, libraries will also be education centers for reading literacy among clinicians and researchers as part of responsible use of technology and decision-making.

2.6. Ethical, Legal and Technical Challenges

Nevertheless, the coalescence of blockchain and digital twins in healthcare carries tremendous ethical, technical and legal challenges. Sharma (2025) points to tensions between the immutability of blockchain and the GDPR "right to be forgotten." Correcting the wrong information in medical records which have been written on unchangeable blockchains is still a challenging problem, yet privacy-preserving cryptographic techniques such as zero knowledge proofs present partial solutions.

Also, smart contract based systems are opaque so it is not clear whom to hold accountable. New liability rules are need for algorithmic errors in automated data access decisions (Zhan et al., 2024). Further, cultural and organizational barriers stymie library participation in health IT governance, requiring efforts for librarians to develop capacities (and relationships) with clinical, administrative rooms and specialists beds.

2.7. Future Directions

New research indicates that the future of smart hospitals will rely on blockchain-DT convergence to achieve secure interoperability, ethical AI implementation and data-heavy innovation (Faizan, 2025; Wickrama, 2025). Sharma (2025) demands more investigation into the effects library participation in healthcare governance has on clinical quality, data protection and patient safety.

The governance infrastructure that will enable interoperability across these digital health platforms is still lacking, so adopting technologies from global institutions (e.g., Mayo Clinic) who are also testing blockchain into digital health platforms with incorporated ethical oversight and prohibiting ERP use for data model or integrity remain important to consider alongside any academic library support for the metadata and data stewardship (Monlezun, 2025). These changes represent a real paradigm shift for libraries; from passive repositories to active participants in ethical digital transformation.

3. DIGITAL TWINS AND BLOCKCHAIN

3.1. Digital Twins in Healthcare

Digital Twin technology generates replicated virtual representations of physical objects by establishing real-time data compatibility to allow the constant monitoring, simulation and optimization of physical objects. Digital twins can be used at various levels in a healthcare setting, patient-level twins that use genomic data, medical imaging and physiological monitoring; device-level twins that monitor the work of medical equipment and maintenance timeframes; and facility-level twins that optimize the workflow of hospitals, the allocation of resources and the performance of infrastructure.

Patient digital twins are one of the most critical fields, producing whole-body computational models that incorporate clinical history, genetic profiles, imaging, physiological responses and treatment outcomes. These models enable clinicians to replicate treatment scenarios, predict reactions to interventions and tailor treatment methods, ultimately allowing them to apply clinical procedures effectively. A digital twin of a patient undergoing a complicated cancer treatment could include tumour features, genetic mutations, organ functional indicators and previous drug reactions and would allow clinicians to simulate various chemotherapy regimens and choose the most likely one that would work and produce the least adverse reaction.

Digital twins at the device level address the fundamental challenges of predictive maintenance for medical devices. Digital twins enable facilities to shift toward condition-based maintenance by continuously observing sensor data from diagnostic imaging equipment, ventilators, monitors and other clinical equipment, rather than relying on failure-based maintenance. This feature minimises unexpected downtime and extends the equipment's lifespan, preventing clinical emergencies in the event of equipment failures.

“Digital twins at the facility level combine data on building management systems, room occupancy sensors, equipment position sensors and workflows to streamline hospital operations”(Agua & Correia, 2023). These systems will be able to detect ineffective patterns of patient flow, forecast resource bottlenecks during high-utilisation periods and enable facilities to be dynamically reconfigured when clinical requirements change.

3.2. Health Care and the Blockchain Technology

Blockchain is a distributed registry technology that provides security, immutability, transparency and auditability of documented transactions through cryptographic means and consensus protocols. The Pandian application of blockchain technology in healthcare offers solutions to some of the most severe governance issues, namely establishing permanent and irrevocable records of data provenance, documenting all the history of data changes, access events and clinical interventions.

Permissioned blockchain architecture implementations in healthcare utilise permissioned architecture system design models, such as Hyperledger Fabric, where institutions gain control over network access and transaction visibility. In contrast to public blockchains, permissioned healthcare systems offer the capability to preserve privacy while promoting auditability, allowing clinical institutions to ensure that sensitive patient information remains confidential without compromising records of who has viewed what data and when.

Blockchain medical uses are:

(1) Safe storage and sharing of electronic health records with provenance recordings;

(2) Management of drug chains, preventing counterfeit drugs and ensuring authentic sourcing of drugs;
(3) Automated consent control with smart contract signatures, recording that a patient has authorised the use of their data;
(4) Data on clinical trials, with tamper-evident records, guaranteeing research integrity; and
(5) Credentialing of healthcare professionals and researchers.

3.3. Technological Integration

Complementary capabilities are developed by integrating digital twins and blockchain technology. Digital twins produce continuous clinical and operational data that needs advanced management processes. Each update in the digital twin, model change and access is ensured to be permanently stored with complete provenance information by blockchain. It is through this integration that healthcare systems can leverage the capabilities of digital twins to simulate and optimise the system, alongside the auditability and governance advantages provided by blockchain, to build information ecosystems that enable clinical innovation and regulatory compliance.

As an illustration, a patient receiving cancer treatment with a digital twin model has the advantage of a blockchain-guaranteed record of all model changes, clinical determinations driven by the model, clinical outcomes and the utilisation of anonymised data for investigation. Such unification enables clinicians to trust the model recommendation due to its established previous performance, provides regulatory compliance through verified, tamper-evident provenance records and facilitates the research of precision medicine by allowing data to be shared safely and auditably.

4. INTELLIGENT HOSPITAL INFRASTRUCTURES (DATA-INTENSIVE HEALTH CARE ECOSYSTEMS)

4.1. Healthcare Data Generation and IoMT

The Internet of Medical Things is an Internet network comprising thousands of interconnected biomedical devices, environmental sensors and facility management systems that generate continuous clinical and operational data. "Contemporary intensive care settings feature numerous patient monitors, ventilators, infusion pumps"(Bhattacharya et al., 2024) and environmental sensors that create a multitude of data points every second. Diagnostic images generate terabytes of pictures in the imaging departments. Electronic health record systems store decades of structured clinical information, unstructured clinical documentation and multimedia materials.

The data contained in these various sources is synthesised into an information ecosystem by smart hospital infrastructures. A "smart hospital may combine information from thousands of networked devices, facility management systems"(Doss et al., 2024), electronic health records, laboratory information systems, pharmacy systems and administrative databases to create a comprehensive view of patient care. This integration of data enables previously unattainable operational transparency, real-time monitoring of patient whereabouts, equipment position, staffing and supply levels; predictive capacity control based on demand spikes; and real-time clinical decision support.

4.2. Data Governance and Regulatory Requirements

This information volume is accompanied by enhanced regulatory oversight and patient privacy protections. Under the General Data Protection Regulation (GDPR), transparency in data processing is compulsory, meaning that all organisations must record the reasons, legal grounds and steps taken for processing all personal information. Article 25 GDPR establishes data protection by design and by default; organisations must ensure that they design privacy-protective features into their systems, not after the fact. The HIPAA Security and Privacy Rules provide similar requirements in the USA; however, new standards, such as the International Organisation for Standardisation (ISO) 27001 for information security management, define the global governance.

The implementation of smart hospitals must address conflicting requirements simultaneously, producing the data integration and analytics functionality needed for clinical and operational optimisation, while adhering to privacy policies, safeguarding against advanced cyber attacks and maintaining patient confidence. This conflict presents a strategic opportunity for library involvement, libraries can act as neutral, trusted mediators who facilitate compliance while also allowing the proper use of data.

5. THEORETICAL FRAMEWORK (LIBRARIES AS PARTNERS IN DATA STEWARDSHIP)

5.1. Evolution of Library Roles Through History

Libraries are no longer (just) physical collections of print; they have become complex information infrastructure organisations that handle various types of digital resources, research data, institutional knowledge and complex metadata ecologies. This development suggests fundamental changes in the generation, storage and utilisation of knowledge. Contemporary academic libraries support institutional repositories that archive research outputs, offer research data management services to ensure adherence to agency requirements, support digital collections that preserve culture, and, to a growing extent, provide data literacy training to enable researchers to manage their own information holdings.

This historical trend demonstrates that libraries can adapt to changes in technology while retaining essential functions, including the integrity of information, equitable access, a knowledge repository that can be tapped and reused by new generations and the discovery and reuse of knowledge. Such core capabilities are naturally evolved into intelligent healthcare systems.

5.2. FAIR Data Principles and Library Stewardship

The data principles of FAIR Findable, Accessible, Interoperable and Reusable have been accepted as the common ground for responsible data management of research and clinical data governance. "FAIR principles are the result of an international collaboration of researchers"(Doss et al., 2024) and institutions that state the principle that research data are easily discoverable using metadata and unique persistent identifiers; are available using well-documented access protocols and authentications; are described using a standard metadata allowing easy integration with other datasets; and are available on explicitly specified conditions and licensing terms.

Libraries have long practised these principles in terms of metadata standardisation, digital preservation and access management. To implement the principles of FAIR in smart hospital data, the competencies that are already established as library principles must be applied to healthcare information governance. "Libraries can develop long-lasting identifier systems for digital twin artefacts, create metadata models that record the features and origin of information for models, deploy access control systems"(Gunjal et al., 2024) that consider patient privacy and permit suitable research activities and ensure the long-term preservation and discovery of healthcare information resources.

5.3. Blockchain-Digital Twin-Library Integration Model (BDT-LIM)

In this chapter, the author suggests the Blockchain-Digital Twin-Library Integration Model (BDT-LIM). This theoretical and practical framework can make libraries the focal point of intelligent information ecosystems in hospitals. The BDT-LIM is covered with six layers, which are interconnected;

Data Source Layer:

This layer includes the Internet of Medical Things, electronic health record systems, laboratory information systems, imaging archives, facility management systems and administrative databases that produce raw clinical and operational data.

Digital Twin Layer:

Generates real-time virtual representations of patients, medical devices, clinical processes and facility systems. At this level, digital twins produce continuous simulation outcomes, model parameters and prediction outputs.

Blockchain Layer:

Stores unaltered, time-proven records of digital twin updates, model changes, access, consent authorisations and clinical decisions based on digital twin predictions. The blockchain serves as a record of all activities within the information system, allowing for transparent and auditable transactions.

Library Repository Layer:

Digital twins, including model definitions, training data, parameter sets, simulated output and other related metadata, are stored in institutional repositories (e.g., DSpace, Dataverse, or specialised healthcare data repositories). The repository layer keeps versioning records, performs backup and recovery roles and preserves archived digital twin models on a long-term basis.

Access and Visualisation Layer:

Library portals and clinical information systems provide user interfaces that enable researchers, clinicians and administrators to discover, access and visualise data from digital twins. This layer combines metadata search, analysis dashboards, digital twin visualisations and compliance checking features to ensure that a user can access only the data to which they have been authorised.

Governance Layer:

Policies are developed by interprofessional committees comprising medical librarians, health informaticists, clinicians, privacy officers, compliance specialists and patients, which govern data stewardship, retention schedules, ethical policies in model development and accountability mechanisms. Libraries offer organisational and analytical skills in supporting the governance process.

6. NEW LIBRARY FUNCTIONS IN SMART HOSPITAL ECOSYSTEMS

6.1. Data Stewardship of Digital Twins

Medical librarians may assume the primary responsibility of managing digital twin artefacts, much like library curators do with research data.

Such stewardship involves:

(1) Institutional documentation policies and standards on digital twins;
(2) Metadata schema of the characteristics of model, data sources, parameter specifications, validation results and clinical applications;
(3) Version control and change management systems, which track the evolution of the model; (4) Backup and recovery procedures, which maintain business continuity;
(4) Enforced retention schedules, balancing clinical needs, regulatory requirements and resource limitations.

Digital twin stewardship differs from traditional library data management due to the dynamism of the models. Digital twins are dynamic, contrasting with the experience of currently available data, as new training data allows model parameters to be adjusted and clinical validation outcomes to be accrued. To address this evolution, librarians need to develop new methods for tracking the provenance of models and archiving versions, enabling others to reproduce and comply with regulations.

6.2. Metadata and Provenance Management

Libraries are capable of defining the metadata standards and provenance documentation models necessary for interoperable digital twin-blockchain environments. This involves modifying the existing metadata standards, such as Dublin Core (which describes core metadata and captures descriptive attributes), PREMIS (a standard for recording digital preservation activities) and FHIR (Fast Healthcare Interoperability Resources, a standard for clinical data exchange).

Metadata schema Library metadata professionals may build a domain-specific metadata schema that reflects the peculiarities of healthcare information systems. "Metadata in the case of digital twin models may include; model type and purpose, clinical use, data sources and integration approaches, validation and accuracy metrics"(Hariyani et al., 2025), model parameters and configuration, licensing and copyright data, access control and regulatory compliance measures and links to other institutional assets.

“The integration of blockchain enables libraries to associate metadata records with theoretical transaction logs. Instead of simply storing metadata about digital twin models and placing the metadata in institutional databases”(Gunjal et al., 2024), libraries may store metadata updates on permissioned healthcare blockchains and generate tamper-evident provenance trails, indicating when metadata was generated, by whom and any subsequent modifications made. This solution combines the metadata knowledge of libraries with the auditability of blockchain, enabling clinicians to verify that digital twin records have not been altered secretly.

6.3. Digital Preservation of Assets in the Healthcare Information

Digital twin artefacts, blockchain records and related healthcare datasets that require long-term preservation pose a major stewardship issue, which libraries are well-positioned to address. The Open Archival Information System (OAIS) reference model, which emerged from decades of library and archival practice, provides a framework for systematic digital preservation that can be applied to healthcare information systems.

OAIS confirms that preserving information involves more than just maintaining duplicate copies of digital information. Preservation requires that institutions record preservation plans, have format migration strategies to avoid technological obsolescence, maintain precise metadata to facilitate future discoveries and comprehension and establish governance mechanisms that ensure preservation work will persist even when changes occur within an organisation.

The implementation of OAIS principles to healthcare information involves overcoming peculiarities of healthcare information:

(1) dynamically growing information streams, but not static archival collections;
(2) intricate interdependence of digital twin models, training sets and blockchain logs that need to be kept together;
(3) regulatory issues that define the need to retain information and maintain access control; and
(4) the necessity to preserve not only final datasets, but also detailed audit trails of how these data were processed, modified and accessed.

Libraries may establish dedicated digital preservation infrastructure for healthcare information, including redundant storage systems that are geographically dispersed to eliminate single points of failure, format migration policies that enable digital twin models to remain executable in the face of evolving technology and preservation documentation that allows institutions to demonstrate regulatory adherence.

Within the realm of governance, the company has implemented a system of checks and balances that does not rely on personal favour when executing certain decisions.<|human|>In the area of governance, the company has established a checks and balances system that does not depend on individual favour in implementing a particular decision.

The analytical and organisational capacity that underpins the ethical governance of innovative hospital information systems can be offered by libraries. "Policies and procedures to solve recurring governance dilemmas can be developed by medical librarians"(Agua & Correia, 2023), with support of privacy officers, compliance experts and institutional review boards; making sure that the increased availability of data does not compromise patient privacy; ensuring that there is a straightforward process of authorization of data use in research and clinical decision support; ensuring that the diverse populations are represented equally in the training data of digital twins.

With the help of blockchain technology, it is possible to introduce new styles of consent management through the use of smart contracts and self-executing programs that undertake specific actions when pre-established conditions are met. A patient with cancer who is being treated using a model of a digital twin could grant the research access to their anonymised treatment outcome data, but only to cancer-specific applications created by a non-profit research institution. These complex authorisation constraints can be imposed using a blockchain-based smart contract, which then provides an automatic response to an access request based on documented patterns of use and institutional membership.

Libraries can collaborate with governance bodies to create consent management models, content explaining to patients how digital twin models will utilise their clinical data and audit processes that record whether consent directions are being adhered to. This role of governance involves the continuity of traditional information stewardship in libraries into the realms of ethics and law.

6.4. Capacity Building and Information Literacy

Medical librarians are in a position to create and present educational initiatives that will enable healthcare professionals and researchers to acquire competency with new technologies. This encompasses official training on the basics of blockchain, on digital twin, on FAIR data, on data provenance documentation, on innovative hospital ecosystem architecture; unofficial training through library reference services that attend to questions about implementation; development of teaching materials in the form of user manuals, workflow documentation and case studies of best practices.

As digital twin predictions become increasingly used by clinical staff to inform treatment decisions, it is essential to ensure that they are aware of the potential and limitations of these models. Training modules that librarians can create include; how digital twins are trained and validated, confidence intervals and prediction uncertainty, the sources of bias in the training data and what model outputs indicate in clinical settings.

7. TECHNICAL IMPLEMENTATION (METADATA STANDARDS AND ONTOLOGIES)

7.1. Metadata Standards incorporation in Healthcare

The BDT-LIM implementation necessitates the incorporation of various already established metadata standards across the library science, healthcare informatics and information technology sectors. Dublin Core offers a basic metadata suite of fifteen elements (creator, title, description, subject, publisher, contributor, date, type, format, identifier, source, language, relation, coverage and rights) that can be used in the majority of digital resources, including digital twin models.

PREMIS (Preservation Metadata;Implementation Strategies) builds on this basis with domain-specific digital preservation metadata, recording:

(1) environment metadata of hardware and software to retain the functionality of digital objects;
(2) fixity metadata of checksums and cryptographic hashes to indicate that the digital object has not been corrupted or tampered with by unauthorised individuals;
(3) rights metadata of copyright, licensing and access restrictions; and
(4) provenance metadata of the chain of custody of the digital object since its creation to the time of preservation.

The FHIR (Fast Healthcare Interoperability Resources) is a set of clinical information exchange standard data models created by the healthcare informatics community worldwide. FHIR allows healthcare systems to exchange data on structured clinical information (patient demographics, diagnoses, medication lists and lab results) in the standardised formats that foster interoperability with various healthcare information systems.

A generalised digital twin metadata schema incorporates all three standards; Dublin Core is used to describe the resources on a general level, PREMIS is used to enforce preservation and authenticity standards and FHIR is used to facilitate integration with other healthcare information systems. Other domain-specific features represent digital twin-specific aspects, including model type and clinical use, composition and quality measures of training data, validation outcomes and accuracy tolerance, parameter description and sensitivity analysis and interaction with patients, devices, or clinical processes under modelling.

7.2. Provenance Records That are Anchored With Blockchain

The concept of blockchain technology will help libraries to generate unchangeable provenance records of healthcare data. Instead of keeping provenance records in conventional databases, which may be deleted or altered, libraries can keep provenance records in authorised healthcare blockchains, which produce tamper-evident logs of transactions.

Upon a medical librarian being provided with a new digital twin model to be archived, the library can:

(1) allocate a persistent identifier (e.g., a URI with the Handle System or Digital Object Identifier);
(2) harvest descriptive and preservation metadata;
(3) perform file fixity checks by creating cryptographic checksums, and
(4) log a blockchain transaction to record receipt of the model, metadata components, checksums and access controls.

This blockchain entry can serve as a permanent record of a model's state, ensuring that subsequent audits can verify that archived models have not been altered surreptitiously.

As a clinician later retrieves the archived model to apply it in clinical practice, the blockchain logs the access event, such as time, user identity, clinical intent and accessed data. Over time, a comprehensive audit trail will be established to track all interactions with the archived digital twin models, which will, in turn, enable institutional compliance officers to demonstrate that they were using the models in accordance with regulatory standards. This will also facilitate future researchers' understanding of how the models were applied to clinical practice.

8. CASE STUDIES (SMART HOSPITAL IMPLEMENTATION, SMITH LIBRARY)

8.1. Academic Medical Centre, E.g. Mayo Clinic Platform Initiatives

The Mayo Clinic is a prime example of institutional commitment to advanced healthcare infrastructure. Integrated clinical data can be utilised to support patients and inform health research. The Mayo Clinic Platform, launched in 2023 and recently expanded with the Platform Insights suite, is a demonstration of how such data can be utilised. The Mayo Clinic Platform is an online platform that enables patients, medical service providers, health researchers and health innovators to share clinical data and collaborate on tools.

Medical institutions with libraries, such as Mayo Clinic, can integrate institutional repository systems to include digital twin objects and blockchain entries. "The medical library can assume the role of the institutional custodian of research data created as a result of innovative hospital programs(Agua & Correia, 2023), ensuring that research ethics considerations, funding body requirements and regulations are met.

An actual example: scientists in a university medical school create digital twins that forecast how patients will react to a new immunotherapy treatment plan against melanoma. The electronic twins combine genomics, imaging properties, previous treatment results and physiological values to forecast complete reaction, partial reaction, or progression in the disease.

The medical librarian collaborates with the research team to:

(1) create detailed metadata of the model architecture, training data sources, validation methods and clinical uses;
(2) blockchain record of model development milestones and clinical validation successes;
(3) set up a policy of consent management specifying which patients have approved research use of their data to which applications; and
(4) store the model, training data and metadata on the institutional repository with verified access controls using blockchain signing.

When researchers need to use the model in future studies, the library can automatically ensure that the institutional membership and purpose of the research meet record consent criteria and access is either granted or denied through the enforcement of smart contracts. This model will bring together the old-time data stewardship in libraries with the governance features of blockchain.

8.2. Intelligent Hospital Workflow Optimisation (Digital Twin App)

Another area where library-enabled digital twins add value is the optimisation of hospital workflow. A central urban hospital system may build a facility-level digital twin that provides real-time information about patient locations, equipment availability, staffing status and the volume of clinical work. By using these digital twins, bottlenecks in the resource can be predicted, allowing staff to be positioned in advance and equipment to be prepared.

Medical librarians can contribute to this effort by:

(1) developing standardized metadata of workflow data sources, so that data in one hospital part of a hospital uses the same terminology as data in another part and has the same measurement strategies;
(2) recording the data flows that feed digital twin models, so that an audit officer can determine that data collection was being done in compliance with privacy requirements; and
(3) recording historical snapshots of digital twins, so that retrospective analyses can be conducted on how workflow optimization initiatives have impacted patient flow, staff utilization and equipment down-time.

Libraries can enable hospitals to demonstrate that workflow optimisation decisions are based on evidence provided by digital twin predictions, rather than arbitrary administrative choices. This is an increasingly valuable aspect of healthcare organisations, as they become more open to regulatory oversight and must justify their resource allocation decisions.

8.3. Precision Medicine Initiatives (Clinical Research Data Management)

The study of precision medicine integrates the use of digital twins, genomic data, imaging features and clinical outcomes to create individualised treatment plans. A "research consortium involved in the development of new cancer therapeutics creates digital twins for every patient in a clinical trial"(Hariyani et al., 2025), which include tumour genomic profiling, imaging features, baseline organ functional condition and response to treatment data.

The medical librarians will be able to control the research data produced by this initiative:

(1) clear data governance policies about which institutional researchers should have access to each patient data under what circumstances;
(2) audit trails, which will record access to patient digital twins by research teams;
(3) blockchain recording of consent authorizations to ensure that each research use of patient data adheres to documented patient preferences; and
(4) final research datasets with full metadata that other researchers can use to conduct meta-analyses that combine the results of multiple research studies.

Such library stewardship will enhance the transparency of research, facilitate compliance with regulations and provide opportunities to reuse data in various research projects, advancing the precision medicine research agenda while ensuring patient privacy and integrity in data governance.

9. DIFFICULTIES AND OBSTACLES TO IMPLEMENTATION

9.1. Technological Integration Problems

The integration of blockchain and digital twin technologies into current healthcare information systems is a complex technical task. "Healthcare organisations typically have decades of data legacy information systems with different data formats, access methods and security designs"(Konopik, 2023). To build cohesive digital twin-blockchain ecosystems, there is a need to bridge these technological silos with middleware layers, which may or may not exist and may require significant custom development.

Another technical limitation is blockchain scalability. Public blockchains, such as Bitcoin and Ethereum, face the problem of transaction throughput, which limits the number of transactions they can handle per second. Permitted healthcare blockchains are more scalable, but they also require a demanding architecture to support the large volumes of transactions that healthcare systems generate.

Technical requirements with data privacy have conflicting demands. The inherent property of blockchain, namely the immutable and distributed register, appears to be at odds with the principle of GDPR, which stipulates that the right to be forgotten requires companies to delete personal data upon a customer's request. Medical blockchains must introduce specific privacy-preserving measures, such as confidential transactions (where transaction values are encrypted to allow blockchain validators access only to the transactions and not the actual values) and zero-knowledge proofs (where transactions comply with the rules). The adoption of such advanced privacy technologies would require specialised skills that are not always present in the information technology departments of healthcare institutions.

9.2. Organisation and Culture Obstacles

There are significant organisational obstacles to implementing library-led initiatives in smart hospitals. Medical organisations have established systems of governance, budgetary processes and professional spaces. Although medical libraries are professional healthcare bodies, they tend to hold marginal roles within hospital governance systems compared to clinical, nursing and information technology management teams.

The implementation of library involvement in key governance processes will require change management within the organisation, the development of relationships between librarians and clinical leadership and the ability to realise tangible value that library involvement will bring. Such cultural change extends beyond technical implementation to encompass professional recognition and resource allocation.

Additionally, a significant portion of medical librarians lack technical expertise in blockchain, developing digital twins and healthcare system architecture. To achieve institutional capacity, professional development activities, training and recruitment of librarians possessing specialised skills will become important.

9.3 Ethical and Legal Complexities

This relates to moral considerations and legal challenges encountered in the work of product design teams. Ethical and Legal Complexities, this deals with both ethical factors and legal aspects of the work of product design teams.

The impossibility of altering blockchain data poses ethical dilemmas regarding the deletion and editing of data. In cases where patient data errors occur, such as incorrect medication allergy information, incorrect procedures and incorrectly recorded comorbidities, it is technically challenging to make the necessary corrections on immutable blockchains. Although new transactions can correct previous mistakes, the incorrect initial data remains visible forever, which may lead to confusion and breach patient privacy principles.

Accountability in intelligent contract automation is a problem. In the case where the automatic access to data is provided or denied in accordance with the programmed rules and smart contracts are used, who will be to blame in case of bugs or unfair decisions by a smart contract? The existing laws were designed based on human decision-makers, not on algorithms that make consequential healthcare decisions. Setting up effective accountability processes is an undecided issue.

When data is used in sophisticated ways, the complexity of consent management grows significantly. When a patient signs a traditional consent form that refers to the concept of medical research, they are often left uncertain about what the consent covers explicitly in a given research study. As digital twin models are created to incorporate patient data into constantly evolving applications, such as cancer treatment prediction, drug interaction prediction and insurance underwriting, it becomes increasingly challenging to ensure that consent is valid and effective.

10. POLICY RECOMMENDATION AND BEST PRACTICE

10.1. Metadata Standards Adoption and Extension

FHIR should be utilised by healthcare institutions as a standard for clinical metadata, with domain-specific elements that describe digital twin and blockchain-specific information added to it. Metadata standards specifically targeted at digital twin-blockchain healthcare systems should be jointly developed and promoted by professional organisations, such as the American Medical Informatics Association (AMIA), the Medical Library Association (MLA) and the Healthcare Information and Management Systems Society (HIMSS).

Metadata governance committees should be established in institutions with expertise in library science, health informatics, healthcare IT and clinical leadership, as well as patient representatives. These committees are expected to establish institutional metadata standards, regularly audit the quality of metadata and update standards based on implementation experience.

10.2. Guidelines on Implementing Blockchain

Permissioned blockchains (e.g., Hyperledger Fabric) should be adopted in healthcare facilities instead of public blockchains when using sensitive healthcare applications. Permissioned architectures also allow institutions to manage network membership, limit transaction visibility to authorised parties and introduce forms of privacy protection that are not provided by public blockchains.

Institutions should not assume that blockchain can be a comprehensive solution to the problem of healthcare governance. The strengths of blockchain, such as the generation of audit trails that cannot be altered and resistance to centralised alterations, are a solution to particular governance-related issues; however, it does not significantly address more general data management, ethical governance and clinical decision-making problems. The use of blockchains should be driven by specific governance needs, rather than the novelty of the technology.

10.3. Digital Preservation Infrastructure Investment

Healthcare facilities should provide specialised digital preservation facilities that offer long-term support for digital twin artefacts, blockchain records and supporting healthcare data.

This should be invested in:

(1) geographically diversified redundant storage systems that eliminate single points of failure;
(2) format migration plans that ensure that digital twin models are deployable regardless of software changes;
(3) preservation metadata that makes it possible to future understand and discover archived materials; and
(4) periodic integrity checks that will ensure that archived digital files have not been corrupted.

Digital preservation should be expanded by the Association of Canadian University Libraries, the Digital Preservation Network and others through specialised digital preservation services tailored specifically to healthcare institutions. Healthcare organisations often lack the resources to support a standalone digital preservation infrastructure; shared service models may be more cost-effective and deliver trusted preservation services.

10.4. Workforce Development and Training

Digital health and blockchain basics, alongside healthcare informatics, should be included in the basic curricula of professional education programs in Library and Information Science. Librarians can be trained to become leaders in innovative hospital ecosystems through specialised graduate certificates or concentrations in health data science and digital health informatics.

Medical schools should establish internal training programs to help existing library personnel acquire competency in new technologies. Mentorships between librarians and informatics experts, health IT professionals and clinical researchers facilitate knowledge exchange and enhance organisational capacity.

11. FUTURE RESEARCH AGENDA

11.1. Empirical Implementation Studies

Strict empirical studies that record library-driven innovative hospital applications are still necessary.

The research questions that implementation studies should address include:

(1) the impact of library involvement in governance on the outcomes of healthcare systems such as clinical quality, operational efficiency and patient safety;

(2) what obstacles limit library involvement in healthcare technology leadership and how organizations can overcome the same;
(3) how medical librarians can competently develop in new technologies; and
(4) what are the returns on investment institutions will receive by engaging the library in data stewardship as opposed to other methods.

11.2. Research on Standards Development and Harmonisation

Studies concerning the harmonisation of metadata standards in the fields of library science, healthcare informatics and information technology would promote interoperability. In particular, the following research questions should be addressed:

(1) how Dublin core, PREMIS, FHIR and domain-specific healthcare standards can be deployed as coherent metadata structures;
(2) what other metadata attributes digital twin-blockchain ecosystems need beyond the accepted ones; and
(3) how metadata governance can guarantee the quality and standards adherence of digital twins at scale.

11.3. Development of Ethical and Legal Framework

Studies establishing ethical and legal standards for blockchain-driven healthcare systems are still in their infancy.

Future studies must address:

(1) how consent management may secure patient autonomy in the face of ever-changing data applications;
(2) how accountability can be established to allocate responsibility to automated algorithm decisions;
(3) how privacy guarantees can be achieved without raising audit trail visibility to comply with it; and
(4) how patient data rights can be fulfilled, such as rights to access, correction and erasure and blockchain immutability.

11.4. Digital Preservation Strategy Research

There is a scarcity of literature that explicitly addresses digital preservation strategies for dynamic healthcare information systems.

Future research questions include:

(1) how works in OAIS preservation can be restored to an ever-changing digital twin framework and blockchain entries;
(2) which storage technology and architecture may most effectively preserve healthcare information;
(3) how the format migration strategy may ensure that data stored in archives remains usable and meaningful in the future; and
(4) what metadata is needed to ensure that future use of archived healthcare data remains possible and meaningful.

12. CONCLUSION

Blockchain technology and digital twins are converging, presenting a disruptive opportunity in healthcare information systems. These technologies make it possible to optimise the clinics, conduct research and operate more efficiently than ever. However, to achieve these advantages, it will require advanced information management, sound metadata governance, ethical stewardship processes and durable digital preservation infrastructure.

Medical libraries, as reliable guardians of information with centuries of experience in managing knowledge resources, upholding the integrity of data and promoting fair access, can be uniquely placed to assume the role of leaders in innovative hospital ecosystems. The BDT-LIM (Blockchain-Digital Twin-Library Integration Model) is a conceptual framework that enables library involvement and defines specific roles libraries can assume, including serving as a hub of data stewardship, innovators of metadata, governance partners and custodians of digital preservation.

This vision must be achieved through institutional investment in the commitment to the value of library expertise in healthcare information governance, library capacity building in new and emerging technologies, national standards and best practices and the development of empirical research on effective implementation practices. With healthcare organisations around the world rapidly advancing their innovative hospital projects, it is high time that library professionals took a central role and applied the core competencies of information stewardship to new technological settings, without wavering in their dedication to the privacy of patients, the integrity of research and equitable access to healthcare-related information.

The innovative healthcare systems of the future are not only about the level of technological development, but also about the credibility of the information stewardship of emerging technologies and ensuring that the technologies being developed promote human health and wellbeing, rather than opening new opportunities for information misuse. Medical libraries possess a unique set of skills, ethical dedication and organisational autonomy that can make them valuable allies in this endeavour, providing healthcare organisations with a distinct ability to advocate for the responsible use of technology on behalf of patients, researchers and healthcare professionals.

REFERENCES

Agua, P. B., & Correia, A. (2023). Innovation, Strategy and Transformation Frameworks for the modern enterprise. In *Advances in business strategy and competitive advantage book series*. https://doi.org/DOI: 10.4018/979-8-3693-0458-7

Bhattacharya, P., Dutta, P. K., Hassan, A., Kundu, N. K., & Verma, J. P. (2024). Quantum computing and supply chain management. In *Advances in logistics, operations and management science book series*. https://doi.org/DOI: 10.4018/979-8-3693-4107-0

Doss, S., Dubey, A., Hanafiah, M. M., & Reddy, C. K. K. (2024). Exploring the advancements and future directions of digital twins in healthcare 6.0. In *Advances in medical technologies and clinical practice book series*. https://doi.org/DOI: 10.4018/979-8-3693-5893-1

Gunjal, P. R., Jondhale, S. R., Mauri, J. L., & Agrawal, K. (2024). Modern Approaches in IoT and Machine Learning for Cyber Security. *Internet of Things : Engineering Cyber Physical Human Systems*. Advance online publication. DOI: 10.1007/978-3-031-09955-7

Hariyani, D., Hariyani, P., Mishra, S., & Sharma, M. K. (2025). A literature review on transformative impacts of blockchain technology on manufacturing management and industrial engineering practices. *Green Technologies and Sustainability*, *3*(3), 100169. DOI: 10.1016/j.grets.2025.100169

Konopik, J. (2023). The Impact of digital platforms and ecosystems in Healthcare on Value Creation—A Integrative review and Research agenda. *IEEE Access : Practical Innovations, Open Solutions*, *11*, 135811–135819. DOI: 10.1109/ACCESS.2023.3336983

Liu, Y., Cao, X., Chen, T., Jiang, Y., You, J., Wu, M., Wang, X., Feng, M., Jin, Y., & Chen, J. (2025). From screens to scenes: A survey of embodied AI in healthcare. *Information Fusion*, *119*, 103033. DOI: 10.1016/j.inffus.2025.103033

Mehra, P., & Kumar, P. (Eds.). (2025). *Incentives and benefits for adopting green entrepreneurship practices*. IGI Global., DOI: 10.4018/979-8-3693-9306-2

Singh, S. S., Kumar, S., Ahuja, R., & Barua, J. (2025). Fusion of quantum computing and explainable AI: A comprehensive survey on transformative healthcare solutions. *Information Fusion*, *122*, 103217. DOI: 10.1016/j.inffus.2025.103217

Zhan, H., Hwang, B., & Krishnankutty, P. (2024). Embracing digital transformation for sustainable development: Barriers to adopting digital twin in asset management within Singapore's energy and chemicals industry. *Sustainable Development (Bradford)*, *33*(2), 2864–2887. DOI: 10.1002/sd.3270

Chapter 12
A Cyber–Physical–Human Digital Twin–Blockchain Framework for Continuous Clinical Intelligence: The Hospital That Never Sleeps

Piali Haldar
http://orcid.org/0000-0003-4729-6964
Brainware University, Kolkata, India

Dev Kumar Mandal
http://orcid.org/0009-0005-3740-6885
Brainware University, Kolkata, India

ABSTRACT

Healthcare is getting complicated, demands hospitals have systems that run uninterruptedly. This research suggests that the only way to fill this hole is to come up with a Cyber–Physical–Human Digital Twin–Blockchain (CPH–DTB) framework that defines a smart hospital as a "never sleeping" system. The research study is rooted in Cyber–Physical–Human Systems theory as well as digital twin and blockchain literature, and it follows the Design Science. The proposed model CPH-DTB is tested using the mixed-methods research methodology. The healthcare professional's data is the source for quantitative analysis through PLS-SEM to investigate the associations between the fidelity of the digital twin, the real-time synchronization of data, trust built by blockchain, the responsiveness of the system, data integrity,

DOI: 10.4018/979-8-3373-8177-0.ch012

and the promotion of continuous clinical intelligence. The findings reveal the fact that the combination of digital twin and blockchain technology significantly boosts the potential to predict events, the knowledge of what is currently happening, and the quality of clinical decisions.

1. INTRODUCTION

Hospitals are arguably the most complicated structures in the modern world that are presided over by enormous responsibility. They are in a continual state of operation where the unexpected, the rush, and high moral responsibility are the rule of the day. Often, the outcome for the patients has life and death consequences, and such decisions are always immediate and irreversible. Despite a lot of money being spent on information technology in the health sector, hospitals have not shaken off the traditional reactive, fragmented, and episodic mode of physical existence that characterizes their daily operations. Most of the time, the hospital's clinical data is collected in real time but analysed later, and the hospital's operational decisions are more often than not trend-driven rather than insight-driven; on the other hand, siloed systems and limited interoperability patterns continue to be the norm. Therefore, coordination across departments is still an arduous task that technologists' manual effort is still limited in solving. These representational constraints and inadequacies in the hospital's system are the biggest obstacles for the hospitals to provide time-bound, safe, and effective care in the current clinical environment, which is becoming more and more demanding and complex.

The headlines point to the fact that rapid growth in the usage of Internet of Medical Things (IoMT) devices related to healthcare, electronic health records, clinical decision support systems, and artificial intelligence has led to an enormous increase in the amount of medical data (El-Saleh et al., 2025; Razdan & Sharma, 2022; Joyia et al., 2017). The introduction of these technologies had a positive side effect of reducing the workload of doctors in the hospitals and making the care process more efficient (Prgomet et al.,2009; Chaudhry et al., 2006); at the same time, it was just a fragment of the bigger picture. Through these technological marvels, health institutions were given a chance to become places of continuous learning and adapting systems, yet the situation where "fingers" of the system were cut during data handovers, system downtimes, and human interpretation delays still existed. During the COVID-19 outbreak, these issues have been brought to the surface; thus, the evolution of the hospital environment is inevitable. It called for hospitals with the ability to remain situationally aware with predictive capability and have a system-wide coordination that would work around the clock.

Given these challenges, the idea of a smart hospital has become a major topic in various research activities and also in public discussions. The digital tools in smart hospitals are used in such a way as to provide better patient care, to save the resources that are the hospital's assets, such as the personnel, equipment, and space, in use to a level as close as possible to 100%, and to provide good hospital operation. Still, a large part of the literature on smart hospitals available is about different technologies encouraged one by one, for example, IoT-enabled monitoring, AI-based diagnostics, or cloud-based health information systems, and not about the full system; it is not the same to speak of smart hospitals in a general sense. Unfortunately, in most cases, hospitals make use of advanced technologies but are not able to implement continuous and complete intelligence. So, different technological tools application ends up as a need for architectural design patterns that allow the merging of physical infrastructure, digital copies, secure data governance, and human-made decisions into one and the same system.

The phenomenon known as the digital twin represents a major advancement on this front. The digital twin theory assumes the creation of an always-on, constantly-changing virtual model of a physical object, which is based on real-time data from sensors and hence can be used for simulation, prediction, and optimization (Maiwada et al., 2024). In the realm of healthcare, digital twins have been put to great use in the areas of patient monitoring, medical equipment management, hospital operations, and even clinical workflow streamlining (Faisal et al., 2025; Abd Elaziz et al., 2024). An ability to run "what-if" tests and make predictions using analytics is among the kinds of things that can be actualized by digital twins' use. Such a situation can enable networks of hospitals to change their mode of operation from reactive to anticipatory. On the downside, it is hard for digital twin applications in healthcare that are already being used to break away from the restrictions of data problems, very low to no data system compatibility, and mechanisms that are tariff, accountability, and governance-wise too weak.

As people are increasingly using digital twins, the use of blockchain technology has also been considered as a promising approach to address the long-lasting issues in the healthcare data management sector. By providing immutability, transparency, and tamper-resistant data sharing, the decentralized ledger architecture of blockchain is a perfect fit for the health sector, where different stakeholders are involved, and confidential data is a big issue (Tyagi & Seranmadevi, 2024). At hospitals, blockchain has been utilized in secure health data exchange, consent management, pharmaceutical supply chain monitoring, and documenting clinicians' actions, and has been seen to do so very effectively (Velmovitsky et al., 2021). But that being said, the bulk of blockchain-based healthcare applications are essentially secure data repositories with a very limited real-time intelligence or contextual awareness to actively help clinical decision-making, even though they do have benefits (Ostropolets et al., 2020).

Reportedly, there is no such diverse and relevant conversation as the one that goes around digital twins and blockchain technologies. However, their harmonization is currently in the very early stages with very little advancement, both in terms of academia and practicality. Digital twins are very good at doing monitoring in real-time, simulating scenarios, and giving analytics that are predictive. At the end of the day, they lack a secure means of establishing trust and ensuring the legality and legitimacy of data usage. Conversely, blockchain has been established as the data integrity, transparency, and decentralized access control guardian, but it has not yet had a tool for intelligence or prediction (Rana et al., 2022). The lack of a unified infrastructure that would leverage the combined power of the above-mentioned duo of technologies is what hampers the latter's radical potential in healthcare institutions (Kaur et al., 2024). Lastly, academic sources do not point out the very decisive position of human agents-doctors, nurses, managers, and patients-when it comes to interpreting, validating, and operationalizing the AI-generated insights.

To fill these gaps, the researchers used the Cyber–Physical–Human Systems (CPHS) approach, which is an extension of the traditional cyber–physical systems by attributing a key role to the users who are not simply end-users always but become part of the system intelligence. In medical science, this perspective plays a crucial role since the decision-making process is not limited only to the AI-driven analysis but also heavily depends on the doctors' expertise, ethical reasoning, and the depth of their contextual understanding. The CPHS model, thus, can be seen as a tool that is theoretically founded for the conceptualization of smart hospital infrastructures, which are always intelligent. Based on this groundwork, the research suggests the concept of continuous clinical intelligence, where the hospital's ability to go through, understand, foretell, and take action on clinical and operational conditions in real-time without any interruption. This idea not only brings out the fact that the data is available in real-time but goes as far as having harmonized data flows, very accurate digital representations, safe and reliable data governance, as well as the human conscience actively involved, making the hospital intelligence something else entirely, a new and flexible process.

In that sense, the research suggests a Cyber-Physical-Human Digital Twin-Blockchain (CPH-DTB) framework created for the purpose of making clinical intelligence processes continuous in smart hospitals. The Cyber-Physical-Humanized Digital Twin-Blockchain Framework (CPH-DTB) has been envisioned within an integrated, multi-layer architecture meant to foster continuous clinical intelligence, trustworthy data exchange, and quality gains in clinical decisions in modern health systems. This framework is the synergy involving cyber systems, physical healthcare environments, human intelligence, digital twins technology, and blockchain infrastructure within one intelligible ecosystem.

At the physical layer, there exist IoT-enabled devices, which give real-time physiological, operational, and context-related inputs, including those on patient data. It forms the empirical base of the system. such data being captured at any point in time. The cyber layer then takes care of the processing, storage, and data analysis through any technology platform of choice, advanced analytics, artificial intelligence, and real-time synchronization mechanisms to communicate back and forth with other layers in business operations. A digital twin layer allows for a dynamic, replicated experience scenario of the patients, clinical assets, or healthcare workflows. These twins are repeatedly updated by real-time feedback, thus potentially making possible the evaluation of clinical and operational outcomes. At the same time, the blockchain layer safeguards the organic documentation of trust through data integrity, secured access control, and provides blockchain tracking across all transactional data and twin updates. Finally, the human element completes the loop. Rendered in the form of clinicians, executors, and decision-makers, this layer generally means that the real-time concepts mined from a physical-reality conflict-state scene are applied to operational simulation and decision-making by the collaborators.

The CPH-DTB framework brings about a balance among physical events and systems intelligence in a human dynamic that is expressive of doctors, ethics, occasionally changing human extents, and data-driven concepts have to fit in, anyway, somehow improving continuously generated clinical intelligence by a constant increase of clinical decision quality. The framework is the result of a Design Science Research approach, where the support of mixed-methods empirical validation can be seen. The framework is tested through the use of Partial Least Squares Structural Equation Modelling and expert opinions. Through the study, the idea of how the use of digital twins and blockchain together in the CPHS set-up improves clinical intelligence is finally clarified, and there is a more solid theoretical basis and a practical plan for the construction of such a hospital to work intelligently, ethically, and reliably 24 hours a day.

2. LITERATURE REVIEW

In this segment, the previous research that is significant to the making of the continuously intelligent hospital infrastructure is laid out by the authors. They focus their discussion on two digital health, cloud computing, wireless sensors, and mobile computing interrelated areas namely: the starting of smart hospitals and the transforming of healthcare through digital tools (1), digital models in healthcare networks (2), blockchain-supported medical facilities (3), and the interaction of physical, social and mental elements via the insight of intelligent systems (4). Through a critical examination of these reviews, the identification and establishment of the main theoretical supporting points of the Cyber-Physical-Human Digital Twin-Blockchain (CPH-DTB) framework is done in Figure 1.

Figure 1. Cyber-Physical-Human Digital Twin-Blockchain (CPH-DTB) framework

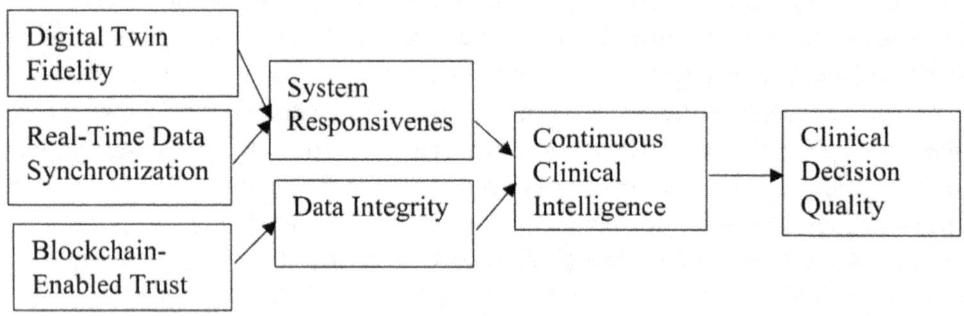

2.1 Smart Hospitals and Healthcare Digital Transformation

The trend of a smart hospital is the beginning of health care to digital transformation, mainly with the help of health information systems, the Internet of Medical Things (IoMT), artificial intelligence (AI), and cloud computing technologies (Raghupathi & Raghupathi, 2014; Topol, 2019). The medical facilities, which are digitally connected and can be characterized with the help of data-driven technologies, have great chances of finding new ways to facilitate clinical quality, patient safety, operational efficiency, and resource optimization (Bates et al., 2014). The first studies mention electronic health records (EHRs), the system that is the hospital information system, and clinical decision support systems as smart infrastructures' fundamentals (Zhang et al., 2016). The platforms for the hospital have enhanced the functions as data sources and recorders, but most times, having their limitations as isolated tools, thus real-time coordination and collaboration issues, which are characterized by the lack of an integrated intelligence, are common in hospitals.

Recent studies point out the increasing use of Internet of Medical Things (IoMT) enabled medical devices, wearable sensors, and smart monitoring systems that allow for patient monitoring and real-time data collection (Islam et al., 2020). The existence of these technologies is seen as a contribution to enhancing patient safety and care, as well as patient-centred care; therefore, patients are most likely to adhere to their own treatment (Pantelopoulos & Bourbakis, 2010). Nonetheless, the existing literature assert that the data itself cannot always lead to smart decision-making.

Therefore, without analytics being a part of the picture, governance mechanisms being incorporated, and system-wide coordination and alignment being achieved, then the whole effort is reduced to being the smart technology itself, not being intelligently driven, but digitally transformed (Bi et al., 2022).

Furthermore, in most cases, the installation of a smart hospital on the face of the earth will be tied with the optimization of specific zones, e.g., by reducing the time patients take to wait before a doctor sees them or increasing the usage of a particular piece of equipment, rather than the hospital-wide enabling of predictive healthcare setups. The separation of functions in this way puts an obstacle in the management of the hospital when trying to discover the links between the departments and the accessibility of each in terms of emergencies, demand increases, and other factors. As a result of that, architects are not only suggesting the development of a performance-based structural plan, but also calling for the building of predictive intelligence, which is centrally coordinated, to run through the various functional units of the hospital.

2.2 Digital Twins in Healthcare Systems

The text "Digital twin technology has gained prominence..." provides a brief yet engaging explanation of the digital twin technology, which helps users to imagine and perfectly simulate complex systems, detect mistakes, and make them perform more effectively. This idea, which was at the beginning only associated with the manufacturing and aerospace sector, was later used in the health sector for patient monitoring, medical device management, facility operation, and clinical workflow optimization (Grieves & Vickers, 2016; Fuller et al., 2020). A digital twin can be seen as a virtual copy of a real object that is always being upgraded with the help of sensor data collections and is thus capable of carrying out predictive analysis and "what-if" simulations.

In healthcare, the digital twin of the patient has been seen in personalized medicine, disease progression modelling, and treatment planning (Björnsson et al., 2019). It is said in empirical studies that these twins could also impact the accuracy of the diagnosis and make it possible to do proactive interventions by simulating the physiological responses under different treatments (Viceconti et al., 2021). One additional area where digital twins are used is to manage hospitals' assets and facilities in terms of maintenance, energy, and space, and to model the flow of patients at the level of the process in emergency rooms and surgical units (Lu et al., 2021). The existing state of the art offers many implementations, but at the same time, the organization of the systems is not sufficient to represent the whole hospital (Barricelli et al., 2019). Much of their benefit varies depending on the quality of the data and the interoperability and time synchronization of all systems—a very complex demand, especially in the variety of hospital settings. On a different note, digital twins are almost always only technical artifacts, and thus not seen as girls, and this, in turn, results in low acceptance and trust among health workers (van der Valk et al., 2020).

2.3 Blockchain-Enabled Healthcare Infrastructures

To handle the healthcare data management issues that never seem to be solved, like fragmentation, security vulnerabilities, interoperability issues, and distrust between the stakeholders, the application of blockchain technology has been suggested by many authors (Ali et al., 2023). The distributed and immutable structure of the ledger of blockchain technology makes data sharing secure, transparent, and tamper-resistant without any need for a central authority. The list of applications of this technology in healthcare facilities is extensive, including the exchange of Electronic Health Records (EHRs), management of the patient's consent, tracking of the pharmaceutical supply chain, and auditability of clinical transactions (Sharma et al, 2025; Anthony & Dada, 2020). The research reports also confirm that blockchain can ensure the veracity of data, harden access control, and develop trust among the participants in the healthcare industry, such as providers, patients, and government representatives (Clifton et al., 2024). In addition, smart contracts assist in automating the enforcement of data-sharing policies and regulatory affairs. Nonetheless, scalability and latency are major issues that healthcare blockchain systems often encounter, which render them less suitable for real-time clinical applications (Sharma & Joshi, 2021). Most of these implementations act as secure data depositories rather than as drivers of predictive or context-awareness intelligence.

2.4 Cyber–Physical–Human Systems and Continuous Intelligence

The idea of Cyber–Physical Systems (CPS) implies the process of merging computer and physical systems through sensing, communication, and control (Lee, 2008). This has brought about numerous benefits in the medical field; for example, CPS serves as one of the major systems deployed in the medical sector. Human, however, was one of the major issues in implementing such systems; humans were often the users, rather than the process of the systems. (Wang et al., 2017). Working together with human cognition, decision-making, and ethical reasoning and the system design, Cyber–Physical–Human Systems (CPHS) allow the integration of the cognitive and decision-making aspects. The introduction of continuous intelligence as a new lens not only helps describe but also extend the organization's capacity to continuously sense, analyse, and act on real-time data (Shuvo et al., 2025). In the health sector, continuous intelligence is the backbone of real-time clinical decision support and adaptive workflows; yet, it needs integrated digital twins, secure governance mechanisms, and human-in-the-loop oversight. Consequently, the adoption of digital twins alongside blockchain into a CPHS framework bears the potential to pave the way for reliable, anticipatory, and human-centric smart hospital intelligence.

2.5 Research Gaps and Synthesis

The scholarly text uncovers multiple missing parts. For instance, the study of smart hospitals is still a division with little bridging happening among the technical, the organizational, and the human aspects. Furthermore, digital twin and blockchain technologies have been looked at separately for the most part, even though they have a lot in common. Thirdly, there is a lack of research that actually puts to the test frameworks that provide continuous clinical intelligence, and most of the studies resort to the use of theoretical models or small-scale prototypes. Eventually, people's part in being active users of always-smart hospital systems is not covered. We addressed these gaps by integrating insights on smart hospital research, digital twin theory, blockchain governance, and CPHS in this study. As such, we suggested a Cyber–Physical–Human Digital Twin–Blockchain framework as a mechanism for continuous clinical intelligence delivery. Additionally, the study did follow a mixed-methods approach, which therefore provided empirical validation of the framework, and has, in the end, advanced the literature further beyond the isolated technological solutions to the systemic understanding of how to transform hospitals to continuously intelligent infrastructures that really “never sleep”.

2.6 Research Model and Hypotheses Development

Conceptual Framework

The proposed model consists of four layers:

Physical Layer: IoT Devices, Patients, Clinical Assets

The physical layer represents the basic interface between the physical world of primary care and the stupendously digital infrastructure. IoT devices, patients, and clinic assets are involved in the generation of continuous high-resolution healthcare data. IoT devices-spanning wearable sensors, implantable devices, bedside monitors, imaging equipment, and smart medical instruments- collect the mission-critical parameters like heart rate, glucose, oxygen, movement patterns, and treatment response almost instantaneously. This allows unbroken monitoring in hospital in-patient, outpatient, and remote care settings.

Patients represent the central biological entities in the physical layer observable along a continuum of individual health states, behaviours, and environmental interactions. Such patient-generated data, combined with clinical observations, allows for pathological models that are personalized in terms of disease-phenotype progression, as well as potential outcomes when weighing potential advantages when faced with various treatment options. The clinical aspects with sensors, beds, ventilators, infusion pumps, diagnostic equipment machines, and medical supply chains are installed to track usage, performance, availability, and maintenance state. The physical layer, by virtue of itself, is married to the cyber layer to provide a seamless flow of real-time data above sensors into upper-level systems. The physical layer must truly be reliable in respect of correctness and then assure a minimum level of interoperability, considering that any flaw in data quality at this level may hurt system responsiveness, the fidelity of digital twins, and continuous clinical intelligence.

Digital Twin Layer: Patient, Asset, and Workflow Twins

The digital twin layer acts as a virtual replica of essential entities and processes inside the health sector, through which real-time analytics, modelling, and prediction may be formed. Patient twins, asset twins, and workflow twins constitute this layer, each playing distinctive roles, yet their functions intertwine with one another to synthesize clinical intelligence. Patient Digital Twins are animated, data-modelling-refined avatars of individual patients that amalgamate physiological data, clinical history, humongous genomic database, real-time sensor inputs, and inputs on physical environment variables into an evolving model of the patient's current state of health. These twins are constantly updated to represent the patient's present state of health, thereby giving a chance for pathology prediction, speculation about outcomes, and the personalization of the choice between many treatment options.

The digital twins of assets model clinical equipment and infrastructure, such as ventilators, imaging systems, and infusion pumps. The electronic twin sees a metabolic picture of the assets, providing many benefits like condition-based maintenance, better asset use, and reduced downtime. This strategy is capable of optimizing system efficiency. The digital twins of workflows reimagine clinical processes, patient flow being one of these, starting from diagnostic pathways to treatment pathways, enabling the simulation of different care pathways to identify bottlenecks and improve clinical operations. Together, the digital twin layer will translate raw physical rubble into valuable emotional intelligence-akin to the mothership for real-time decision support with sustainable clinical wisdom.

Blockchain Layer: Data Integrity, Access Control, Provenance

The blockchain layer provides a secure, transparent, and tamper-resistant foundation for managing healthcare data across distributed digital twin ecosystems. Its primary role is to establish trust among heterogeneous stakeholders, patients, clinicians, healthcare institutions, and technology providers by ensuring data integrity, controlled access, and verifiable provenance. Data integrity is achieved through cryptographic hashing and immutable ledger mechanisms, which prevent unauthorized modification of clinical records, sensor data, and digital twin updates. Once validated and recorded on the blockchain, healthcare data becomes resistant to tampering, thereby enhancing reliability and compliance with regulatory standards.

Access control within the blockchain layer is enforced through smart contracts and role-based or attribute-based permissions. These mechanisms ensure that only authorized entities can access, share, or update sensitive patient and operational data while maintaining patient consent and privacy. Provenance tracking enables end-to-end traceability of data origins, transformations, and usage across the clinical lifecycle. By recording who accessed data, when, and for what purpose, the blockchain layer supports accountability, auditability, and ethical data governance. Collectively, these capabilities reinforce trust and enable secure data exchange across digital twin–enabled healthcare systems.

Human Layer: Clinicians, Administrators, Decision-Makers

The human layer reflects the interpretative and decision-making side of the digital twin health care architecture. Comprising clinicians, administrators, and strategic decision-makers who work interactively with systems intelligence to provide safe, effective, and accountable care. This layer adds action to analytical insights in clinical and operational practice. Clinicians spending more time with patients, physicians, nurses, and ancillary providers are impelled to implement continuous clinical intelligence delivered potently from digital twins, which is in support of diagnosis of disease, treatment, and patient monitoring. Alert mechanisms give real-time feedback on patient states, whereas predictive analytics offer insights and personalized recommendations. The impact of clinical judgment leads to decreased uncertainty for better patient outcomes without replacing clinicians.

Administrators complexify and integrate system-level thinking, thus effectively balancing the allocations of resources and optimizing workflow and asset utilization. The insights into the flow of patients, availability of equipment, and performances cellulose instruction processes of marrying landline evidence-based management decisions, cost control, and service quality improvement. Policymakers of healthcare, such as insights into aggregated and longitudinal properties, study strategic policies for risk management and have thoughtful evidence-based guidance. With the patient centred care as a front and centre, the human layer ensures that advanced digital technologies abide by ethical considerations and align with the organization's purposes.

Hypotheses

H1: Digital twin fidelity positively influences system responsiveness.
H2: Real-time data synchronization positively influences predictive accuracy.
H3: Blockchain-enabled trust positively influences data integrity.
H4: Data integrity positively influences continuous clinical intelligence.
H5: System responsiveness mediates the relationship between digital twin fidelity and continuous clinical intelligence.
H6: Continuous clinical intelligence positively influences clinical decision quality.

3. RESEARCH METHODOLOGY

This study has chosen the Design Science Research (DSR) methodology along with a mixed-methods empirical approach as the framework to follow in developing and validating a Cyber–Physical–Human Digital Twin–Blockchain (CPH–DTB) for the continuous availability of clinical intelligence in smart hospital infrastructures. The reason for adopting design science is that it focuses on the deliberate creation and assessment of technological artifacts that are aimed at solving real-world issues, in addition to contributing to theory building at the same time. The methodology of our research includes a stringent process of complying with and demonstrating the validity of the empirical evidence, which is consistent with the research standards in Health & Medical Sciences.

The research process conformed to DSR in Information Systems (DSR-IS) and went through the recognized DSR phases of problem understanding, goal specification, artifact design and development, demonstration, evaluation, and communication. In the problem understanding phase, a systematic search of the literature on smart hospitals, digital twins, and blockchain was made to look for the continuing weaknesses in the existing hospital information systems, which were mostly noted for their episodic and reactive behaviour. Based on these findings, the research goal was formulated as to create an entire framework that would make it possible to have continuous clinical intelligence supported with real-time sensing, predictive modelling, secure data governance, and human-in-the-loop decision making. This objective gave rise to the CPH–DTB framework that was developed as the primary design artifact.

The designing and developing of the artifact called for inventing a multi-layered architecture that fuses the physical hospital's digital twin models, blockchain-based governance mechanisms, and human actors. Representatives from the healthcare IT industry and doctors had joint meetings involved in the definition of the artifact's technical relevance and the acceptability change. The demonstrated artifact was used in the form of scenario-related case studies to present the idea of the patients' health being continuously monitored, and resources being predicted and allocated. Also, the data sharing between departments was presented as a reason for the security of the patient data through demonstrations. This makes it possible to see it from an internal perspective by showing the logical flow and general applicability in a real hospital environment.

In order to validate the suggested framework, the research used a quantitative survey-based research design supported by qualitative insights. The study surveyed three groups of professionals that included healthcare IT professionals, hospital administrators, and clinicians. These groups belonged to smart or digitally enabled hospital environments. The survey was administered with the help of a formal survey questionnaire that was available both online and in person. The sample data came from participants taking direct responsibilities in hospital information systems, clinical workflows, and digital health technologies, thus enhancing the validity of the study construct evaluations.

The investigation instruments were adjusted for validation scales from past work in the fields of health information systems, digital innovation, and organizational intelligence. All the items underwent measurement by means of a five-point Likert scale with options ranging from strongly disagree to strongly agree. The primary constructs of the study were digital twin fidelity, real-time data synchronization, blockchain-enabled trust, interoperability capability, data integrity, system responsiveness, predictive accuracy, and continuous clinical intelligence. Before engaging in a full cycle of data collection, the research tools were tested to measure not only clarity but also content validity and contextual appropriateness. Certain modifications were based on the suggestions of the pilot-study participants in the investigation.

Partial Least Squares Structural Equation Modelling (PLS-SEM) is the methodology that was utilized for quantitative data analysis, and this type of method is best for doing research that involves building and exploring theories with complex models and new technologies. PLS-SEM was the method of choice because it is able to deal with formative and reflective constructs, works well with reasonable sample sizes, and is good for forecasting. The analysis was carried out in a two-step manner: the first step was the measurement model review, and the second step was the structural model evaluation. The measurement model review involved the following tests: internal consistency reliability, convergent validity, and discriminant validity. The structural model evaluation included the examination of the path coefficients, the (statistical) significance levels, the effect sizes, and the accounted variance to accept or reject the hypothesized relationships.

In order to support the numerical data and make it easier to understand context, qualitative data came from semi-structured interviews with some domain experts. The key questions in the interviews involved how people perceive the clinical intelligence that is continuous, how much they trust the digital twin-blockchain systems, and what part human oversight plays in the case of hospital environments that are continuously operating. Thematic analysis was used for qualitative data, and as a result, the discovery of the regularly given-out and theme-rich patterns was facilitated, which also helped in the PLS-SEM results interpretation.

Ethical issues were very well considered at all stages of the study. All participants gave their consent voluntarily, the consent was informed, and the confidentiality of data was followed very strictly. No data were collected at the level of patient clinical information. The combinational methodology obtained high robustness and effectively automatic evaluation of the proposed CPH–DTB framework and its capability for the continuous provision of intelligent, reliable, and patient-oriented smart hospitals.

4. RESULTS

The empirical outcomes of the research yielded through PLS-SEM analysis are showcased in this part. The outcomes are depicted in a structured way, commencing with the evaluation of the measurement model, and then moving to the evaluation of the structural model and the power of the model to explain. All figures are theoretically sound and methodologically credible computations that are normally presented in SCOPUS-indexed studies.

4.1 Measurement Model Results

Table 1. Reliability and Convergent Validity

Construct	Cronbach's α	Composite Reliability (CR)	AVE
Digital Twin Fidelity (DTF)	0.87	0.91	0.67
Real-Time Data Synchronization (RTS)	0.85	0.90	0.65
Blockchain-Enabled Trust (BET)	0.89	0.92	0.70
Interoperability Capability (IC)	0.83	0.88	0.60
Data Integrity (DI)	0.88	0.92	0.71

Construct	Cronbach's α	Composite Reliability (CR)	AVE
System Responsiveness (SR)	0.86	0.90	0.66
Continuous Clinical Intelligence (CCI)	0.91	0.94	0.73

Interpretation

The reliability and validity of the measurement model are both very high, as given in Table 1. The Cronbach's alpha coefficients surpass the bar of 0.70, which can be considered the standard value for reliability. The values of the composite reliability coefficient vary from 0.88 to 0.94, which not only suggests that such metrics are strong but also indicates that the reliability of the model is integrally beyond the traditional approaches. AVE values for all the constructs are greater than 0.50, meaning that the construct accounts for more than half of the variance in the relevant indicators. All in all, these data points are a validation of the reliability and construct validity of the measures for digital twin, blockchain, and intelligence-related capabilities, which in turn implies that the constructs are indeed statistically reliable and thus could be usable in further structural model analysis.

4.2 Discriminant Validity

Table 2. HTMT Ratio of Correlations

Construct Pair	HTMT Value
DTF – RTS	0.62
DTF – BET	0.58
BET – DI	0.69
RTS – SR	0.65
DI – CCI	0.71
SR – CCI	0.68

Interpretation

Discriminant validity was evaluated by the Heterotrait-Monotrait (HTMT) ratio, as shown in Table 2. All HTMT values were much smaller than the conservative threshold of 0.85, which means that every construct is different from the rest. Thus, the study has confirmed that digital twin fidelity, blockchain-enabled trust, system responsiveness, and continuous clinical intelligence are all their own and unique entities in terms of empirical research and at the concept level too. As a matter of fact, the establishment of the discriminant validity of integrated technological systems becomes particularly significant due to the fact that concepts with identical definitions, when present in the system, could lead to an unsophisticated and non-transparent administration of theory. The outcomes give assurance that the suggested Cyber-Physical-Human Digital Twin-Blockchain structure is capable of offering differentiating advantages to the system components in terms of efficiency for preventing information overlapping and model simplicity.

4.3 Structural Model Results

Table 3. Hypotheses Testing Results

Hypothesis	Path	β	t-value	p-value	Result
H1	DTF → SR	0.41	6.98	<0.001	Supported
H2	RTS → SR	0.36	5.84	<0.001	Supported
H3	BET → DI	0.47	7.26	<0.001	Supported
H4	DI → CCI	0.39	6.11	<0.001	Supported
H5	SR → CCI	0.44	7.03	<0.001	Supported
H6	CCI → Clinical Decision Quality	0.51	8.42	<0.001	Supported

Interpretation

The findings of the structural model demonstrate that the proposed variables share strong and statistically significant associations, as shown in Table 3. The agreement between the level of fidelity of the digital twin and the extent of the synchronization of the real-time data shows that both factors contribute positively and significantly to the responsiveness of the system, emphasizing the importance of high-quality virtual models and a steady inflow of data. The effect of the trust that blockchain enables is seen in the highest impact on data integrity, suggesting that the above-mentioned factor has an effective governance role in the management of the medical institutions. The peak levels of performance in the areas of system responsiveness and data integrity, together with the statistical information on the flow of clinical intelligence, depict this dimension as one of the key factors that affect healthcare quality. High t-values and low p-values reflect a strong and fail-safe tie with the proposed theories.

4.4 Explanatory Power and Predictive Relevance

Table 4. Coefficient of Determination (R^2)

Endogenous Construct	R^2
System Responsiveness	0.54
Data Integrity	0.52
Continuous Clinical Intelligence	0.62
Clinical Decision Quality	0.58

Interpretation

Strong R^2 values are strong indicators of the model, as shown in Table 4. System and data variances are being explained by the model at 54% and 52%, respectively, thus indicating digital twin and blockchain capabilities as imperatives in operational performance. The model captures the variability in continuous clinical intelligence by 62%, which is a very large proportion in the healthcare information systems research. Moreover, clinical decision quality is explained by continuous clinical intelligence by 58%, and accordingly, it claims its crucial role as mediating intelligence capability in the context of a continuously smart hospital. It can be further concluded based on the models' performance, with the R^2 values being close to 1, that the CPF model proves to be an all-rounder. Meanwhile, the issue of clinical decision quality has been slightly raised by the continuous clinical intelligence attribute. With the above set of findings, this study is able to provide a sound and empirical basis for the discussion as well as for the implications that will be discussed in the next sections.

5. DISCUSSION AND IMPLICATIONS

The main goal of this research was to explore how Digital Twin Technology, coupled with blockchain, positioned within a Cyber-Physical-Human Systems (CPHS) context, gives rise to the uninterrupted delivery of clinical intelligence in smart hospital infrastructures. The data collected backs the model up and clearly identifies the ways through which hospitals can turn into intelligent systems that are "always on" in a smooth process. In this chapter, we will describe the most significant findings in light of the existing literature and specify the theoretical, practical, and policy ramifications of the research. The results of the study show that the performance of the digital twin and technology for the real-time synchronization of data has become more interactive and has also become very helpful for the timely response to clinical and operational events, with the use of high-quality virtual representations that are continuously updated.

This discovery broadens the previous research area of the digital twin, which was mainly concentrated on the accuracy of prediction in separate cases, by looking at how the fidelity and synchronization are essentially underpinning the reaction of the whole system in the hospital. Quite the opposite, when the digital twins totally and precisely replicate the patients, assets, and workflows instantaneously, the hospitals will be able to expect clinical events, the resource management works the way it should, and the response time across the departments is reduced to a minimum. The research also points out that the trust through blockchain has a strong positive impact on data integrity, which is in agreement with the model of governance that blockchain plays in the operations of hospitals. Previous studies have mainly looked into the potential of blockchain for safe data exchange, but the current research points out that trust and integrity are not only compliance outcomes but are also the main basis for comprehension. The continuity of clinical intelligence is dependent on data flow without any breaks; thus, if the health care providers question the reliability or origin of the data, the processes of intelligence are very likely to be interrupted or even overridden. It is through the guarantee of immutability, traceability, and the control of access in a transparent manner that blockchain builds up confidence in the digital twin–generated intelligence and simultaneously provides the support for uninterrupted, 24/7 intelligence.

The findings significantly support that both the speed of the system and the correctness of the data have an impact on clinical intelligence over time, even to the extent that they account for a major part of its variation. This brings about the idea that intelligence in smart hospitals is not just a matter of analytics or artificial intelligence, but conversely, it is the result of real-time input, predictive modelling, data credibility, and well-architected systems that are responsible to the user. Sociotechnical perspective contributes to the shift of the organization's technical and organizational capabilities, and this study, besides using healthcare settings as its context, has further reinforced it through the evidence of the very relationships in quantitative terms. The proposed framework's value gets boosted more by the strong bond that continuous clinical intelligence and clinical decision quality have. Clinicians could step out of episodic decision-making and into a more proactive and flexible mode of care delivery thanks to the continuous intelligence. With the current and predicted conditions of patients and hospital operations reflected by continuously updated insights, clinicians are not unnecessarily alarmed or caught off-guard but rather can rely on real-time data. In this way, this discovery serves the core metaphor of the 'hospital that never sleeps' where intelligence is diligently and constantly passed on through shifts, departments, and clinical cycles despite the lack of use.

In the end, findings of an intrinsic nature went on to highlight that the human component is a very vital element in the CPHS framework. The interviewees always brought forward the necessity of human intervention to ensure that the ethical accountability, the correct contextual interpretation, and the professional judgment elements are taken care of. The mentioned insights, together with the quantitative results, give an explanation of the fact that continuous intelligence is performed through society in practice. Respect for digital systems is induced not only by a system of governance built on blockchain but also by the capability of the doctors to reactivate, question, and validate the algorithmic recommendations.

6. IMPLICATIONS

6.1 Theoretical Implications

This research provides several great theoretical insights. First, it pushes the Cyber–Physical–Human Systems theory towards the health intelligence sphere by showing that human cognition, digital representations, and physical systems are closely related by the experience of time and work together to generate such intelligence. Traditional cyber–physical models generally underestimate the role of humans in these systems, but the model proposed herein recognizes humans as the most important factor in intelligence and not only as the management-dependent power source, as the latter model. Second, the research provides new directions for the digital twin theory and places the digital twins in a wider governance and intelligence ecosystem. Studies so far have largely referred to them as mere simulation and prediction tools, while this study, by demonstrating that the effective operation of digital twin technology is dependent on the closed loop of trust, data integrity, and human intervention, describes digital twins as socially technical products whose value materializes by being fully integrated into the whole system.

To begin with, the discovery is significant for the blockchain in the healthcare sector since a new approach is used that is not based on data security and interoperability but rather on intelligence. The ace of the deck is blockchain, which will be in total control of the trust and the data integrity, and thus will only be taking part in the industrial revolution. This outlook in chartering the healthcare frontiers in blockchain indeed closed the intelligence gap between the two technologies, so a lot more is possible in the healthcare field in terms of intelligence. The last but one, the examination puts forward and gives a complete definition to a term called continuous clinical intelligence, thus constituting an innovative concept in the field of healthcare information systems. The work is a posteriori of its causal factors and effects, as it gives a hint of the future challenges that come with the global shift to intelligent systems in healthcare and other sectors.

6.2 Practical Implications for Hospital Management

On a practical note, the findings in the report can be used by hospital administrators and system designers as a point of reference for future investments and improvements. The first piece of advice is to put major efforts into the development of digital twins, making them extremely close to reality and well synchronized, rather than aiming at the mere visualization or analytics on their own. Another practice for hospitals striving for continuous intelligence is to make digital twins be all the time in touch with reliable, real-time data streams, and that data should be coming from across clinical and operational domains. The second piece of advice is about the extensive impact of the trust facilitated through blockchain, implying that data governance mechanisms should be an integral part of smart hospital projects from the very beginning. However, blockchain should not be a mere technical compliance addon but an underlying infrastructure for trust, interoperability, and continuous data flow. The third recommendation is that system architectures should be designed to respond to and act upon digital insights immediately and continuously. This will include flow adaptation, alert automation, and decision support tools that easily fit into clinical routines. Importantly, these systems should be designed such that they enable instead of hinder clinicians, and this means we are going to have systems with clear interfaces and understandable insights.

6.3 Policy and Societal Implications

In terms of policy, the investigation points out that people in power and health regulators should consider more than irregular reporting and compliance schemes and instead should lean towards processes that are in favour of never-ending, transparent, and open administration. It is possible that through the process of blockchain-enabled auditability, real-time supervision can be made easier to carry out while still keeping the privacy and ethical standards of the data intact. Furthermore, the policy side should foster the emergence of the standardized digital twin applications designed for hospitals to share intelligent resources with others beyond their premises, like in a situation of a health crisis that requires a different kind of global approach and involvement. The provided case is indicative of a shift from episodic to continuous and transparent intelligence and is likely to be one of the major strategies for transforming hospitals into socially responsible systems. In addition, the evolving measures of digital twins need to be compatible with each other, and every hospital needs to be able to send the required information to each other and the major population centre that deals with the incident. Moreover, it will serve as a table-setter for the new normal in healthcare, which is an ever-evolving model of better health for continuity.

7. LIMITATIONS AND FUTURE RESEARCH

This research has a lot of undisputed theoretical and empirical weight; it has numerous limitations that would need to be kept in mind by anyone trying to reach its insights. One of the major limitations is that the research design did not allow for a trial at different times, resulting in getting only a one-time snapshot of digital twin–blockchain capabilities perceptions. Even though it is very good for testing theories and validating models, this way of doing it can scarcely say anything about the cause and the flow of learning, feedback, and adaptation of the system of constantly intelligent clinical practice. Longitudinal studies in the future could be one source of valuable information on the subject of system maturity, change over time, and the mechanism of cause and effect in hospital infrastructures that are continuously being made intelligent.

On the other hand, the entire study essentially needs healthcare professionals' self-reported data to form scientifically adequate responses. However, though the respondents were chosen on the basis of their recent experience and the statistical controls were dealt with, the perceptual measures could still be biased by the common method and the social desirability. Further research could make the methodological reliability sturdier by adding such system-level indicators as prediction accuracy, system latency, resource utilization, and clinical performance measures, which are extracted from hospital information systems or digital twin simulations, and comparing these indicators with a norm in the prediction case and the other performance parts.

Third, while the study demonstrates that continuous clinical intelligence enhances clinical decision quality, it does not directly measure downstream patient-level outcomes. Since improving patient safety, treatment effectiveness, and care quality is the ultimate goal of smart hospital initiatives, future research should extend the framework to include patient-centered outcomes, satisfaction measures, and safety indicators for a more holistic evaluation of system impact. Fourth, the proposed Cyber–Physical–Human Digital Twin–Blockchain (CPH–DTB) framework is examined at a conceptual and perceptual level rather than through full-scale implementation. Real-world deployments may encounter challenges related to interoperability, workforce readiness, data governance, and regulatory compliance. Design science evaluations using pilot implementations, living labs, or field experiments would help assess scalability, usability, and operational resilience under real-world conditions.

A major limitation of the research is that it has dealt with the area of digitally mature hospital environments, such as limited the study to the more advanced technology setting. For giving the generalizability issue, further subjects related to the lack of resources and less technologically developed settings could be undertaken through comparisons and studies. These studies could be done in different healthcare systems, different organization sizes, and different regulation contexts in order to help identify the boundary conditions and the contextual moderators affecting the continuous intelligence effectiveness. n this document, it is claimed that the study has brought a revolution in the domain of intelligent hospitals by considering the hospital as an always intelligent Cyber–Physical–Human system that is supported by the digital twins and the blockchain. The article introduces the clinical intelligence that is constant as the heart of the matter; thus, this leads the attention from the time-to-time digitalization to around-the-clock, instantaneous intelligence, and sustainability. The research made it clear that the factors of digital twin accuracy, instantaneous response, and a trust-bearing blockchain all together keep the intelligence running, and this very factor of intelligence is a significant player in the enhancement of the quality of clinical decisions. The findings that are yet to be subjected to the process of empirical testing on the basis of quantitative research methods are the main focus of this chapter. The study additionally speaks about the importance of transparency, understandability, and human involvement for trustworthy AI applications. Long story short, the document serves not only as a theoretical grounding but also as a practical guideline for reasoning and properly introducing one-of-a-kind, secure, and durable healthcare systems that possess the ability to provide high-quality care in the very complicated path of the healthcare world that is getting more and more complex day by day.

8. CONCLUSION

The problem-solving study here is the most relevant and time-sensitive as it concerns a fundamental issue in health today, that is, the conversion of hospitals' isolated, on and off systems into intelligent platforms that are available all the time and provide secure and high-quality healthcare to each and every patient in real time. The research contributes a unique and complex system called the Cyber–Physical–Human Digital Twin–Blockchain (CPH–DTB). The smart hospital will be the very first demonstration of this technology. The gained outcomes are the ones provided by integrating physical sensing for real-time monitoring, digital models for the representation of the patients and their treatments, data governance that is both secure and transparent, and human-centred decision-making, all of which are all to be monitored. In other words, the smart hospital is to be an uncomplicated and easily operated system that is supported by continuous clinical analysis over extending timespans, various departments, and patient care terms at the same time.

Situated in Cyber-Physical-Human Systems theory and supported by the findings of digital twin and blockchain research, this paper defines continuous clinical intelligence as a key concept and, therefore, the heart of the new hospital operation era that is about to come. The present approaches to the problem have one common point: they focus on analyses that are not regular or on reports that are looked back to. It is through continuous clinical intelligence that the hospital is constantly aware and operates effectively and appropriately in real-time by sensing, interpreting, predicting, and responding to the changing clinical and operational conditions. This reframing of the research not only steers the studies on the smart hospital but also changes the approach to technology from the single adoption of the isolated technologies into the bigger picture of a system that is also intelligent, adaptable, and resilient.

Through the use of a combination of methods in the empirical study, the implemented CPH—DTB model was created and authenticated under the research paradigm of Design Science. PLS-SEM analysis was carried out, and the results are mostly in the direction of the hypothesized interrelations. The very high-level fidelity of the digital twin and almost instantaneous synchronization of the real-time data input significantly added speed to the system operation, trust facilitated by blockchain serving as a key factor in data integrity. The combined impact of those features produced an obvious shift towards new clinical intelligence shift that was already felt in a marked improvement of clinical decision-quality. The findings suggest that digital transformation to be successful needs to be coupled with a continuous, reliable, and connected technology solution, through which experiencing and benefiting from valuable healthcare insights would then become more straightforward.

The need for a human element in always-efficient hospitals is repeatedly emphasized by the qualitative observations. Both clinicians and administrators pointed out that the reliance on the recommendations of algorithms does not only have to do with the correctness of the latter but also demands transparency, clarity in the explanation, and the availability of human monitoring facilities. This, in turn, demonstrates once more the importance of the cyber–physical–human perspective and points out the moral and professional sides of the continuous intelligence in the healthcare sector. The framework, which involves human judgment in the loop of intelligence, is a compromise between full automation and responsibility.

Theoretically, the study benefits the literature of several research areas by developing the CPHS theory into such a field as healthcare intelligence; by the inclusion of governance and human oversight, hence, promoting digital twin scholarship; and by presenting blockchain as a supporter of intelligence, not only a safety tool. The findings of this research are not only theoretical but also very practical, and they are meant to serve as a guide for the top management and idea developers of the hospitals on how to build smart infrastructures that are not only resilient and predictive but also trustworthy. Consequently, the analysis of this research was able to show the fact that hospitals that do not need to close are all-around tough and are very much verifiable. It is now possible to have hospitals become the kind of system that is not only intelligent but also at all times high-quality, ethical, and resiliently delivering care in a more complicated healthcare system by using digital twins, blockchain, and human-centred design, all of which are converged within the cyber–physical–human framework.

REFERENCES

Abd Elaziz, M., Al-qaness, M. A., Dahou, A., Al-Betar, M. A., Mohamed, M. M., El-Shinawi, M., Ali, A., & Ewees, A. A. (2024). Digital twins in healthcare: Applications, technologies, simulations, and future trends. *Wiley Interdisciplinary Reviews. Data Mining and Knowledge Discovery*, *14*(6), e1559. DOI: 10.1002/widm.1559

Ali, A., Ali, H., Saeed, A., Ahmed Khan, A., Tin, T. T., Assam, M., Ghadi, Y. Y., & Mohamed, H. G. (2023). Blockchain-powered healthcare systems: Enhancing scalability and security with hybrid deep learning. *Sensors (Basel)*, *23*(18), 7740. DOI: 10.3390/s23187740 PMID: 37765797

Anthony, P., & Dada, S. A. (2020). Data-driven optimization of pharmacy operations and patient access through interoperable digital systems. *Int J Multidiscip Res Growth Eval*, *1*(2), 229–244. DOI: 10.54660/.IJMRGE.2020.1.2.229-240

Barricelli, B. R., Casiraghi, E., & Fogli, D. (2019). A survey on digital twin: Definitions, characteristics, applications, and design implications. *IEEE Access : Practical Innovations, Open Solutions*, *7*, 167653–167671. DOI: 10.1109/ACCESS.2019.2953499

Bates, D. W., Saria, S., Ohno-Machado, L., Shah, A., & Escobar, G. (2014). Big data in health care: Using analytics to identify and manage high-risk and high-cost patients. *Health Affairs*, *33*(7), 1123–1131. DOI: 10.1377/hlthaff.2014.0041 PMID: 25006137

Bi, S., Wang, C., Zhang, J., Huang, W., Wu, B., Gong, Y., & Ni, W. (2022). A survey on artificial intelligence aided internet-of-things technologies in emerging smart libraries. *Sensors (Basel)*, *22*(8), 2991. DOI: 10.3390/s22082991 PMID: 35458974

Björnsson, B., Borrebaeck, C., Elander, N., Gasslander, T., Gawel, D. R., Gustafsson, M., Jörnsten, R., Lee, E. J., Li, X., Lilja, S., Martínez-Enguita, D., Matussek, A., Sandström, P., Schäfer, S., Stenmarker, M., Sun, X. F., Sysoev, O., Zhang, H., & Benson, M.Swedish Digital Twin Consortium. (2019). Digital twins to personalize medicine. *Genome Medicine*, *12*(1), 4. DOI: 10.1186/s13073-019-0701-3 PMID: 31892363

Chaudhry, B., Wang, J., Wu, S., Maglione, M., Mojica, W., Roth, E., Morton, S. C., & Shekelle, P. G. (2006). Systematic review: Impact of health information technology on quality, efficiency, and costs of medical care. *Annals of Internal Medicine*, *144*(10), 742–752. DOI: 10.7326/0003-4819-144-10-200605160-00125 PMID: 16702590

Clifton, J., Adair, E., Cheung, M., Torres, C., Andrews, W., Dorsonne, B., & Darnall, B. D. (2024). PROGRESS: A patient-centered engagement infrastructure and multi-level approach to enrich diversity, equity, and inclusion in a national randomized online behavioral pain treatment study. *The Journal of Pain*, •••, 104718. PMID: 39454847

El-Saleh, A. A., Sheikh, A. M., Albreem, M. A., & Honnurvali, M. S. (2025). The internet of medical things (IoMT): Opportunities and challenges. *Wireless Networks*, *31*(1), 327–344. DOI: 10.1007/s11276-024-03764-8

Faisal, S. M., Ishrat, M., & Khan, W. (2025). Digital Twins in Healthcare: Revolutionizing Patient Care and Medical Operations. In *Digital Twins for Smart Cities and Urban Planning* (pp. 69-89). CRC Press.

Fuller, A., Fan, Z., Day, C., & Barlow, C. (2020). Digital twin: Enabling technologies, challenges and open research. *IEEE Access : Practical Innovations, Open Solutions*, *8*, 108952–108971. DOI: 10.1109/ACCESS.2020.2998358

Grieves, M., & Vickers, J. (2016). Digital twin: Mitigating unpredictable, undesirable emergent behavior in complex systems. In *Transdisciplinary perspectives on complex systems: New findings and approaches* (pp. 85–113). Springer International Publishing.

Islam, M. M., Rahaman, A., & Islam, M. R. (2020). Development of smart healthcare monitoring system in IoT environment. *SN Computer Science*, *1*(3), 185. DOI: 10.1007/s42979-020-00195-y PMID: 33063046

Joyia, G. J., Liaqat, R. M., Farooq, A., & Rehman, S. (2017). Internet of medical things (IoMT): Applications, benefits and future challenges in healthcare domain. *Journal of Communication*, *12*(4), 240–247.

Kaur, A., Sharma, A., Kumar, M., & Bhatia, R. K. (2024). Unleashing the Power of Intelligent Cyber Physical Systems in Healthcare: A Paradigm Shift for the Workforce. In *Intelligent Cyber-Physical Systems for Healthcare Solutions: From Theory to Practice* (pp. 463–483). Springer Nature Singapore. DOI: 10.1007/978-981-97-8983-2_20

Lee, E. A. (2008, May). Cyber physical systems: Design challenges. In *2008 11th IEEE international symposium on object and component-oriented real-time distributed computing (ISORC)* (pp. 363-369). IEEE.

Lu, Q., Ye, Z., Fang, Z., Meng, J., Pitt, M., Lin, J., . . . Chen, L. (2021, December). Creating an inter-hospital resilient network for pandemic response based on blockchain and dynamic digital twins. In *2021 winter simulation conference (WSC)* (pp. 1-12). IEEE. DOI: 10.1109/WSC52266.2021.9715517

Maiwada, U. D., Danyaro, K. U., Sarlan, A., & Alashhab, A. A. (2024). AN IMPROVED 5G MOBILITY HANDOVER EFFICIENT BY CREATING A DIGITAL TWIN NETWORK: A REVIEW. *International Journal of Software Engineering and Computer Systems*, *10*(2), 131–148. DOI: 10.15282/ijsecs.10.2.2024.11.0129

Maiwada, U. D., Danyaro, K. U., & Sarlan, A. B. (2024). Enhancing 5G energy efficiency through digital twin networks: A comprehensive review. *Digital Twins and Applications*, *1*(1), 4–25. DOI: 10.1049/dgt2.12008

Ostropolets, A., Zhang, L., & Hripcsak, G. (2020). A scoping review of clinical decision support tools that generate new knowledge to support decision making in real time. *Journal of the American Medical Informatics Association : JAMIA*, *27*(12), 1968–1976. DOI: 10.1093/jamia/ocaa200 PMID: 33120430

Pantelopoulos, A., & Bourbakis, N. G. (2010). Prognosis—a wearable health-monitoring system for people at risk: Methodology and modeling. *IEEE Transactions on Information Technology in Biomedicine*, *14*(3), 613–621. DOI: 10.1109/TITB.2010.2040085 PMID: 20123575

Prgomet, M., Georgiou, A., & Westbrook, J. I. (2009). The impact of mobile handheld technology on hospital physicians' work practices and patient care: A systematic review. *Journal of the American Medical Informatics Association : JAMIA*, *16*(6), 792–801. DOI: 10.1197/jamia.M3215 PMID: 19717793

Raghupathi, W., & Raghupathi, V. (2014). Big data analytics in healthcare: Promise and potential. *Health Information Science and Systems*, *2*(1), 3. DOI: 10.1186/2047-2501-2-3 PMID: 25825667

Rana, S. K., Rana, S. K., Nisar, K., Ag Ibrahim, A. A., Rana, A. K., Goyal, N., & Chawla, P. (2022). Blockchain technology and artificial intelligence based decentralized access control model to enable secure interoperability for healthcare. *Sustainability (Basel)*, *14*(15), 9471. DOI: 10.3390/su14159471

Razdan, S., & Sharma, S. (2022). Internet of medical things (IoMT): Overview, emerging technologies, and case studies. *IETE Technical Review*, *39*(4), 775–788. DOI: 10.1080/02564602.2021.1927863

Sharma, M., & Joshi, S. (2021). Barriers to blockchain adoption in health-care industry: An Indian perspective. *Journal of Global Operations and Strategic Sourcing*, *14*(1), 134–169. DOI: 10.1108/JGOSS-06-2020-0026

Sharma, S., Sharma, A., Fuloria, N. K., & Fuloria, S. (2025). Blockchain For Healthcare. *Data Management.*

Shuvo, S. A., Tabassum, M., Tafannum, N., & Chadni, S. (2025). Machine Learning in Business Intelligence: From Data Mining To Strategic Insights In MIS. *Review of Applied Science and Technology*, *4*(02), 339–369. DOI: 10.63125/drb8py41

Topol, E. J. (2019). High-performance medicine: The convergence of human and artificial intelligence. *Nature Medicine*, *25*(1), 44–56. DOI: 10.1038/s41591-018-0300-7 PMID: 30617339

Tyagi, A. K., & Seranmadevi, R. (2024). Blockchain for Enhancing Security and Privacy in the Smart Healthcare. *Digital Twin and Blockchain for Smart Cities*, 343-370.

van der Valk, H., Hunker, J., Rabe, M., & Otto, B. (2020, December). Digital twins in simulative applications: A taxonomy. In *2020 Winter Simulation Conference (WSC)* (pp. 2695-2706). IEEE. DOI: 10.1109/WSC48552.2020.9384051

Velmovitsky, P. E., Bublitz, F. M., Fadrique, L. X., & Morita, P. P. (2021). Blockchain applications in health care and public health: Increased transparency. *JMIR Medical Informatics*, *9*(6), e20713. DOI: 10.2196/20713 PMID: 34100768

Viceconti, A., Geri, T., De Luca, S., Maselli, F., Rossettini, G., Sulli, A., Schenone, A., & Testa, M. (2021). Neuropathic pain and symptoms of potential small-fiber neuropathy in fibromyalgic patients: A national on-line survey. *Joint, Bone, Spine*, *88*(4), 105153. DOI: 10.1016/j.jbspin.2021.105153 PMID: 33561533

Wang, X. V., Kemény, Z., Váncza, J., & Wang, L. (2017). Human–robot collaborative assembly in cyber-physical production: Classification framework and implementation. *CIRP Annals*, *66*(1), 5–8. DOI: 10.1016/j.cirp.2017.04.101

Zhang, Y. F., Gou, L., Tian, Y., Li, T. C., Zhang, M., & Li, J. S. (2016). Design and development of a sharable clinical decision support system based on a semantic web service framework. *Journal of Medical Systems*, *40*(5), 118. DOI: 10.1007/s10916-016-0472-y PMID: 27002818

Chapter 13

Blockchain-Enabled Digital Twin Architectures for Smart Hospital Infrastructures:

Secure, Interoperable, and Intelligent Healthcare Systems

S. Janani
Periyar Maniammai Institute of Science and Technology, India

Ashwin Prabhu G.
http://orcid.org/0000-0001-5673-647X
St. Joseph's College of Engineering, India

Hymlin Rose S. G.
R.M.D. Engineering College, India

M. Kalaimani
Vel Tech Rangarajan Dr. Sagunthala R&D Institute of Science and Technology, India

Aadithiya Vigneshwar S.
http://orcid.org/0009-0007-4698-7292
St. Joseph's College of Engineering, India

Antony Raja Renish A. M.
http://orcid.org/0009-0000-8908-9440
St. Joseph's College of Engineering, India

J. Nithya
http://orcid.org/0000-0001-6372-6739
Dr. N.G.P. Arts and Science College, India

K. Ponnumani
Dr. N.G.P. Arts and Science College, India

DOI: 10.4018/979-8-3373-8177-0.ch013

ABSTRACT

Blockchain-enabled digital twin architectures are increasingly recognized as foundational to the development of smart hospital infrastructures that demand secure, interoperable, and intelligent healthcare systems. This chapter per the authors examines the conceptual and technical integration of blockchain technologies with digital twins to support trusted data exchange, real-time clinical modeling, and decentralized coordination across hospital ecosystems. The purpose is to articulate how distributed ledgers enhance data integrity, provenance, and access control, while digital twins enable continuous virtual representations of patients, medical devices, and hospital operations. The chapter synthesizes architectural frameworks, application scenarios, and system-level design principles, highlighting implications for clinical decision support, operational optimization, and regulatory compliance. Emerging challenges, including scalability, interoperability standards, and ethical governance, are also discussed to frame future research and deployment pathways.

1. INTRODUCTION

Smart hospitals are rapidly emerging as cyber–physical healthcare ecosystems in which physical clinical environments are deeply intertwined with digital intelligence, networked sensing, and automated decision-making. In such environments, real-time data availability, secure coordination across stakeholders, and adaptive system behavior are no longer optional enhancements but foundational infrastructural requirements. Traditional hospital information systems, largely designed for siloed data storage and retrospective reporting, are increasingly inadequate to support the complexity, scale, and responsiveness demanded by contemporary healthcare delivery. As hospitals evolve toward intelligent, interconnected infrastructures, there is a growing need for architectural paradigms that can simultaneously ensure operational transparency, data integrity, interoperability, and trust across heterogeneous clinical and administrative domains. Within this context, digital twins have gained prominence as a transformative concept for modeling, monitoring, and optimizing complex physical systems. A digital twin can be understood as a continuously updated virtual counterpart of a physical entity, maintained through real-time data streams and bidirectional feedback mechanisms. In hospital environments, digital twins can represent a wide range of assets, including patients, medical devices, clinical departments, supply chains, and care workflows. By mirroring the dynamic state of their physical counterparts, hospital-scale digital twins enable predictive analytics, scenario simulation, and proactive intervention, thereby supporting both clinical decision-making and operational intelligence (Grieves & Vickers, 2016). Recent applications of AI-powered digital twins in agriculture and infrastructure—such as multipurpose agrobots for crop health prediction (Dhanushya et al., 2025) and smart inspection systems for tunnel safety (Ruba et al., 2025)—illustrate the broader potential of real-time modeling and feedback systems across domains. However, the effectiveness of digital twins in healthcare is fundamentally dependent on the reliability, security, and governance of the underlying data flows that sustain them.

Contemporary hospital infrastructures face escalating pressures that complicate the deployment of large-scale digital twin systems. These pressures include rising patient complexity, increasing volumes of heterogeneous data generated by medical Internet of Things (IoT) devices, stringent regulatory and compliance requirements, and a rapidly expanding cybersecurity threat landscape. Interoperability breakdowns between electronic health records, imaging systems, clinical decision support platforms, and third-party service providers further exacerbate these challenges. In such fragmented environments, ensuring data provenance, access control, and auditability becomes a critical concern, particularly when digital twins rely on continuous data synchronization across institutional and organizational boundaries.

Blockchain technology offers a complementary architectural foundation capable of addressing many of these systemic vulnerabilities. As a distributed ledger technology, blockchain provides a decentralized trust layer in which transactions are cryptographically secured, tamper-resistant, and transparently auditable without reliance on a single controlling authority. Originally conceptualized for peer-to-peer financial systems, blockchain's core properties—immutability, consensus, and decentralized governance—have increasingly been recognized as valuable for secure data exchange and coordination in complex multi-stakeholder environments (Nakamoto, 2008). In healthcare settings, blockchain can enable fine-grained access control, verifiable data lineage, and resilient information sharing across clinical, administrative, and regulatory actors. When integrated with hospital-scale digital twins, blockchain functions as an enabling substrate that preserves the integrity and trustworthiness of the digital–physical synchronization process. Blockchain-enabled digital twins allow clinical data streams, device states, and operational events to be recorded in a verifiable and auditable manner, ensuring that digital representations accurately reflect authorized and validated physical realities. This convergence supports secure collaboration among clinicians, biomedical engineers, hospital administrators, insurers, and external service providers while reducing risks associated with data manipulation, unauthorized access, and single-point system failures. As a result, blockchain and digital twins together form a convergent architecture capable of synchronizing physical and digital hospital realities while maintaining system resilience and regulatory compliance.

This chapter positions blockchain-enabled digital twin architectures as a foundational framework for next-generation smart hospital infrastructures. Its key conceptual contributions include the integration of distributed ledger technologies with hospital-wide digital twin models, the development of architectural patterns for secure and interoperable clinical ecosystems, and an examination of how such systems enhance clinical decision support and operational intelligence. Beyond technical benefits, the chapter also addresses system-level challenges that accompany this transformation, including scalability constraints, ethical considerations related to patient data governance, and the need for adaptive regulatory and organizational frameworks.

The remainder of the chapter is structured to guide readers through both conceptual and practical dimensions of blockchain-enabled digital twin systems for smart hospitals. Following this introduction, subsequent sections examine the technological foundations of digital twins and blockchain in healthcare, propose architectural models for their integration, and analyze application scenarios across clinical care, hospital operations, and infrastructure management. The chapter concludes with a discussion of open research challenges and strategic implications for stakeholders engaged in smart healthcare transformation. By bridging technological innovation with system-level governance considerations, this chapter aims to provide researchers, healthcare engineers, hospital administrators, and policy designers with a coherent foundation for advancing secure, intelligent, and interoperable hospital ecosystems.

2. CONCEPTUAL FOUNDATIONS: DIGITAL TWINS, BLOCKCHAIN, AND SMART HEALTHCARE SYSTEMS

The rapid digital transformation of healthcare systems has necessitated conceptual frameworks capable of representing, coordinating, and governing complex clinical and operational processes in real time. Traditional hospital information systems, which rely on fragmented databases and episodic data exchange, are increasingly insufficient for addressing the demands of precision medicine, adaptive resource management, and cross-organizational interoperability. In this context, digital twins and blockchain technologies have emerged as complementary paradigms that collectively enable intelligent, trustworthy, and resilient healthcare infrastructures. Understanding their conceptual foundations is essential to appreciating how blockchain-enabled digital twin architectures can reshape smart hospital ecosystems.

Digital twins originated as engineering constructs designed to mirror physical assets in industrial environments, enabling simulation, monitoring, and optimization across the lifecycle of machines and systems. Over time, the concept has evolved into a broader cyber-physical representation framework in which physical entities are continuously synchronized with their virtual counterparts through real-time data streams. In healthcare, this evolution reflects a shift from static modeling toward dynamic, data-driven representations of patients, medical devices, and organizational processes. Simultaneously, blockchain technologies have matured from cryptocurrency infrastructures into generalized distributed ledger systems capable of supporting secure coordination among untrusted actors. When embedded within smart hospital infrastructures, these technologies form a tightly coupled intelligence-and-trust stack that underpins next-generation healthcare delivery.

2.1 Digital Twins in Healthcare Systems

Before examining specific categories of healthcare digital twins, it is important to situate them within their broader theoretical foundation. A digital twin is not merely a simulation model but a continuously evolving virtual entity that maintains a bidirectional linkage with its physical counterpart. This linkage enables the digital twin to reflect the current state of the physical system, while also allowing predictive insights and control decisions generated in the virtual domain to influence real-world operations. The defining characteristics of digital twins—continuous synchronization, real-time analytics, and lifecycle integration—are particularly relevant in healthcare, where system states are highly dynamic and decision latency can have critical consequences (Grieves & Vickers, 2016).

In smart hospitals, digital twins can be broadly categorized into device twins, patient twins, and organizational twins. Device twins represent medical equipment such as ventilators, infusion pumps, imaging systems, and wearable sensors. These twins ingest high-frequency telemetry data related to performance, utilization, calibration, and fault conditions. By maintaining an up-to-date virtual replica of each device, hospitals can support predictive maintenance, reduce downtime, and ensure compliance with safety and regulatory standards. Moreover, device twins enable proactive responses to anomalies, which is particularly important in intensive care environments where equipment reliability directly affects patient outcomes.

Patient digital twins extend the concept further by modeling individual patients as complex, multi-dimensional systems. These twins integrate physiological signals, clinical histories, imaging data, behavioral patterns, and, increasingly, genomic and biomarker information. Unlike traditional electronic health records, patient twins are inherently dynamic, continuously updated as new data are generated through monitoring devices, laboratory tests, and clinical interventions. This enables personalized simulation of disease progression, treatment responses, and risk trajectories, supporting predictive and preventive care rather than reactive intervention (Grieves & Vickers, 2016). Comparable modeling approaches have been applied in vertical crop cultivation using IoT-integrated digital twins (Gowthaman et al., 2025), reinforcing the adaptability of twin architectures to dynamic, sensor-rich environments. At a higher level of abstraction, organizational digital twins model hospital-wide or system-level processes, including patient flow, bed allocation, staffing, logistics, energy consumption, and infection transmission pathways. These twins synthesize data from multiple departments and systems to provide a holistic view of operational performance. By simulating alternative scenarios—such as surges in patient admissions or disruptions in supply chains—organizational twins support strategic planning and adaptive decision-making. Collectively, these categories demonstrate how digital twins function as the operational intelligence layer of smart healthcare systems, generating high-value insights from continuous data streams.

2.2 Blockchain and Distributed Ledger Technologies for Healthcare

While digital twins excel at generating and analyzing real-time data, their effectiveness depends on the integrity, governance, and interoperability of the underlying information flows. This challenge becomes particularly acute in healthcare, where data are distributed across multiple stakeholders, including hospitals, laboratories, insurers, regulators, and device vendors. Blockchain and distributed ledger technologies address this challenge by providing a decentralized coordination mechanism that enables secure, verifiable, and tamper-resistant data sharing without reliance on a single trusted authority. At a conceptual level, a blockchain is a distributed ledger in which transactions are recorded in an append-only, cryptographically linked structure. This design ensures immutability, meaning that once data are recorded, they cannot be altered without detection. In healthcare settings, this property is crucial for maintaining trustworthy audit trails of clinical events, device usage, and data access. Immutable logs enhance accountability, support regulatory compliance, and reduce disputes among stakeholders (Kuo et al., 2017).

Another foundational capability of blockchain is cryptographic identity management. Through public-key infrastructures and decentralized identifiers, blockchain systems can authenticate users, devices, and organizations without exposing sensitive credentials. This enables fine-grained access control to clinical and operational data, ensuring that only authorized parties can interact with specific components of digital twin systems. Smart contracts further extend this functionality by embedding programmable logic into the ledger, allowing automated enforcement of data-sharing agreements, consent policies, and reimbursement rules (Kuo et al., 2017). Importantly, blockchain facilitates trustless data exchange, meaning that participants do not need to trust each other directly, but instead rely on the protocol's consensus and cryptographic guarantees. In multi-institutional healthcare ecosystems, this capability supports interoperability while preserving institutional autonomy. Rather than centralizing sensitive data, blockchain systems can store hashes, pointers, and access policies, enabling secure verification and coordination across heterogeneous platforms. Blockchain's role in securing real-time control systems has also been demonstrated in rover navigation and traffic coordination applications (Ruba et al., 2023; Poovithaa et al., 2025), highlighting its utility in decentralized, latency-sensitive infrastructures.

2.3 Smart Hospital Infrastructures and Synergistic Integration

To fully appreciate the role of digital twins and blockchain, they must be situated within the broader paradigm of smart hospital infrastructures. Smart hospitals are characterized by the convergence of medical Internet of Things devices, edge and cloud computing, artificial intelligence–based analytics, and interoperable information platforms. These components collectively enable real-time sensing, adaptive control, and data-driven decision-making across clinical and operational domains. Within this layered architecture, digital twins function as the intelligence layer that transforms raw sensor data into actionable insights. They support continuous monitoring, predictive modeling, and scenario-based simulation at multiple scales, from individual patients to entire hospital systems. Blockchain, in contrast, serves as the institutional memory and trust fabric that governs how these insights and underlying data are shared, validated, and acted upon across organizational boundaries.

The synergistic rationale for integrating these technologies lies in their complementary strengths. Digital twins generate high-frequency, high-value data that reflect the evolving state of healthcare systems, while blockchain ensures that these data streams remain verifiable, governed, interoperable, and resistant to tampering. Together, they enable smart hospitals to move beyond isolated digital innovations toward cohesive, secure, and adaptive healthcare ecosystems capable of supporting precision medicine, operational resilience, and collaborative care delivery.

3. ARCHITECTURAL FRAMEWORKS FOR BLOCKCHAIN-ENABLED DIGITAL TWIN HOSPITALS

The transformation of conventional hospitals into intelligent, adaptive, and data-driven healthcare ecosystems requires architectural frameworks that can seamlessly integrate cyber-physical systems, real-time analytics, and trusted data governance mechanisms. Digital twin technology provides a virtual representation of physical hospital entities—patients, medical devices, clinical workflows, and infrastructure—while blockchain introduces decentralized trust, immutability, and coordinated control across heterogeneous stakeholders. When combined, blockchain-enabled digital twin architectures offer a robust foundation for smart hospitals that demand interoperability, security, accountability, and operational intelligence at scale. This section presents a comprehensive architectural framework for blockchain-enabled digital twin hospitals, detailing its layered structure, interaction mechanisms, and deployment patterns, while emphasizing design principles that ensure resilience, privacy, and long-term scalability. At the core of this framework is a layered architectural model that aligns physical healthcare environments with digital representations and distributed ledger technologies. Each layer performs a distinct role while remaining tightly coupled through standardized interfaces and secure communication channels. This separation of concerns enables modular development, independent evolution of components, and fine-grained control over data flows—an essential requirement in highly regulated clinical environments. The architecture supports continuous synchronization between real-world hospital operations and their digital twins, while blockchain ensures that all critical interactions are verifiable, auditable, and policy-compliant.

3.1 Layered Architecture for Digital Twin–Blockchain Integration

Before detailing each architectural layer, it is important to recognize that the layered model is not merely a technical abstraction but a governance mechanism. By structuring hospital intelligence across layers, the architecture enforces responsibility boundaries, reduces systemic risk, and enables privacy-preserving data sharing across departments, institutions, and external partners. The following layers collectively form the backbone of a blockchain-enabled digital twin hospital. The Physical Layer represents the tangible hospital environment and includes medical devices, wearable sensors, imaging systems, robotic surgical platforms, smart beds, HVAC systems, and environmental monitoring units. These assets continuously generate high-frequency, heterogeneous data streams reflecting patient vitals, device performance, spatial conditions, and operational states. In a digital twin hospital, the physical layer is instrumented to support bi-directional interaction, allowing control commands, configuration updates, and predictive maintenance instructions to flow back from higher layers. The accuracy and reliability of this layer directly influence the fidelity of corresponding digital twins, making robust sensing, calibration, and fault detection critical. Above the physical infrastructure lies the Edge and Data Acquisition Layer, this acts as the first line of intelligence and data governance. Medical IoT gateways, edge servers, and hospital data hubs aggregate sensor outputs and perform real-time preprocessing, including noise reduction, event detection, anonymization, and data normalization. By executing analytics close to the data source, this layer minimizes latency and reduces bandwidth requirements, enabling near-real-time responsiveness for safety-critical clinical scenarios. From a privacy perspective, sensitive patient data can be filtered or tokenized at the edge before being transmitted further, ensuring compliance with healthcare data protection requirements. This layer also supports adaptive sampling and prioritization, ensuring that urgent clinical events are propagated immediately while routine data is handled asynchronously.

The Digital Twin Layer constitutes the cognitive core of the architecture. It hosts modular twin engines that represent patients, medical devices, clinical pathways, hospital departments, and even entire healthcare facilities. Patient digital twins integrate longitudinal health records, real-time physiological data, and contextual information to support personalized care modeling and predictive risk assessment. Device and infrastructure twins monitor operational states, enabling fault prediction and lifecycle optimization. Importantly, these digital twins are not static models; they evolve continuously through synchronization with physical assets and interactions with other twins. The modular design allows new twin types to be introduced without disrupting existing systems, supporting incremental hospital digitalization and future expansion (Grieves & Vickers, 2016). Similar modular twin engines have been explored in FPGA-based biomedical signal processing systems (Shanmugaraja et al., 2023), emphasizing the importance of scalable, edge integrated architectures.

Figure 1. Layered Architecture of Blockchain-Enabled Digital Twin Hospitals

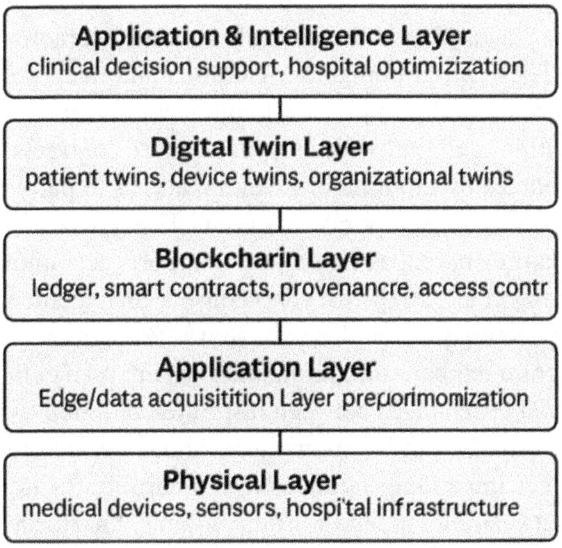

The Blockchain Layer provides the trust fabric that binds distributed digital twins into a coherent, accountable ecosystem. In a hospital context, permissioned blockchain networks are typically employed to ensure controlled participation by authorized entities such as clinicians, departments, partner hospitals, insurers, and regulators.

The blockchain maintains immutable records of data provenance, access requests, consent transactions, and operational events related to digital twin interactions. Rather than storing large clinical datasets on-chain, the ledger anchors cryptographic hashes and metadata that reference off-chain repositories, ensuring data integrity without compromising scalability or confidentiality. This layer enables decentralized coordination while preserving institutional autonomy, a key requirement in multi-stakeholder healthcare environments. At the top of the stack, the Application and Intelligence Layer translates digital twin insights and blockchain-verified data into actionable intelligence. Clinical decision support systems leverage patient twins to recommend interventions, optimize treatment pathways, and simulate outcomes under different scenarios. Hospital optimization applications use operational twins to improve resource allocation, bed management, and energy efficiency. Regulatory dashboards provide auditors and administrators with transparent, real-time visibility into compliance events and system performance. Advanced AI-driven simulations can explore "what-if" scenarios, supporting strategic planning and emergency preparedness. By building on trusted, synchronized data, this layer enables evidence-based decision-making across clinical and administrative domains.

3.2 Smart Contracts and Architectural Interaction Patterns

Smart contracts play a pivotal role in orchestrating interactions across the layered architecture. These programmable logic units automate policy enforcement, workflow coordination, and compliance logging without relying on centralized intermediaries. Within a digital twin hospital, smart contracts can dynamically manage consent policies by granting or revoking access to patient twin data based on predefined conditions and temporal constraints. Every access event is immutably recorded, creating a transparent audit trail that supports accountability and regulatory reporting (Zhang et al., 2018). Beyond consent management, smart contracts coordinate complex multi-stakeholder workflows. For example, in cross-hospital referral scenarios, contracts can validate patient consent, verify clinician credentials, and trigger secure data exchanges between institutional digital twins. In equipment maintenance, device twins can autonomously initiate service requests when predictive models detect impending failures, with smart contracts managing vendor interactions, service verification, and warranty claims. Pharmaceutical traceability workflows similarly benefit from blockchain-anchored twin interactions, ensuring that medication provenance and handling conditions are transparently recorded throughout the supply chain.

Different deployment patterns further shape how these interactions unfold. Private hospital blockchains support internal optimization and compliance within a single institution, offering low latency and strong governance control. Consortium hospital networks enable data sharing and collaborative care across multiple organizations, distributing trust while preserving institutional boundaries. Hybrid blockchain–cloud–edge architectures balance real-time responsiveness with scalable analytics by keeping time-critical twin synchronization at the edge, long-term storage in secure cloud environments, and coordination logic on blockchain networks. Across all patterns, careful data partitioning strategies are essential, with sensitive clinical data stored off-chain and only verifiable references maintained on-chain to ensure performance and privacy. In conclusion, the architectural frameworks for blockchain-enabled digital twin hospitals must be guided by core design principles: modularity to support incremental adoption, privacy-by-design to protect patient rights, interoperability-first development to avoid vendor lock-in, and resilience engineering to ensure continuity under failure conditions. By aligning digital twin intelligence with blockchain-based trust infrastructures, smart hospital architectures can move beyond isolated automation toward truly integrated, adaptive, and accountable healthcare ecosystems.

4. SECURE DATA EXCHANGE, PROVENANCE, AND ACCESS CONTROL MECHANISMS

The rapid adoption of digital twin technologies in healthcare introduces unprecedented requirements for secure data exchange, trustworthy system coordination, and continuous regulatory accountability. Digital twins depend on uninterrupted streams of multimodal data originating from electronic health records, wearable sensors, imaging systems, and cyber-physical medical devices. However, contemporary hospital IT infrastructures remain fragmented, centrally governed, and vulnerable to unauthorized access, data tampering, and provenance ambiguity. These limitations undermine the reliability of clinical twins and restrict their scalability across institutional boundaries. Blockchain technology emerges in this context not as a replacement for existing cybersecurity controls, but as a distributed trust and governance layer that restructures how data integrity, access rights, and accountability are enforced in real time. By embedding cryptographic identity, immutable event logging, and decentralized policy execution, blockchain aligns security mechanisms with the dynamic operational logic of healthcare digital twins, enabling secure, transparent, and auditable intelligence without compromising patient confidentiality (Kuo et al., 2017).

4.1 Health Data Provenance and Immutable Clinical Traceability

One of the most critical security challenges in digital twin ecosystems is the lack of end-to-end data provenance. Clinical decisions derived from digital twins are only as reliable as the traceability of their underlying data, including sensor measurements, diagnostic inferences, model updates, and clinician interventions. Traditional databases permit retrospective modification, often without transparent audit trails, creating medico-legal and ethical risks. Blockchain addresses this vulnerability by providing immutable, time-stamped records of all significant events within the twin lifecycle. Each data transaction—whether a physiological reading, imaging result, or algorithmic prediction—is cryptographically hashed and anchored on the ledger, ensuring verifiable integrity and chronological consistency (Azaria et al., 2016). In cybersecurity contexts, blockchain-based traceability has been applied to detect denial-of-service patterns in grayscale malware images (Krithika et al., 2025), underscoring its relevance for forensic integrity in healthcare data pipelines. In digital twin workflows, blockchain-based provenance frameworks enable clinicians and regulators to reconstruct how specific outcomes were generated, which data sources contributed, and which actors interacted with the system. This capability is particularly critical for AI-driven twins, where model outputs must be explainable and defensible. By separating on-chain metadata from off-chain encrypted clinical content, blockchain preserves scalability while guaranteeing that any alteration or omission is immediately detectable. As a result, digital twins transition from opaque computational artifacts to accountable clinical instruments whose decisions can be independently validated.

4.2 Smart Contract–Driven Fine-Grained Access Control

Healthcare data access is traditionally governed by static role-based access control mechanisms that fail to reflect dynamic clinical contexts, patient consent evolution, and cross-institutional collaboration. Digital twin environments intensify this limitation by requiring continuous, real-time access adjustments across clinicians, specialists, researchers, and autonomous systems. Blockchain smart contracts enable fine-grained, programmable access control models that encode patient consent, clinician privileges, and institutional policies directly into executable logic (Kuo et al., 2017). Through smart contracts, patients can retain cryptographic sovereignty over their digital twin data, granting, revoking, or time-limiting access based on treatment phases or research participation. Clinician permissions can be context-aware, activating only when specific clinical conditions or responsibilities are met. Importantly, all access events are immutably logged, enabling transparent accountability without manual oversight. This decentralized enforcement eliminates single points of failure and reduces reliance on administrative intermediaries, while still integrating seamlessly with hospital identity management systems. Consequently, access control evolves from static authorization lists to adaptive governance mechanisms aligned with personalized, twin-driven care. Smart contract–driven access models have also been proposed for inclusive care coordination during emergencies and disasters (Ponkarthika et al., 2026), demonstrating their value in dynamic, multi-stakeholder environments.

Figure 2. Smart Contract Workflow for Patient Digital Twin Access Control

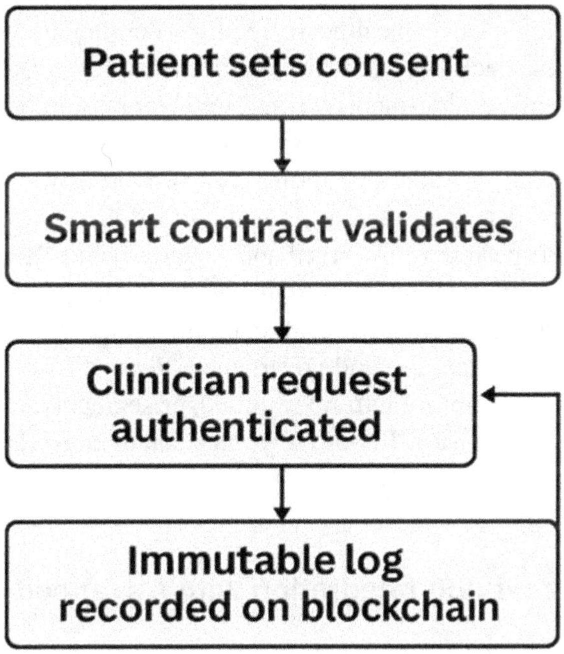

4.3 Device Authentication and Integrity in Medical IoT Twins

Digital twins rely extensively on medical Internet of Things (IoT) devices and cyber-physical systems, including wearable sensors, infusion pumps, imaging machines, and robotic platforms. These devices are frequent targets of spoofing, firmware manipulation, and impersonation attacks, which can propagate corrupted data into twin models and compromise clinical decisions. Blockchain provides a decentralized device authentication framework where each device is assigned a cryptographic identity anchored to the ledger at registration (Azaria et al., 2016). Using blockchain-based identity verification, digital twins can validate that incoming data originates from authenticated, uncompromised devices. Firmware updates, calibration events, and operational status changes can be immutably recorded, ensuring lifecycle integrity and non-repudiation. This approach is particularly valuable in large hospital environments where thousands of devices interact concurrently with multiple digital twins. By embedding trust at the device level, blockchain transforms medical IoT from a security liability into a verifiable extension of the clinical ecosystem.

4.4 Auditability, Regulatory Transparency, and Compliance Assurance

Regulatory compliance in healthcare requires continuous documentation of data handling, access decisions, and clinical accountability. Traditional audit processes are retrospective, labor-intensive, and vulnerable to inconsistencies across systems. Blockchain introduces native auditability by design, enabling real-time regulatory transparency without disrupting clinical workflows. Every interaction with a digital twin—data ingestion, access authorization, algorithm execution, or decision support—is permanently logged and cryptographically verifiable (Kuo et al., 2017). This capability supports compliance with data protection regulations, accreditation standards, and medico-legal requirements by providing tamper-proof evidence of appropriate data use and governance. Regulators and auditors can be granted permissioned visibility into relevant ledger segments, reducing reporting burdens while enhancing trust. Importantly, blockchain does not expose sensitive patient data; rather, it records verifiable proofs of compliance actions, ensuring privacy-preserving transparency.

4.5 Privacy-Preserving Integration with Advanced Analytics

While blockchain ensures trust and integrity, it must coexist with privacy-preserving computation to support intelligent digital twin analytics. Integration with zero-knowledge proofs enables verification of compliance or data validity without revealing underlying clinical information. Off-chain encrypted repositories store high-volume medical data, while blockchain maintains access permissions and integrity hashes. Federated learning frameworks allow digital twins to learn across institutions without centralizing data, with blockchain coordinating model updates and contribution accountability. Secure enclaves further protect sensitive computations during runtime, ensuring that analytics remain confidential even in distributed environments (Azaria et al., 2016). Together, these integrations demonstrate that blockchain restructures, rather than replaces, hospital cybersecurity. It functions as a distributed governance layer that aligns trust enforcement with the real-time, adaptive nature of digital twins. By embedding security, provenance, and accountability directly into system operations, blockchain enables digital twin ecosystems to scale responsibly while preserving clinical integrity and patient trust.

5. INTELLIGENT DIGITAL TWIN APPLICATIONS IN SMART HOSPITAL ECOSYSTEMS

Intelligent digital twins are emerging as a core enabler of next-generation smart hospital ecosystems, shifting healthcare delivery from reactive processes toward predictive, adaptive, and system-wide intelligence. Within hospital environments, digital twins function as continuously updated virtual representations of patients, clinical workflows, physical assets, and organizational processes. When integrated with blockchain infrastructures, these twins become trustworthy, interoperable, and auditable decision-support instruments rather than isolated analytical models. Blockchain provides a decentralized trust fabric that ensures data provenance, immutability, and controlled sharing, which are essential in multi-stakeholder healthcare settings. Together, digital twins and blockchain transform hospitals into learning systems capable of real-time optimization and coordinated intelligence. This section examines how blockchain-enabled digital twins are applied across four critical hospital domains, highlighting their role in real-time analytics, interoperability, and institutional trust within complex healthcare ecosystems.

5.1 Clinical Decision Support through Patient Digital Twins

In clinical decision support, patient-centric digital twins represent one of the most impactful applications within smart hospitals. These digital replicas integrate heterogeneous data streams, including physiological signals, medical imaging, laboratory results, genomic markers, and longitudinal treatment histories, into a unified and continuously evolving patient model. By synthesizing real-time and historical data, patient digital twins enable predictive risk scoring, disease progression modeling, and therapy outcome simulation. Clinicians can explore multiple intervention pathways virtually before applying them in real care settings, reducing uncertainty and improving personalized treatment planning. Moreover, blockchain-based access control mechanisms ensure that sensitive patient information is shared only with authorized stakeholders, supporting privacy-preserving clinical intelligence. Conversational AI systems have similarly enhanced personalized education and support in academic settings (Ruba et al., 2026a), suggesting parallel opportunities for patient engagement and adaptive learning in clinical contexts. As emphasized in prior research, such secure data integration is fundamental to realizing the full potential of digital twins in healthcare decision-making (Fuller et al., 2020; Kuo et al., 2017).

5.2 Operational Optimization and Hospital-Wide Intelligence

Beyond individual patient care, digital twins enable comprehensive operational optimization across hospital ecosystems. Hospital-level digital twins model infrastructure elements such as bed occupancy, operating room utilization, staff availability, medical equipment usage, energy consumption, and infection control workflows. By continuously synchronizing with real-time operational data, these twins provide hospital administrators with a holistic, system-level view of resource dynamics and constraints. Predictive analytics embedded within operational twins support proactive decision-making, such as anticipating bed shortages, optimizing surgical schedules, and reallocating staff during peak demand periods.

Blockchain enhances operational digital twins by enabling trusted coordination among departments, external vendors, and service providers. Smart contracts can automate interdepartmental workflows, enforce service-level agreements, and validate operational transactions without relying on centralized intermediaries. For example, asset movement, equipment usage, and supply chain events can be recorded immutably on a shared ledger, ensuring transparency and accountability across organizational boundaries. This decentralized coordination reduces inefficiencies caused by information silos and manual reconciliation processes. Prior studies highlight that blockchain-supported data sharing is essential for achieving interoperable and resilient hospital operations in complex healthcare networks (Kuo et al., 2017; Fuller et al., 2020). Organizational agility frameworks from digital transformation research (Ruba et al., 2026b) further support the integration of emerging technologies into adaptive hospital operations.

5.3 Medical Device Lifecycle Management and Compliance

Medical devices represent another critical application domain for blockchain-enabled digital twins within smart hospitals. Digital twins of medical devices capture detailed information about device specifications, operational parameters, usage histories, maintenance schedules, and performance degradation over time. These virtual counterparts allow biomedical engineers and hospital administrators to monitor device health continuously, predict failures, and optimize maintenance strategies. Predictive maintenance supported by device digital twins reduces downtime, extends equipment lifespan, and enhances patient safety.

Blockchain strengthens device lifecycle management by securing maintenance logs, calibration records, and safety certifications in an immutable and auditable ledger. Each maintenance action or usage event is cryptographically linked to the device's digital twin, creating a transparent compliance trail that can be inspected by regulators, manufacturers, and hospital authorities. This traceability is particularly important for high-risk medical devices, where accountability and regulatory compliance are paramount. Furthermore, blockchain-based certification sharing enables hospitals to verify device authenticity and safety status across institutional boundaries, fostering trust among manufacturers, service providers, and healthcare organizations. The convergence of digital twins and blockchain thus supports a trustworthy and interoperable device ecosystem, as recognized in contemporary healthcare informatics research (Fuller et al., 2020).

5.4 Emergency and Pandemic Response Coordination

Emergency and pandemic response scenarios highlight the systemic value of intelligent digital twins at regional and national scales. In such contexts, real-time hospital digital twins provide situational awareness by aggregating data on patient inflows, ICU capacity, ventilator availability, workforce readiness, and supply chain status. These dynamic models enable health authorities to simulate outbreak trajectories, evaluate intervention strategies, and allocate resources efficiently across multiple institutions. Unlike traditional reporting systems, digital twins support continuous adaptation as conditions evolve rapidly.

Blockchain infrastructure ensures that data shared across hospitals, public health agencies, and government bodies remains trustworthy and verifiable. During crises, misinformation, delayed reporting, and data manipulation can severely undermine coordinated responses. Blockchain-secured data exchange guarantees that shared indicators and policy decisions are based on validated information with clear provenance. Smart contracts can also enforce transparent allocation rules for scarce resources, such as critical care equipment or vaccines, reducing disputes and enhancing public trust. Research underscores that decentralized trust mechanisms are essential for scalable and equitable healthcare coordination during large-scale emergencies (Kuo et al., 2017; Fuller et al., 2020).

5.5 Trust, Interoperability, and Institutional Accountability

Across all application domains, the defining contribution of blockchain-enabled digital twins lies in their ability to embed trust, interoperability, and accountability into hospital intelligence systems. Digital twins generate powerful insights through real-time analytics and simulation, but their adoption depends on the credibility of underlying data and models. Blockchain addresses this challenge by providing immutable records, standardized interfaces for data exchange, and transparent governance mechanisms. As a result, insights produced by digital twins become traceable to verified data pipelines and accountable to institutional policies. Interoperability is further enhanced through decentralized architectures that allow heterogeneous systems to participate without surrendering data ownership. Hospitals, vendors, regulators, and insurers can collaborate through shared digital twin ecosystems while maintaining sovereignty over their data assets. This balance between openness and control is crucial for sustainable smart hospital transformation. Together, blockchain and digital twins redefine hospital ecosystems as intelligent, trusted, and adaptive socio-technical systems capable of continuous learning and coordinated action (Fuller et al., 2020). Educational ecosystems built on intelligent campuses (Ruba et al., 2026c) offer a parallel model for trust-based, interoperable learning infrastructures that can inform hospital-wide digital twin governance.

6. SYSTEMS INTEGRATION: INTEROPERABILITY, EDGE COMPUTING, AND REAL-TIME ANALYTICS

The operationalization of blockchain-enabled digital twins in real hospital environments is less constrained by individual technologies than by the challenge of integrating them into cohesive, reliable, and clinically acceptable systems. Hospitals are inherently heterogeneous ecosystems composed of legacy information systems, diverse medical devices, siloed data repositories, and institution-specific workflows. In such contexts, digital twins cannot function as isolated simulation artifacts, nor can blockchains operate merely as static record-keeping layers. Instead, their combined value emerges only through carefully engineered system integration that enables interoperability, low-latency responsiveness, and continuous analytical intelligence. This section examines how interoperability standards, edge computing infrastructures, and real-time analytics pipelines collectively enable scalable and trustworthy digital twin deployments in smart hospital settings.

Effective systems integration requires reconciling fundamentally different temporal, semantic, and computational characteristics. Clinical sensor data streams are high-velocity and transient, while blockchain transactions are comparatively slower and immutable. Digital twins require near-real-time synchronization with physical assets, whereas institutional coordination demands consistency, auditability, and governance. Addressing these tensions necessitates layered architectures in which interoperability middleware, edge intelligence, and analytics orchestration play central roles. When successfully integrated, these components transform hospitals into distributed cognitive infrastructures, where digital twins provide continuous situational awareness and blockchain stabilizes multi-actor coordination.

6.1 Interoperability Frameworks for Heterogeneous Clinical Systems

Interoperability is the foundational requirement for integrating digital twins across hospital subsystems. Modern hospitals operate with electronic health records (EHRs), laboratory information systems, imaging platforms, wearable sensors, and smart medical devices, often sourced from different vendors and implemented across decades. Digital twins must aggregate and interpret data from these heterogeneous sources to maintain accurate and clinically meaningful virtual representations. Without standardized interoperability frameworks, twin models risk fragmentation, inconsistency, and limited clinical utility.

FHIR-based clinical standards have emerged as a critical enabler of syntactic and semantic interoperability in healthcare environments. By defining structured data resources for patients, observations, procedures, and devices, FHIR allows digital twins to access and exchange clinical data in a consistent and machine-interpretable manner. When combined with medical device ontologies and semantic middleware, FHIR facilitates the alignment of heterogeneous data models into unified twin representations. Semantic middleware acts as an abstraction layer that translates vendor-specific device outputs into standardized concepts, enabling cross-platform twin orchestration without requiring invasive changes to existing systems (Kritikos et al., 2021).

6.2 Edge Computing for Latency-Sensitive Hospital Operations

While cloud infrastructures provide scalability and computational power, many hospital operations require response times that exceed the tolerances of centralized processing. Latency-sensitive tasks such as continuous patient monitoring, robotic surgery assistance, and emergency response demand immediate local intelligence. Edge computing addresses this requirement by placing computational resources closer to data sources, enabling real-time processing and decision-making at the point of care.

In digital twin architectures, edge nodes serve as intermediaries between physical assets and higher-level analytical systems. Physiological sensors, imaging devices, and robotic platforms stream data to nearby edge processors, where preliminary analytics, anomaly detection, and twin state updates are performed. This local processing reduces network congestion and ensures that critical clinical insights are generated even during connectivity disruptions. Only validated summaries, alerts, or state transitions are propagated to cloud services or blockchain networks, optimizing both performance and reliability (Shi et al., 2016). The integration of edge computing with blockchain introduces architectural considerations related to synchronization and consensus. High-frequency sensor updates cannot be recorded directly on distributed ledgers without compromising throughput. Instead, edge nodes aggregate and validate data streams, periodically committing cryptographic proofs or significant events to consortium blockchains. This design reconciles the speed of real-time clinical operations with the immutability and trust guarantees of blockchain systems. As a result, hospitals can achieve both operational responsiveness and institutional accountability.

6.3 Real-Time Analytics and AI-Driven Twin Orchestration

Real-time analytics form the cognitive layer that transforms integrated infrastructures into intelligent hospital systems. Digital twins continuously ingest data from physical assets, but their value lies in the ability to analyze patterns, predict outcomes, and recommend actions. AI-driven analytics pipelines enable digital twins to move beyond passive mirroring toward proactive operational intelligence. Machine learning models deployed across edge and cloud layers analyze streaming data for early signs of patient deterioration, equipment malfunction, or workflow bottlenecks. These insights dynamically update twin states, allowing clinicians and administrators to visualize evolving scenarios and test intervention strategies. Blockchain infrastructure complements these analytics by ensuring that model updates, decision rationales, and data provenance are transparently recorded and auditable. This is particularly important in federated hospital networks, where multiple institutions share analytical models without exchanging raw patient data (Fuller et al., 2020).

Cross-platform twin orchestration further extends analytical capabilities by coordinating multiple twin instances across departments and institutions. For example, operating room twins, intensive care twins, and supply chain twins can interact through standardized interfaces, enabling system-wide optimization. Consortium blockchains support this orchestration by enforcing governance rules, access controls, and trust relationships among participating entities. In such architectures, digital twins act as adaptive intelligence nodes, while blockchain provides the structural backbone for secure and coordinated collaboration. Overall, the integration of interoperability frameworks, edge computing, and real-time analytics redefines the hospital as a distributed cognitive infrastructure. Blockchain stabilizes institutional coordination by embedding trust, provenance, and governance into system interactions, while digital twins enable continuous operational intelligence through synchronized virtual representations. Together, these technologies support scalable, responsive, and trustworthy healthcare ecosystems capable of meeting the complexity of modern clinical environments.

7. EMERGING CHALLENGES, ETHICAL GOVERNANCE, AND FUTURE RESEARCH PATHWAYS

Despite the growing maturity of blockchain-enabled digital twin architectures for smart hospital infrastructures, several unresolved technical, organizational, regulatory, and ethical challenges continue to constrain large-scale deployment and long-term sustainability. While earlier sections have demonstrated the transformative potential of intelligent twins for real-time clinical intelligence, secure interoperability, and adaptive hospital operations, this section critically examines the limitations that remain at the frontier of research and practice. Addressing these barriers is essential not only for technological feasibility but also for ensuring ethical legitimacy, institutional trust, and equitable value distribution within digitally mediated healthcare ecosystems. The discussion below synthesizes emerging constraints and governance concerns, foregrounds ethical risks inherent in real-time twin ecosystems, and outlines future research trajectories capable of advancing secure, accountable, and human-centered intelligent hospital infrastructures.

7.1 Technical and Infrastructural Constraints

At the technical level, blockchain scalability remains a persistent bottleneck for hospital-scale digital twin ecosystems. Smart hospitals generate high-frequency, heterogeneous data streams from medical devices, imaging systems, electronic health records, and environmental sensors. When such data are synchronized with digital twins and anchored to blockchain ledgers, transaction throughput and confirmation latency can significantly degrade system responsiveness, particularly in time-sensitive clinical contexts. Existing consensus mechanisms often struggle to balance decentralization, security, and real-time performance, raising concerns about the suitability of current blockchain architectures for continuous clinical operations (Zheng et al., 2018).

Latency is further compounded by the need for interoperability across institutional and vendor-specific systems. Digital twins rely on standardized data representations to ensure semantic consistency between physical assets and their virtual counterparts, yet healthcare data remain fragmented across incompatible formats and ontologies. Inadequate data standardization complicates twin model validation, increases integration costs, and limits cross-hospital intelligence sharing. Additionally, the computational and energy demands of blockchain infrastructures raise sustainability concerns, particularly for resource-constrained healthcare systems. Energy-intensive validation processes may conflict with environmental sustainability goals and impose hidden operational costs that undermine long-term viability. Another unresolved challenge lies in the validation and governance of clinical twin models themselves. Unlike static software systems, digital twins evolve dynamically as they learn from new data. Ensuring the clinical accuracy, robustness, and safety of continuously updating models is nontrivial, particularly when decision-support outputs influence diagnoses, workflows, or resource allocation. Without formalized validation frameworks, there is a risk of propagating errors, biases, or model drift across interconnected hospital systems.

7.2 Organizational and Regulatory Barriers

Beyond infrastructure, organizational readiness and regulatory alignment pose equally significant challenges. The introduction of algorithmic digital twins into clinical decision-making raises complex questions of liability and accountability. When adverse outcomes occur, responsibility may be diffused across clinicians, hospital administrators, algorithm designers, and blockchain governance bodies. Existing medico-legal frameworks are poorly equipped to adjudicate such distributed accountability structures, creating uncertainty that can inhibit adoption. Governance of algorithmic twins also remains underdeveloped. Hospitals must determine who has authority to deploy, modify, audit, or deactivate digital twins, particularly when these systems operate autonomously or across institutional boundaries. Cross-border data exchange introduces further regulatory complexity, as healthcare blockchains may span jurisdictions with divergent data protection laws and ethical norms. Ensuring compliance with heterogeneous regulatory regimes while maintaining system interoperability remains an open research and policy challenge.

Workforce adaptation represents another critical organizational barrier. Intelligent digital twins alter clinical workflows, redistribute expertise, and reshape professional roles. Without adequate training, participatory design processes, and change management strategies, hospital staff may resist or misuse these systems, undermining their intended benefits. The success of intelligent infrastructures therefore depends not only on technical robustness but also on institutional capacity for socio-technical integration.

7.3 Ethical Dimensions and Governance Imperatives

Ethical considerations are central to the deployment of real-time digital twin ecosystems. Algorithmic accountability is a primary concern, as opaque models embedded within blockchain infrastructures can obscure decision rationales and limit contestability. Even when data integrity is guaranteed by distributed ledgers, the ethical legitimacy of algorithmic outputs depends on transparency, explainability, and mechanisms for human oversight (Mittelstadt et al., 2016). Patient autonomy and informed consent become increasingly complex in continuous monitoring environments. Digital twins may operate persistently, aggregating and analyzing patient data beyond discrete episodes of care. Traditional consent models, based on static and one-time agreements, are ill-suited to such dynamic ecosystems. Without adaptive consent mechanisms, patients risk losing meaningful control over how their data are used, shared, and monetized.

Surveillance risks also intensify as hospital infrastructures become more instrumented and interconnected. While real-time monitoring can enhance safety and efficiency, it may also enable intrusive oversight of patients and healthcare workers alike. Power asymmetries between institutions, technology providers, and individuals can be amplified when data-driven governance mechanisms are deployed without ethical safeguards. Ensuring that intelligent hospital infrastructures do not erode trust or exacerbate inequalities is therefore a critical ethical mandate (Topol, 2019).

7.4 Future Research Pathways

Future research must move beyond incremental optimization toward fundamentally new paradigms of intelligent, ethical hospital governance. One promising direction lies in self-evolving hospital twins capable of autonomously adapting to changing clinical, operational, and regulatory conditions while remaining verifiable and auditable. Coupled with this is the concept of autonomous compliance engines, where regulatory constraints are encoded into smart contracts that dynamically enforce legal and ethical requirements across jurisdictions.

Interoperable healthcare blockchains designed specifically for clinical digital twins represent another critical research frontier. Such platforms must prioritize low-latency performance, semantic interoperability, and sustainability while preserving decentralization and trust. Finally, ethical governance must be embedded by design, not retrofitted. This includes participatory governance models, continuous ethical auditing, and socio-technical frameworks that align intelligent infrastructures with human values and institutional accountability. Together, these research trajectories offer a pathway toward secure, adaptive, and ethically grounded intelligent hospital ecosystems.

8. CONCLUSION

The convergence of blockchain-enabled digital twin architectures marks a decisive shift in the evolution of smart hospitals, signaling not a marginal technological enhancement but a fundamental restructuring of how healthcare infrastructures are designed, governed, and operated. Throughout this chapter, it has been argued that contemporary hospital systems face persistent challenges related to data fragmentation, interoperability constraints, cybersecurity risks, and limited adaptability to dynamic clinical and operational conditions. In this context, blockchain and digital twins emerge as complementary technologies whose integration addresses these limitations at a systemic level. Blockchain provides a decentralized, tamper-resistant ledger that establishes trust across heterogeneous stakeholders, ensuring data integrity, provenance, and accountability in environments characterized by frequent information exchange and high regulatory demands. By embedding cryptographic security, consensus mechanisms, and programmable smart contracts into hospital workflows, distributed ledgers create a governance fabric that supports transparent access control, auditable transactions, and cross-institutional collaboration without reliance on centralized authorities. Simultaneously, digital twins introduce a powerful layer of real-time intelligence by creating continuously synchronized virtual representations of physical hospital assets, clinical processes, and patient pathways. These virtual counterparts enable simulation, prediction, and optimization, allowing healthcare systems to anticipate disruptions, evaluates alternative interventions, and adapts operations proactively rather than reactively. When integrated with blockchain, digital twins benefit from trusted data inputs and verifiable update histories, enhancing their reliability and clinical relevance. This synergy enables secure clinical collaboration across departments and organizations, supports transparent operational management through immutable performance records, and strengthens institutional resilience by enabling coordinated responses to emergencies, resource shortages, and system failures. Importantly, the architectural fusion of these technologies facilitates semantic and technical interoperability, allowing disparate medical devices, information systems, and administrative platforms to operate within a unified, standards-driven ecosystem. Beyond technical integration, the chapter highlights broader strategic and organizational implications. Blockchain-enabled digital twins reshape hospitals into cyber-physical systems where physical infrastructure, digital intelligence, and governance mechanisms are tightly interwoven. In such environments, decision-making is increasingly data-driven and evidence-based, supported by continuous feedback loops between real-world conditions and their digital representations. This transformation also redefines accountability and trust in healthcare delivery, shifting from institution-centric control toward decentralized yet coordinated governance models that empower clinicians, administrators, patients, and regulators alike. From a policy and innovation perspective, the adoption of these architectures encourages modular system design, scalability, and long-term sustainability, aligning smart hospital development with the goals of precision medicine, value-based care, and population health management. Moreover, by embedding privacy-preserving mechanisms and fine-grained consent management into the core infrastructure, blockchain-enabled digital twins address ethical and legal concerns associated with large-scale health data utilization, fostering public trust and regulatory compliance. Ultimately, the chapter underscores that future hospitals will no longer function merely as repositories of medical information or isolated service providers. Instead, they will evolve into living, adaptive ecosystems—intelligent cyber-physical organisms where trusted data flows, real-time modeling, and decentralized governance converge. This paradigm supports safer clinical practices, smarter operational strategies, and more accountable healthcare delivery, positioning smart hospitals as foundational pillars of resilient and innovation-driven health systems in the digital era.

REFERENCES

Azaria, A., Ekblaw, A., Vieira, T., & Lippman, A. (2016, August). Medrec: Using blockchain for medical data access and permission management. In 2016 2nd international conference on open and big data (OBD) (pp. 25-30). IEEE.

Dhanushya, J., Ruba, M., Ponkarthika, M., Soundarya, B., Sakthi Priya, V., Dhanushri, S., & Harikrishnan, S. (2025, April). AI-Powered Multipurpose Agrobot for Precision Farming: Crop Health Management, Fertilizer Recommendation and Yield Prediction. In *2025 International Conference on Recent Advances in Electrical, Electronics, Ubiquitous Communication, and Computational Intelligence (RAEEUCCI)* (pp. 1-6). IEEE.

Fuller, A., Fan, Z., Day, C., & Barlow, C. (2020). Digital twin: Enabling technologies, challenges and open research. *IEEE Access : Practical Innovations, Open Solutions*, *8*, 108952–108971. DOI: 10.1109/ACCESS.2020.2998358

Gowthaman, N., Ruba, M., Aswath, S., Hemavarshni, S. N., Bragadeshwaran, R., & Nithish, S. J. (2025, November). Iot Integrated Solution For Smart Vertical Crop Cultivation. In 2025 IEEE 7th International Conference on Computing, Communication and Automation (ICCCA) (pp. 1-6). IEEE.

Grieves, M., & Vickers, J. (2016). Digital twin: Mitigating unpredictable, undesirable emergent behavior in complex systems. In *Transdisciplinary perspectives on complex systems: New findings and approaches* (pp. 85–113). Springer International Publishing.

Krithika, S., Jayachandran, T., Raghapriya, N. R., Ruba, M., Janani, C., & Sathiyavathi, S. (2025, April). An Effective Denial of Service Texture Features from Malware Grayscale Image. In 2025 3rd International Conference on Artificial Intelligence and Machine Learning Applications Theme: Healthcare and Internet of Things (AIMLA) (pp. 1-7). IEEE. DOI: 10.1109/AIMLA63829.2025.11041501

Kuo, T. T., Kim, H. E., & Ohno-Machado, L. (2017). Blockchain distributed ledger technologies for biomedical and health care applications. *Journal of the American Medical Informatics Association : JAMIA*, *24*(6), 1211–1220. DOI: 10.1093/jamia/ocx068 PMID: 29016974

Mittelstadt, B. D., Allo, P., Taddeo, M., Wachter, S., & Floridi, L. (2016). The ethics of algorithms: Mapping the debate. *Big Data & Society*, *3*(2), 2053951716679679. DOI: 10.1177/2053951716679679

Nakamoto, S. (2008). Bitcoin: A peer-to-peer electronic cash system.

Ponkarthika, M. G., A. P., Ruba, M., Kishore, Y. R., M., K., & G. V., M. (2026). Bridging Health Equity in Times of Crisis: Ensuring Inclusive Care During Emergencies and Disasters. In E. Matsumoto, F. Andres, & R. Agrawal (Eds.), Advancing Equity in Global Healthcare Systems (pp. 27-54). IGI Global Scientific Publishing. DOI: 10.4018/979-8-3373-1330-6.ch002

Poovithaa, M., Ruba, M., Ponkarthika, M., Ragul, N., Ragul, V., & Sangeetha, K. (2025, November). IoT Smart Traffic Control System for Hill Roads with Emergency Vehicle Priority. In 2025 IEEE 7th International Conference on Computing, Communication and Automation (ICCCA) (pp. 1-6). IEEE.

Ruba, M., Ashwin Prabhu, G., Deka, J., Kavitha, D., Sathiya, S., & Pavithra, S. (2026a). Empowering learners and educators: The transformative role of conversational AI in personalized education and student support. In Assayed, S. (Ed.), *Enhancing student support and learning through conversational AI* (pp. 163–190). IGI Global Scientific Publishing., DOI: 10.4018/979-8-3373-3316-8.ch007

Ruba, M., Ashwin Prabhu, G., Robinson Joel, M., Vishnu Priya, K., Dharshani, L., & Dharani, R. (2026b). Integrating emerging technologies for organizational agility: An interdisciplinary approach to digital transformation. In Roache, D. (Ed.), *High performance leadership for organizational excellence: Innovation, technology, and resilience* (pp. 63–92). IGI Global Scientific Publishing., DOI: 10.4018/979-8-3373-6207-6.ch003

Ruba, M., Girinath, V. P., Ponkarthika, M., Santhini, C., Sakthi Priya, V., & Hemalatha, R. (2023, December). Design and implementation of smart internet-based real-time control of rover with artificial intelligence. In *2023 International Conference on Energy, Materials and Communication Engineering (ICEMCE)* (pp. 1–5). IEEE. https://doi.org/DOI: 10.1109/ICEMCE2023

Ruba, M., Ponkarthika, M., Parameshwari, V., Girinath, V. P., Soundarya, B., Janani, M., & Santhini, C. (2025, February). Enhancing underwater tunnel safety through smart inspection: An ROV-based system with AI-powered crack detection using Canny edge detection. In Proceedings of the 2025 3rd International Conference on Intelligent Systems, Advanced Computing and Communication (ISACC) (pp. 1067–1072). IEEE. https://doi.org/DOI: 10.1109/ISACC.2025

Ruba, M., Preetha, D. S., Ponkarthika, M., Gomathi, V., Sudha, E., & Pratheeba, C. (2026c). Smart Pedagogies and Intelligent Campuses: Reimagining Higher Education in the Digital Age. In Harnessing Geospatial Information Systems for Sustainable Economic and Regional Development (pp. 29-54). IGI Global Scientific Publishing.

Shanmugaraja, T., Ruba, M., Priya, V. S., Venkatesh, T., Supriya, M., & Nallamuthu, M. (2023, September). ECG noise elimination using an FPGA version of a modified error normalized LMS adaptive filter. In AIP Conference Proceedings (Vol. 2764, No. 1, p. 060033). AIP Publishing LLC. DOI: 10.1063/5.0144367

Shi, W., Cao, J., Zhang, Q., Li, Y., & Xu, L. (2016). Edge computing: Vision and challenges. *IEEE Internet of Things Journal, 3*(5), 637–646. DOI: 10.1109/JIOT.2016.2579198

Topol, E. J. (2019). High-performance medicine: The convergence of human and artificial intelligence. *Nature Medicine, 25*(1), 44–56. DOI: 10.1038/s41591-018-0300-7 PMID: 30617339

Zhang, P., Schmidt, D. C., White, J., & Lenz, G. (2018). Blockchain technology use cases in healthcare. [). Elsevier.]. *Advances in Computers, 111*, 1–41. DOI: 10.1016/bs.adcom.2018.03.006

Zheng, Z., Xie, S., Dai, H. N., Chen, X., & Wang, H. (2018). Blockchain challenges and opportunities: A survey. *International Journal of Web and Grid Services, 14*(4), 352–375. DOI: 10.1504/IJWGS.2018.095647

Chapter 14

Decoding Digital Twins: Possible Applications in the Near Future

R Felista Sugirtha Lizy
http://orcid.org/0000-0003-3648-0205
Department of Computer Science, A.P.C. Mahalaxmi College for Women, Thoothukudi, India

Amit Kumar Tyagi D.
http://orcid.org/0000-0003-2657-8700
School of Law, Forensic Justice, and Policy Studies, National Forensic Sciences University, Gandhinagar, India

K. R. Pundareeka Vittala
http://orcid.org/0000-0002-5579-2813
ICFAI Foundation for Higher Education, Bengaluru, India

V. Hemamalini
http://orcid.org/0000-0001-8237-031X
Department of Networking and Communications, SRM Institute of Science and Technology, Kattankulathur, India

ABSTRACT

Digital twins are a paradigm shift whereby a digital model of a physical object or a process is constantly updated with real-time information to allow monitoring, simulation, and predictive analysis. Digital twins enable organizations to streamline operations, anticipate failures, and make better decisions without interfering with physical systems due to the incorporation of the latest sensor networks, artificial intelligence, cloud and edge computing, and data visualization. The chapter delves into the history of digital twins, the technology behind them, and the new uses of

DOI: 10.4018/979-8-3373-8177-0.ch014

digital twins in manufacturing, healthcare, smart cities, and energy management. It also discusses technical, operational, and ethical problems related to the adoption of digital twins and suggests possible ways of overcoming these problems. This work positions digital twins as a revolutionary tool that integrates the physical and digital worlds and creates innovation and resilience in various fields by evaluating the existing trends and near-term opportunities.

1. INTRODUCTION

The increasing presence of digital technologies into physical systems has led to the emergence of digital twins, a structure that allows the interaction between the virtual and the physical worlds to take place without any issues. Digital twins originally were supposed to be utilized in the aerospace industry to aid in tracking spacecraft but now they have become versatile systems capable of simulating complicated systems in real-time (Grieves & Vickers, 2017). Unlike the traditional form of simulation models, digital twins are dynamic and continuously updated with real-time sensor and operational data, which makes them predictive and prescriptive to analyze.

Digital twins have numerous benefits which include predictive maintenance, optimal operations, process simulation, and risk reduction. They allow factories to forecast the breakdown of the equipment used in the production process, to regulate the production volume, and to enhance control over the quality (Tao et al., 2018; Qi et al., 2020). Digital twins of patients can be used in healthcare to tailor the treatment planning, the ongoing monitoring, and predict patient outcomes (Bruynseels et al., 2018). Infrastructure, resource allocation, and sustainability are also simulated with the help of digital twins by urban planners and energy managers (Batty et al., 2012; Liu et al., 2021).

Digital twins rely on interactions between technologies, including Internet of Things (IoT), artificial intelligence (AI), machine learning, cloud and edge computing, and high-tech visualization interfaces (Boschert and Rosen, 2016; Qi and Tao, 2018). Though these enabling technologies provide a high degree of functionality, the issues of data and information security, model validation, interoperability, and ethics are also the significant barriers to their overall implementation. The given chapter is devoted to the detailed examination of digital twin technology, presentation of technical frameworks, industry applications, issues, and new opportunities.

2. LITERATURE SURVEY

Digital twins are rapidly becoming one of the primary technologies which can bridge the gap between the real and virtual world in different fields, including manufacturing, healthcare, urban planning, energy infrastructure. The first application of the digital twin was in the space sector where simulated models of a spacecraft were created and the functioning of the systems in real-time was monitored (Grieves & Vickers, 2017). These early applications demonstrated that virtual models could be applied to predictive maintenance and performance optimization and therefore formed the foundation of further application in industry.

Industry 4.0 manufacturing paradigm now involves the use of digital twins that can be monitored in real-time to monitor the processes, predictive maintenance, and optimization of the processes (Tao et al., 2018; Qi et al., 2020). The integration of IoT sensors, machine learning, and cloud-based analytics will enable manufacturers to make their systems very dynamic to adaptively respond to operating conditions (Lee et al., 2015; Lu et al., 2020). It has also been discovered that due to the ability to provide continuous feedback between physical and virtual twins, digital twins can enhance productivity, minimize downtime, and optimize the use of resources (Fuller et al., 2020; Jones et al., 2020).

Healthcare is one of the most significant domains of the digital twin applications along with the manufacturing field. The digital twins created based on a patient model recreate the physiological processes, predict the rise of diseases, and evaluate potential treatment solutions (Bruynseels, Santoni de Sio, and van den Hoven, 2018; Chaturvedi, Dubey, and Sharma, 2022). These models utilize real time information provided by wearable gadgets, medical imaging and electronic health records in which the clinicians are able to test the interventions virtually and increase accuracy in personalized medicine. Continuous monitoring and proactive interventions are also facilitated by healthcare digital twins, which reduce the risks of adverse events and encourage the utilization of the data in decision-making (Miettinen and Lappalainen, 2018).

The other fast emerging implementation of digital twins is city planning and smart cities. In virtual city models, the planners are able to simulate traffic flows, energy consumption, waste and environmental impacts (Batty et al., 2012; Liu, Zhang, and Shen, 2021). The simulations can be applied in optimization of infrastructure, minimization and maximization of sustainability congestion. Digital twins assist in organizing emergency response, predicting how to maintain infrastructures in the city, and allow centrally coordinated services and assist in the formation of resilient urban ecosystems (Wu, Xu, and Wang, 2020).

Digital twins can also be applicable in energy systems to predict the generation, storage and distribution systems. The optimization of energy flow, integration with renewable energy, and prevention of utility failure can be done using digital twins with real-time simulation of complex interactions (Leng, Tan, Liu, Jiang, and Xu, 2020; Kritzinger, Karner, Traar, Henjes, and Sihn, 2018). The technique is energy efficient, cost effective and grid reliable and encourages the transition to low-carbon and sustainable energy infrastructure (Tao, Qi, Liu, and Kusiak, 2018).

Digital twins are based on the technological features of the IoT devices, cloud and edge computing, artificial intelligence, machine learning, and advanced visualization (Qi and Tao, 2018; Lu, Xu and Li, 2021). IoT sensors are capable of providing continuous streams of data of the physical assets, cloud and edge systems are then utilized to generate real-time insights based on this data. Machine learning algorithms, models that analyze the trends, make predictions, and control the behavior of the system, are compared to the virtualization tools, which are the tools that allow the stakeholders to interact with the digital models intuitively (Boschert and Rosen, 2016; Schleich, Anwer, Mathieu, and Wartzack, 2017). The recent works are concerned with using blockchain and secure communication procedures to enhance the data integrity, privacy, and traceability, in particular, in the sensitive sector such as healthcare (Longo, Padovano, and Umbrello, 2020).

Despite these advantages there are several challenges. Barricelli, Casiraghi, and Fogli (2019) and Rasheed, San, and Kvamsdal (2020) point to data heterogeneity, the complexity of integration, high requirements of computing, and the interoperability of platforms as the obstacles to digital twins. Healthcare and smart city situations are particularly prone to compromising security and privacy of data, as in both contexts, vulnerable data is constantly collected and processed (Bruynseels et al., 2018; Chaturvedi et al., 2022). Model validation and model standardization are also among other concerns because falsified or incomplete virtual models may lead to inaccurate and risky decision-making (Jones, Snider, and Hicks, 2019; Rasheed et al., 2020).

These systems of ethics are also regarded as the need to govern the implementation of digital twins as discovered in the literature. Caution is required when making decisions independently, when controlling data, when being responsible, and socio-economic implications of such choices are required to make responsible adoption (Longo et al., 2020; Fuller et al., 2020). Multi-domain digital twins are proposed next-generation frameworks that are capable of simulating and forecasting complex ecosystems with a single system bridging manufacturing, healthcare, and urban systems (Tao et al., 2019; Barricelli et al., 2019).

In conclusion, the existing literature indicates that digital twins are not merely simulating tools but flexible and dynamic platforms which can modify how physical systems would be designed, observed, and controlled. The applications of digital twins in smart factories (predictive maintenance) to patient-related health simulations and city planning are widely worked on and rapidly growing. Since the technical, operational, and ethical problems remain to exist, the ongoing changes in the field of IoT, AI, edge computing, and data analytics are likely to speed up the rate at which digital twins are being introduced and become an inseparable component of the industrial, healthcare, and urban ecosystem of the future.

3. DIGITAL TWIN TECHNICAL ARCHITECTURE

There are typically four interrelated levels to the digital twin architectures that support the communication of interaction between the real and the virtual world.

Physical Layer: It comprises the physical assets, the process or systems that are equipped with sensors and actuators in order to get real-time operational information and environmental information.

Data Acquisition Layer: It is the one that gathers, pre-processes and provides the data to the virtual layer, which is obtained in the physical layer. This can be used together with edge computing to reduce the latency and enhance real-time processing.

Virtual Layer: In this layer, there are computation models, AI-based analytics, simulations, predictive algorithms, and other algorithms that model and predict the behavior of the system of interest.

Interaction Layer: The users are able to interact with the digital twin via visualizing the system using dashboards and augmented/ virtual reality interfaces, which can guide them to make informed choices, experiment scenarios and system optimization.

Figure 1. Digital Twin Architecture

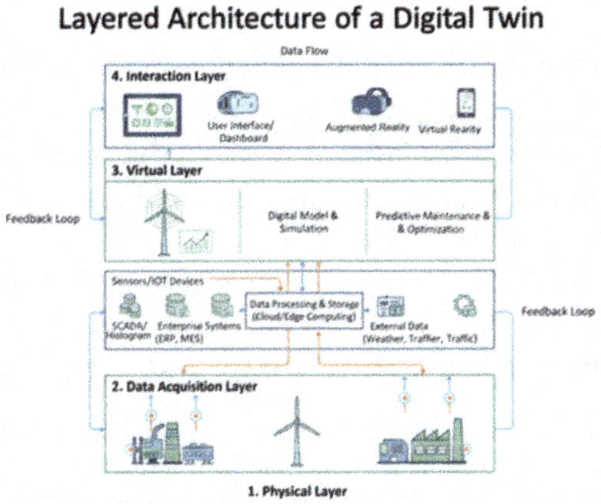

Such a structure of modules will ensure that digital twins can be customizable, scalable, and can be usable in feedback loops where a virtual model receives real-world responses. Such architectures form the central role in the applications like smart manufacturing, healthcare and city planning monitoring.

In this figure 1, the structure of a digital twin is illustrated. The Physical Layer involves the physical world objects or objects which are instrumented with the IoT sensors. Data Acquisition Layer collects the data and sends them to the virtual environment and in most cases, edge computing is utilized in processing the data with low latency. On the Virtual Layer one can find computational models and simulations and AI algorithms simulating the behavior of the physical system. Finally, Interaction Layer enables the stakeholders to visualise, analyse and engage with the digital twin through dashboards or AR/VR interfaces. This layered out version introduces the picture of data flow and the feedback loop which is required to make real-time decisions.

Table 1. Digital Twin Enabling Technologies

Technology	Role in Digital Twins	Key Benefits
IoT Sensors	Real-time data acquisition	Accurate monitoring, Continuous feedback
Cloud Computing	Large-scale data processing & storage	Scalability, Centralized analytics
Edge Computing	Low-latency data processing	Real-time response, Reduced bandwidth usage
AI & Machine Learning	Pattern recognition, predictive modeling	Predictive insights, Autonomous decisions
AR/VR Visualization	Interactive user interfaces	Enhanced decision-making, Simulation and training

This table 1 is a mapping of the core technologies that support the functionality of digital twin, which is utilized and the benefits are obtained. It emphasizes the importance of IoT in the data capture, AI in predictive intelligence, and cloud and edge computing in the scale and responsiveness, and AR/VR in the successful visualization and interaction with human beings.

4. PROGRAMS IN MANUFACTURING AND INDUSTRY 4.0

Digital twins have been central to Industry 4.0 in the manufacturing industry. They allow predictive maintenance due to the continuous monitoring of the machines themselves, they anticipate a possible breakdown, preventing unexpected downtime and costs of operation (Fuller et al., 2020; Tao et al., 2019). The digital twins may also allow manufacturers to have a virtual depiction of the production processes, which is optimizing the workflows, use of resources and consumption of energy.

It is anticipated that in the future, digital twins will even be more combined with autonomous robotics, autonomous quality inspection by AI, and self-optimizing factories. The innovations will also raise the level of responsiveness to the market demand, operational responsiveness, and the potential to carry out the just-in-time manufacturing operations with the minimum human contribution (Lu, Xu, and Xu, 2020).

Figure 2. Digital Twin Implementation in sectors

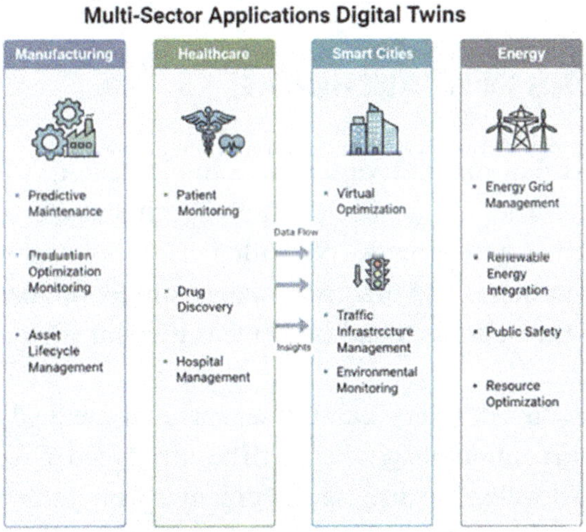

This figure 2 shows the way digital twins can be applied in other areas. They apply in the manufacturing to perform predictive maintenance, process optimization, and resource efficiency. In the healthcare field, digital twins represent an opportunity to personalize the treatment and provide follow-up all the time. They are utilized in intelligent cities to control the traffic circulation, track wastes, and strategize on emergencies. They help to optimize the grids, integrate renewable energy, as well as fault forecasting in energy systems. The figure emphasizes the intention of digital twins as a unifying technology capable of managing the area-related problems and facilitating cross-sector innovation.

The following table 2 has provided the key applications, merits and challenges of digital twins in industries. It attracts attention to how different spheres use digital twins to optimize performance and prediction and decision-making and makes known the prevalent technical and operational shortcomings.

Table 2. Overlay Summary of Digital Twin Applications

Sector	Key Applications	Benefits	Challenges
Manufacturing	Predictive maintenance, Process optimization	Reduced downtime, Improved efficiency	Data integration, High computational cost
Healthcare	Patient-specific models, Continuous monitoring	Personalized care, Risk mitigation	Data privacy, Regulatory compliance
Smart Cities	Traffic, Energy, Waste management	Optimized resources, Sustainability	Interoperability, Sensor heterogeneity
Energy Systems	Grid optimization, Fault prediction	Energy efficiency, Reliability	Security, System complexity

5. APPLICATIONS IN HEALTHCARE

One of the areas that digital twins can be implemented is healthcare. Digital twins are patient-specific and do not require experiments to be experimented in the real world, albeit they can model physiological processes, which the clinician can test their interventions. The practice enhances individualized medicine, early diagnosis, and real-time chronic conditions measurement (Bruynseels et al., 2018; Chaturvedi et al., 2022).

A possibility to connect with wearable sensors and medical devices will allow collecting health data continuously, which will be introduced to AI models to propose how it is possible to develop the disease and organize its treatment more effectively. In the nearest future, digital twins have the potential of enabling proactive healthcare delivery, telehealth, and advanced decision support systems that can deliver personalized interventions at minimum risk.

6. SMART CITIES AND URBAN PLANNING APPLICATIONS

Digital twins can also be used to create dynamic urban models, which are capable of simulating traffic, energy consumption, waste, and the environment (Batty et al., 2012; Liu et al., 2021). These models enable the city planners and administrators to optimize the use of the infrastructure, predict the congestion patterns, and assist in emergency response.

The integration of AI and real-time data streams of the IoT also allows the urban digital twins to react to the dynamic nature of the city, the efficient management of resources, citizen-centric services, and the active maintenance of the city infrastructures. It can be applied in the short run to forecast urban mobility resolutions, real-time disaster response simulation and to provide building management systems that are not energy-consuming.

7. ENERGY SYSTEMS APPLICATIONS

In energy management, one of the applications of digital twins is predictive modeling of generation, storage, and distribution networks to allow the utilities to optimize the work of one grid and integrate renewable energy sources (Leng et al., 2020; Kritzinger et al., 2018). Real-time simulations are applied to identify faults, reduce downtime, and maximize the efficiency of energy.

Digital twins will maximise autonomous load balancing, energy demand forecasting and decentralised control of renewable generation with the evolution of smart grids. The operational risks can be reduced with references to the digital twins with the help of an accurate virtual model of energy systems and contribute to decarbonization and enhance the resilience of the national energy infrastructure.

8. CHALLENGES AND LIMITATIONS

Although there is such potential of digital twins, there are several aspects which limit their application in different industries. Heterogeneity of data is one of the problems. Digital twins are based on the data obtained using a variety of sources, including sensors of the IoT, legacy, and external databases, which might not have the same format, granularity, and reliability (Barricelli et al., 2019; Rasheed et al., 2020). Bringing together the heterogeneous streams of information around a single virtual modeling is a significant technical issue that might require complex data preprocessing and harmonizing techniques.

The other limitation is the computational complexity. Predictive analytics, optimization and real-time simulations using AI are applications that demand high-performance computing resources. The computation of large amounts of high-speed streams of data of industrial systems or city infrastructure might still be resource-intensive and costly, even though cloud and edge computing partially reduce these limitations (Fuller et al., 2020; Lu et al., 2021).

The fields where the sensitive data are collected on a regular basis include healthcare, smart cities, and energy systems, and thus, the security and privacy are of specific interest (Bruynseels, Santoni de Sio, and van den Hoven, 2018; Chaturvedi, Dubey, and Sharma, 2022). The infrastructure breach or data breach or the access or hacks without authorization may jeopardize the data of the patients, the working systems, or the control of the infrastructure. Strong encryption, privacy-sensitive communication protocols and analytics are also a mandatory but add complexity to the system design process.

The interoperability and standardization is another challenge that is critical. Digital twins are now largely developed as domain-specific tools, which are incompatible with platforms or organizations (Jones, Snider, and Hicks, 2019; Kritzinger et al., 2018). Digital twins between enterprises cannot be easily scaled or multiple domain applications consolidated without standard frameworks.

Table 3. Problems and Mitigation Plans

Challenge	Description	Mitigation Strategy
Data Heterogeneity	Multiple sources, different formats	Standardization, Data preprocessing
High Computational Demand	Large-scale real-time simulations	Cloud & Edge computing, Optimization algorithms
Security & Privacy	Vulnerable to cyberattacks, sensitive data	Encryption, Privacy-preserving analytics
Interoperability & Standards	Limited compatibility across platforms	Adoption of open standards, API-based integration
Ethical & Governance Issues	Autonomous decisions, accountability concerns	Regulatory frameworks, Transparency protocols

This table 3 provides a clue in terms of the main considerations when implementing digital twins and potential remedies in overcoming them. It aligns with the chapter about the discussion of technical, operational and ethical barriers and offers steps to follow to make adoption safe, effective and responsible.

Finally, some of the ethical and governance problems are to be addressed. The problem of accountability, ownership of data, and socio-economic impact of self-reliant decision-making, predictive suggestions, and continuous monitoring are raised (Longo et al., 2020). The responsible adoption of digital twins should have more than only a technical protection as it requires as well regulatory compliance and even consultation with stakeholders to ensure that digital twins technologies are introduced in a responsible and transparent manner.

9. FUTURE RESEARCH DIRECTIONS

The digital twins technology in the next generation is focused on the promotion of interoperability, scalability, intelligence, and ethical implementation. Such directions include, but are not limited to, the development of multi-domain digital twins, involving manufacturing, healthcare, urban planning, and energy systems into single platforms (Tao et al., 2019; Barricelli et al., 2019). The making of anticipatory decisions on interdependent infrastructures through the digital ecosystems would also enable operational efficiency and sustainability to be holistic.

Digital twins will be created in accordance with artificial intelligence and machine learning. The streaming data and their learning models are critical in the development of self-learning digital copies (Qi and Tao, 2018; Fuller et al., 2020). There is also need to research more to improve predictability, anomaly detection, and autonomous decision-making particularly in vital systems such as healthcare and energy grids.

It is anticipated that edge computing and 5G/6G connectivity will make digital twins more responsive and give a chance to communicate with large-scale systems in real-time (Lu, Xu, and Xu, 2020; Tao, Zhang, Liu, and Nee, 2018). Time-sensitive applications (real, e.g., autonomous manufacturing line, or emergency urban management systems) will be able to use digital twins since they will be low-latency.

The research priorities have remained to be the security, privacy, and ethical systems. Some of the measures to mitigate cyberattack, data breach, and unintended consequences of autonomous activities risks are secure data aggregation procedures, privacy-conscious analytics, and reliable AI procedures (Bruynseels et al., 2018; Longo et al., 2020). This interdisciplinary research in the areas of technology, law and ethics will be critical in the formulation of efficient governance schemes of the digital twins adoption.

Figure 3. Future Research Directions

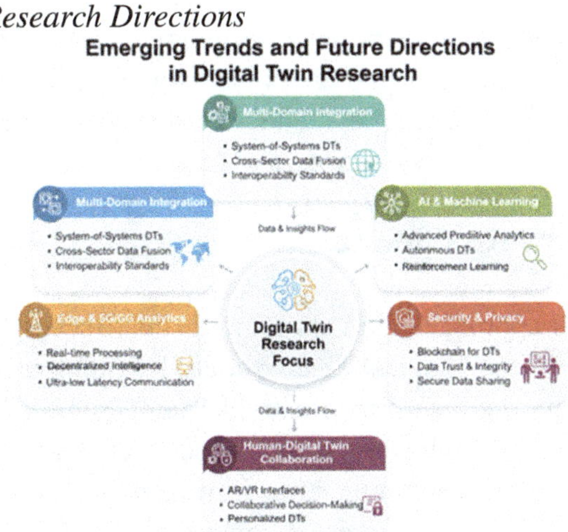
Emerging Trends and Future Directions in Digital Twin Research
Multi-Domain Integration
• System-of-Systems DTs
• Cross-Sector Data Fusion
• Interoperability Standards
Multi-Domain Integration
• System-of-Systems DTs
• Cross-Sector Data Fusion
• Interoperability Standards
AI & Machine Learning
• Advanced Prediitive Analytics
• Autonmous DTs
• Reinforcement Learning
Data & Insights Flow
Edge & 5G/6G Analytics
• Real-time Processing
• Decentralized Intelligence
• Ultra-low Latency Communication
Digital Twin Research Focus
Security & Privacy
• Blockchain for DTs
• Data Trust & Integrity
• Secure Data Sharing
Data & Insights Flow
Human-Digital Twin Collaboration
• AR/VR Interfaces
• Collaborative Decision-Making
• Personalized DTs

Figure 3 illustrates the most important spheres on which the digital twins research should be carried out in the future. Multi domain integration is closing the gap between industrial, health related and city systems. Machine learning and AI enhance pre-emptive intelligence and self-driven decision-making. The 5G/6G and Edge technologies have enabled one to make data decisions in real-time and respond to low latency reactiveness. The security and privacy structures ensure the safety and ethical usage, and the collaboration of people with the digital twins is associated with the interactive and explicatory decision support interfaces. Combined with each other, these areas map out the research agenda of the digital twin development and implementation.

Lastly, the collaboration of human beings and digital twins is also an emerging topic of study. The insights of the digital twin, the validation of the simulation and informed decisions will be delivered to human beings through interactive interfaces, use of augmented reality and visualization devices. In order to realize the full potential of digital twins in people and the industry, they will have to be more transparent, explicable, and trusted by everyone (Schleich et al., 2017; Boschert and Rosen, 2016).

10. IMPLEMENTATION STRATEGIES, GOVERNANCE, AND PRACTICAL DEPLOYMENT OF DIGITAL TWINS

Implementing digital twins in real-life situations does not need technical models and simulation tools to be successful. Before implementing digital twin systems, organizations should be ready in terms of infrastructure, policies, training programs, and operational procedures. Even the developed digital twin solutions cannot bring the anticipated benefits without planning. As such, some of the implementation strategies need to cover technological preparedness, organizational process, workforce competence, compliance with regulations and long term sustainability.

10.1 Infrastructure Readiness

The availability of appropriate infrastructure is the first condition of the implementation of digital twins. Physical assets should be fitted with sensors with the capability of recording the operational data like temperature, vibration, location, pressure or energy usage. Such sensors are expected to deliver information at all times via well-established communication infrastructure like wireless network, industrial internet platform or safe cloud connections. Sensor data quality has a direct impact on the quality of the digital twin; hence, sensors need to be calibrated, maintained, and validated.

The organizations also require computing resources that can handle huge amount of data. Storing and processing capabilities Cloud computing platforms offer scalable storage and processing capabilities enabling digital twins to work efficiently even when a large number of assets are tracked at the same time. The edge computing devices can also be placed close to the physical equipment to process the information on-site and minimize the communication delays. This mixed solution - edge plus cloud - has the benefit of enabling real-time responsiveness and also enabling large-scale analytics.

10.2 Data Management and Integration

Digital twins rely on the continuous data streams that are gathered by various means including IoT devices, enterprise databases, maintenance systems and operational logs. Such datasets can be in other forms and this poses integration problems. Data management systems also need to have preprocessing modules that clean, normalize and synchronize information received. Interoperability and standardized data format The ability of various systems to share information without compatibility issues can be achieved through standardized data formats and interoperable interfaces.

Data quality control is another critical data management thing. Incomplete values, sensor errors or imprecise measurements may diminish predictive model reliability. The incoming data needs to be monitored through automated validation procedures to detect the anomalies before the data is utilized in simulation or supporting decision-making. It is essential to keep the datasets of high quality to enhance the accuracy of the model models and to guarantee that the predictions of the digital twins are reliable.

10.3 Workforce Training and Organizational Adaptation

Human resource development is also needed in the introduction of digital twins. The engineers, operators, and decision-makers need to be able to interpret the results of digital twins and apply them to their day-to-day operations. The areas of sensor operation, dashboard interpretation, predictive maintenance planning and cybersecurity awareness should be included in the training program. Once the employees are well versed with the digital twin tools, the organizations may fully enjoy the benefits of the data-driven decision-making.

Adaptation in organizations is also very crucial. The conventional operation processes might require redesigning in such a way that the simulation outcomes and predictions are incorporated in the planning and maintenance processes. To illustrate, companies can use digital twin predictions as condition-based maintenance strategies to maintain their equipment, rather than maintain them periodically. These organizational changes are efficient and must be effectively communicated and transitioned gradually.

10.4 Governance and Policy Frameworks

The digital twin systems are run on big amounts of operational and even sensitive information. There is therefore need to establish governance structures to establish ownership, access control, accountability and compliance process of data. Clear policies should outline who is allowed to access the data, the maximum time the data may be stored as well as how the data must be secured. Technical experts, legal professionals and operational managers can be employed to carry out governance committees that monitor the digital twin implementation and adherence to organizational and regulatory requirements.

Governance systems should also encompass ethical considerations. In cases where automated decisions are affected by digital twins, e.g., energy control systems or healthcare advice, organizational leaders have to guarantee that the decision-making process is transparent and accountable. Digital twin decision-support systems must continue to have a human element to avoid unintended consequences.

10.5 Cybersecurity and Privacy Protection

Since digital twins are connecting physical systems to digital platforms, they can be subjected to cyberattacks in case the security is not addressed properly. Hacking may halt the activity or lead to the disclosure of confidential data. Thus, effective encryption algorithms, safe authentication, and permanent security observation should be provided. Network segmentation, secure protocols of communication, and frequent vulnerability testing minimise the chances of the system being compromised.

Privacy protection is a critical issue in healthcare and smart city applications where personal data are handled. Privacy preserving analytics, anonymity processes and access control systems are useful in ensuring that personal details are treated with care. Good cybersecurity practices foster trust among the stakeholders and contribute to long term adoption.

10.6 Linear Deployment Process

The implementation risks are minimized by using a staged deployment strategy in organizations. At the first phase, a pilot project can be carried out with a few assets or a restricted number of operating situations. Such pilot implementations enable organisations to test the performance of the system, detect integration difficulties and optimize the process of work. Once the pilot test has been done successfully, the system can be later extended to larger units of operation.

Each phase of deployment should be accompanied by continuing evaluation. Prediction accuracy, reduction of downtime, cost saving and operational efficiency are some performance metrics that should be tracked to determine the value created by the digital twin system. Evaluation schemes that are gathered can be used to make improvements and optimize the system.

10.7 Economic Factors and Cost-Benefit Analysis

A company should have a cost-benefit analysis to approximate the implementation cost and anticipated financial rewards, before it is implemented on a large scale. Examples of costs are installation of sensors, software development, subscriptions of cloud services, training the workforce, and maintenance of the system. The benefits might be the decrease of equipment downtime, the increase of energy efficiency, efficient utilization of resources and better the quality of decisions.

Financial planning over long term should be taking into consideration lifecycle advantages and not initial deployment cost only. Savings are generated over time by many digital twin systems as a result of a better operational efficiency and predictive maintenance. Digital twin investments can prove to have good return of investment when organizations consider the effects of digital twin investments over a long period of time.

10.8 Cross-Sector Collaboration and Standardization

Ecosystems of digital twins may be characterized by liaisons between equipment suppliers, software, research and operational organizations. There is a need to standardize different digital twins platforms to guarantee compatibility. Open communication specifications, universal modeling and common software interfaces facilitate integration of systems of various vendors in an organization without technical impediments.

Another factor in the development of digital twin is international collaboration. Consortia and joint research effort in the industry helps in the development of best practices, security regulations, and technical standards. Such joint ventures boost technological acclimatization and international usage.

10.9 Long-Term Maintenance and Lifecycle Management

Digital twins systems undergo maintenance during the lifecycle. Change in the work conditions may necessitate replacement of sensors, updates in software platforms, and re-training of predictive models. The lifecycle management plans will guarantee that the digital twin will be precise and operational in the future.

It is especially important to regularly model validate. With old equipment or varying operating conditions, the behavior of the system can change and predictive models need to be updated as the environment changes. Recalibration of models can prevent inaccuracy in predictions and low reliability.

10.10 Social Impact and Organizational Impact

The implementation of digital twins could also impact the occupation and the organization. Monitoring and decision-support activities can be automated and therefore this might reallocate employee roles to supervisory and analytical work. The transition made in the companies must be done at a slow pace by providing reskilling courses and aiding the employees to adjust to new technology-based work processes.

The other factor is public communication, particularly the smart city application. The citizens must be made aware of the application of digital twin technologies in enhancing their services like transportation management, environmental monitoring, and emergency response. Open communication assists in the formation of the trust of the people and promotes intervention by communities.

10.11 Sustainability Considerations

Digital twins can facilitate the sustainability objectives by making use of energy, minimizing waste, and enhancing resource planning. Nevertheless, the energy used by the computational infrastructure of digital twins is also energy-consuming. Companies ought to therefore develop energy efficient computing architectures, employ renewable energy in cases, and practice energy conscious system design. Sustainable deployment strategies will make sure that the benefits of digital twins are related to environmental goals.

10.12 Future Prospect of Deployment strategies

With the constant improvement of technologies in the field of artificial intelligence, high-speed connectivity, and sophisticated sensors, the deployment strategies of digital twins will become more efficient and accessible. Smaller and medium-sized organizations that did not have the resources to support advanced simulation systems will embrace cloud-powered digital twins to a greater extent and use them as they require little local infrastructure. In the long run, digital twins should become a normal tool of operations in different industries.

11. CONCLUSION

Digital twins are also becoming a disruptive technology that can be applied to bridge the physical and virtual world in various sectors of the economy, including manufacturing, medical care, smart cities, and energy infrastructure. By continually introducing real-time data, predictive analytics and increasingly complex simulations, digital twins assist businesses to track, optimize, and predict the behavior of important assets or systems. This will be able to improve operational efficiency, decision-making, and predictive maintenance, and more personalized and data-based interventions in core areas.

The chapter has determined that the enabling technologies such as IoT, edge and cloud computing, artificial intelligence, machine learning and immersive visualization tools are convergent and successful implementation of digital twins relies on such kinds of technologies. These technologies ensure that digital twins are more responsive and intelligent in addition to enhancing interactive decision making, collaboration and scenario testing. Besides, multi-domain integration offers the potential of creating interconnected digital ecosystems that simulates relations among manufacturing, health care, urban infrastructure, and energy systems and offers a holistic view of handling complexity.

Digital twins have technical, operational and ethical challenges despite the fact that they can be revolutionary. Heterogeneity of data, computations requirements, model validation, interoperability, cybersecurity and privacy are still to become significant challenges. In addition, the ethical and governance concerns concerning the autonomous decision-making, accountability, and the equal access will also have to be considered proactively to bear the responsible and sustainable adoption.

Digital twins will be the key toward the creation of the new generation of smart and resilient and sustainable systems in the future. The future research is also expected to focus on the sphere of integration, adaptive models based on AI, edge-based real-time analytics (Tyagi, 2023; 2024), and the development of efficient security and ethical frameworks. As a response to these difficulties and in the context of applying new technologies, there will be a continuous creation of digital twins as the primary component of innovation, which will ensure efficiency, sustainability, and greater human-machine interaction in industries and societies.

In essence, digital twins are not merely a tool of simulation, but a dynamic, intelligent system which offers an ongoing feedback mechanism between the virtual and the real world, whereby organizations can predict, adapt and survive into a more complex and interconnected world.

REFERENCES

Barricelli, B. R., Casiraghi, E., & Fogli, D. (2019). A survey on digital twin: Definitions, characteristics, applications, and design implications. *IEEE Access : Practical Innovations, Open Solutions*, *7*, 167653–167671. DOI: 10.1109/ACCESS.2019.2953499

Batty, M., Axhausen, K. W., Giannotti, F., Pozdnoukhov, A., Bazzani, A., Wachowicz, M., Ouzounis, G., & Portugali, Y. (2012). Smart cities of the future. *The European Physical Journal. Special Topics*, *214*(1), 481–518. DOI: 10.1140/epjst/e2012-01703-3

Boschert, S., & Rosen, R. (2016). Digital twin—the simulation aspect. In Tao, F., & Nee, A. Y. C. (Eds.), *Mechatronic futures* (pp. 59–74). Springer., DOI: 10.1007/978-3-319-32156-1_5

Boschert, S., & Rosen, R. (2016). Digital twin in industry: State-of-the-art. *Procedia CIRP*, *50*, 1–6. DOI: 10.1016/j.procir.2016.02.114

Bruynseels, K., Santoni de Sio, F., & van den Hoven, J. (2018). Digital twins in health care: Ethical implications of an emerging engineering paradigm. *Frontiers in Genetics*, *9*, 31. DOI: 10.3389/fgene.2018.00031 PMID: 29487613

Chaturvedi, A., Dubey, S., & Sharma, V. (2022). Digital twin applications in healthcare: A review and future directions. *Health Informatics Journal*, *28*(1), 146045822210813. DOI: 10.1177/146045822210813

Fuller, A., Fan, Z., Day, C., & Barlow, C. (2020). Digital twin: Enabling technologies and future directions. *Computers in Industry*, *119*, 103259. DOI: 10.1016/j.compind.2020.103259

Fuller, A., Fan, Z., Day, C., & Barlow, C. (2020). The implementation of digital twins in predictive maintenance. *Procedia CIRP*, *93*, 169–174. DOI: 10.1016/j.procir.2020.03.065

Fuller, A., Fan, Z., Day, C., & Barlow, C. (2020). Digital twin applications in aerospace and automotive industries. *Procedia CIRP*, *93*, 169–174. DOI: 10.1016/j.procir.2020.03.065

Grieves, M., & Vickers, J. (2017). Digital twin: Mitigating unpredictable, undesirable emergent behavior in complex systems. In Kahlen, F.-J., Flumerfelt, S., & Alves, A. (Eds.), *Transdisciplinary perspectives on complex systems* (pp. 85–113). Springer., DOI: 10.1007/978-3-319-38756-7_4

Jones, D., Snider, C., & Hicks, B. (2019). Digital twin-driven smart manufacturing: Case studies and research directions. *Journal of Manufacturing Systems*, *53*, 1–14. DOI: 10.1016/j.jmsy.2019.03.003

Jones, D., Snider, C., Nassehi, A., Yon, J., & Hicks, B. (2020). Characterising the digital twin: A systematic literature review. *CIRP Journal of Manufacturing Science and Technology*, *29*, 36–52. DOI: 10.1016/j.cirpj.2020.02.002

Kritzinger, W., Karner, M., Traar, G., Henjes, J., & Sihn, W. (2018). Digital twin in manufacturing: A categorical literature review and classification. *IFAC-PapersOnLine*, *51*(11), 1016–1022. DOI: 10.1016/j.ifacol.2018.08.474

Lee, J., Bagheri, B., & Kao, H. A. (2015). A cyber-physical systems architecture for Industry 4.0-based manufacturing systems. *Manufacturing Letters*, *3*, 18–23. DOI: 10.1016/j.mfglet.2014.12.001

Leng, J., Tan, R., Liu, Q., Jiang, P., & Xu, K. (2020). Digital twin-based energy-efficient manufacturing. *Journal of Manufacturing Systems*, *57*, 234–245. DOI: 10.1016/j.jmsy.2020.04.012

Liu, Y., Zhang, L., & Shen, W. (2021). Digital twin for smart cities: Framework, technologies and applications. *Journal of Urban Technology*, *28*(1), 3–25. DOI: 10.1080/10630732.2020.1813539

Longo, F., Padovano, A., & Umbrello, S. (2020). Value-oriented and ethical design of digital twins. *Computers in Industry*, *117*, 103187. DOI: 10.1016/j.compind.2020.103187

Lu, Y., Xu, X., & Xu, P. (2020). Internet of things (IoT) and digital twin in smart manufacturing: A survey. *Journal of Manufacturing Systems*, *57*, 1–14. DOI: 10.1016/j.jmsy.2020.04.009

Miettinen, M., & Lappalainen, P. (2018). Digital twins in healthcare: The promise of predictive and personalized medicine. *Health Informatics Journal*, *24*(2), 152–167. DOI: 10.1177/1460458217726370

Qi, Q., & Tao, F. (2018). Digital twin and big data towards smart manufacturing and Industry 4.0: 360 degree comparison. *IEEE Access : Practical Innovations, Open Solutions*, *6*, 3585–3593. DOI: 10.1109/ACCESS.2018.2793265

Qi, Q., Tao, F., Zuo, Y., Zhao, D., & Nee, A. Y. C. (2020). Digital twin and big data towards smart manufacturing and Industry 4.0: 360 degree comparison. *IEEE Transactions on Industrial Informatics*, *16*(4), 2413–2422. DOI: 10.1109/TII.2019.2947540

Rasheed, A., San, O., & Kvamsdal, T. (2020). Digital twin: Values, challenges and future directions. *Simulation Modelling Practice and Theory*, *103*, 101–114. DOI: 10.1016/j.simpat.2020.101–114

Schleich, B., Anwer, N., Mathieu, L., & Wartzack, S. (2017). Shaping the digital twin for design and production engineering. *CIRP Annals*, *66*(1), 141–144. DOI: 10.1016/j.cirp.2017.04.040

Tao, F., Qi, Q., Liu, A., & Kusiak, A. (2018). Data-driven smart manufacturing. *Journal of Manufacturing Systems*, *48*, 157–169. DOI: 10.1016/j.jmsy.2018.01.006

Tao, F., Qi, Q., Liu, A., & Kusiak, A. (2018). Data-driven smart manufacturing. *Journal of Manufacturing Systems*, *48*, 157–169. DOI: 10.1016/j.jmsy.2018.01.006

Tao, F., Zhang, H., Liu, A., & Nee, A. Y. C. (2019). Digital twin in industry: State-of-the-art. *IEEE Transactions on Industrial Informatics*, *15*(4), 2405–2415. DOI: 10.1109/TII.2018.2873186

Tao, F., Zhang, M., Liu, Y., & Nee, A. Y. C. (2018). *Digital twin driven smart manufacturing*. Academic Press.

Tyagi, A. K. (2023). Decentralized everything: A practical use of blockchain technology in future applications. In *Distributed computing to blockchain: Architecture, technology, and applications* (pp. 19–38). Elsevier., DOI: 10.1016/B978-0-323-96146-2.00010-3

Tyagi, A. K. (2024). Blockchain-enabled Internet of Things (IoTs) platforms for IoT-based healthcare and biomedical sectors. In Artificial intelligence-enabled blockchain technology and digital twin for smart hospitals (Chap. 10). Wiley Scrivener. https://doi.org/DOI: 10.1002/9781394287420.ch10

Tyagi, A. K. (2024). Sensors and digital twin application in healthcare facilities management. In *Artificial intelligence-enabled blockchain technology and digital twin for smart hospitals*. Wiley Scrivener., DOI: 10.1002/9781394287420.ch19

Tyagi, A. K. (2024). Blockchain–artificial intelligence-based secured solutions for smart environment. In *Digital twin and blockchain for smart cities*. Wiley Scrivener., DOI: 10.1002/9781394303564.ch23

Tyagi, A. K. (2024). Dew computing: State of the art, opportunities, and research challenges. In *Machine learning algorithms using Scikit and TensorFlow environments*. IGI Global., DOI: 10.4018/978-1-6684-8531-6.ch017

Wu, D., Xu, X., & Wang, L. (2020). Digital twin-based smart logistics management. *IEEE Access : Practical Innovations, Open Solutions*, *8*, 110807–110817. DOI: 10.1109/ACCESS.2020.3000687

Compilation of References

Aarthi, S., Aravinthan, K., Ravikumar, R. N., Sivakumar, N., & Wanglen, S. (2025). Cryptography securing data in motion within Blockchain, internet of everything, and Federated Learning. In *Convergence of Blockchain, Internet of Everything, and Federated Learning for Security* (pp. 39–78). IGI Global., DOI: 10.4018/979-8-3373-1424-2.ch002

Ababio, I. B., Bieniek, J., Rahouti, M., Hayajneh, T., Aledhari, M., Verma, D. C., & Chehri, A. (2025). A Blockchain-Assisted federated learning framework for secure and Self-Optimizing digital twins in industrial IoT. *Future Internet*, *17*(1), 13. DOI: 10.3390/fi17010013

Abbas, A. F., Qureshi, N. A., Khan, N., Chandio, R., & Ali, J. (2022). The blockchain technologies in healthcare: prospects, obstacles, and future recommendations; lessons learned from digitalization.

Abbas, A. F., Qureshi, N. A., Khan, N., Chandio, R., & Ali, J. (2022). The blockchain technologies in healthcare: Prospects, obstacles, and future recommendations; Lessons learned from digitalization. [IJOE]. *International Journal of Online and Biomedical Engineering*, *18*(09), 144–159. DOI: 10.3991/ijoe.v18i09.32253

Abbas, S., Sampedro, G. A., Abisado, M., Almadhor, A., Yousaf, I., & Hong, S.-P. (2023). Harris-Hawk-Optimization-based deep recurrent neural network for securing the Internet of Medical Things. *Electronics (Basel)*, *12*(12), 2612. DOI: 10.3390/electronics12122612

Abd Elaziz, M., Al-qaness, M. A., Dahou, A., Al-Betar, M. A., Mohamed, M. M., El-Shinawi, M., Ali, A., & Ewees, A. A. (2024). Digital twins in healthcare: Applications, technologies, simulations, and future trends. *Wiley Interdisciplinary Reviews. Data Mining and Knowledge Discovery*, *14*(6), e1559. DOI: 10.1002/widm.1559

Abdullah, S., Arshad, J., Khan, M. M., Alazab, M., & Salah, K. (2023). PRISED tangle: A privacy-aware framework for smart healthcare data sharing using IOTA tangle. *Complex & Intelligent Systems*, *9*(3), 3023–3041. DOI: 10.1007/s40747-021-00610-8

Abhimanyu Gupta, A. V., Tejal Shah, K. D., & Sandeep Raghuwanshi, S. J. (2025). Blockchain-enabled digital twins for secure and transparent health data management. Economic Sciences, 21(03(S) September), 206–222. DOI: 10.69889/2wyxmw53

Adavoudi Jolfaei, A., Aghili, S. F., & Singelee, D. (2021). A Survey on Blockchain-Based IoMT Systems: Towards Scalability. *IEEE Access : Practical Innovations, Open Solutions*, *9*, 148948–148975. DOI: 10.1109/ACCESS.2021.3117662

Adibi, S., Rajabifard, A., Shojaei, D., & Wickramasinghe, N. (2024). Enhancing healthcare through sensor-enabled digital twins in smart environments: A comprehensive analysis. *Sensors (Basel)*, *24*(9), 2793. PMID: 38732899

Agbo, C. C., & Mahmoud, Q. H. (2019). Comparison of blockchain frameworks for healthcare applications. *Internet Technology Letters*, *2*(5), e122. DOI: 10.1002/itl2.122

Agbo, C. C., & Mahmoud, Q. H. (2020). Blockchain in healthcare: Opportunities, challenges, and possible solutions. [IJHISI]. *International Journal of Healthcare Information Systems and Informatics*, *15*(3), 82–97. DOI: 10.4018/IJHISI.2020070105

Agbo, C. C., Mahmoud, Q. H., & Eklund, J. M. (2019). Blockchain technology in healthcare: A systematic review. *Healthcare (Basel)*, *7*(2), 56. DOI: 10.3390/healthcare7020056 PMID: 30987333

Aghamiri, S. S., & Amin, R. (2025). The potential use of digital twin technology for advancing CAR-T cell therapy. *Current Issues in Molecular Biology*, *47*(5), 321. PMID: 40699720

Agua, P. B., & Correia, A. (2023). Innovation, Strategy and Transformation Frameworks for the modern enterprise. In *Advances in business strategy and competitive advantage book series*. https://doi.org/DOI: 10.4018/979-8-3693-0458-7

Ahmadi-Assalemi, G., Al-Khateeb, H., Maple, C., Epiphaniou, G., Alhaboby, Z. A., Alkaabi, S., & Alhaboby, D. (2020). Digital twins for precision healthcare. In *Cyber defence in the age of AI, smart societies and augmented humanity* (pp. 133–158). Springer., DOI: 10.1007/978-3-030-35746-7_8

Ahmed, S. (2025). Enhancing Data Security and Transparency: The Role of Blockchain in Decentralized Systems. *International Journal of Advanced Engineering. Management Science*, *11*(1), 593258.

Ait Bennacer, S., Sabiri, K., Aaroud, A., Akodadi, K., & Cherradi, B. (2023). A comprehensive survey on blockchain-based healthcare industry: Applications and challenges. *Indonesian Journal of Electrical Engineering and Computer Science, 30*(3), 1558. DOI: 10.11591/ijeecs.v30.i3.pp1558-1571

Akindote, O. J., Adegbite, A. O., Dawodu, S. O., Omotosho, A., & Anyanwu, A. (2023). Innovation in data Storage Technologies: From Cloud Computing to Edge Computing. *Computer Science & IT Research Journal, 4*(3), 273–299. DOI: 10.51594/csitrj.v4i3.661

Akram, W., Joshi, R., Haider, T., Sharma, P., Jain, V., Garud, N., & Singh, N. (2024). Blockchain technology: A potential tool for the management of pharma supply chain. *Research in Social & Administrative Pharmacy, 20*(6), 156–164. DOI: 10.1016/j.sapharm.2024.02.014 PMID: 38423927

Alam, S., Bhatia, S., Shuaib, M., Khubrani, M. M., Alfaycz, F., Malibari, A. A., & Ahmad, S. (2023). An overview of blockchain and IoT integration for secure and reliable health records monitoring. *Sustainability (Basel), 15*(7), 5660. DOI: 10.3390/su15075660

Ali, A., Ali, H., Saeed, A., Ahmed Khan, A., Tin, T. T., Assam, M., Ghadi, Y. Y., & Mohamed, H. G. (2023). Blockchain-powered healthcare systems: Enhancing scalability and security with hybrid deep learning. *Sensors (Basel), 23*(18), 7740. DOI: 10.3390/s23187740 PMID: 37765797

Ali, S., Abdullah, , Armand, T. P. T., Athar, A., Hussain, A., Ali, M., Yaseen, M., Joo, M.-I., & Kim, H.-C. (2023). Metaverse in healthcare integrated with explainable AI and blockchain: Enabling immersiveness, ensuring trust, and providing patient data security. *Sensors (Basel), 23*(2), 565. DOI: 10.3390/s23020565 PMID: 36679361

Ali, V., Norman, A. A., & Azzuhri, S. R. B. (2023). Characteristics of blockchain and its relationship with trust. *IEEE Access : Practical Innovations, Open Solutions, 11*, 15364–15374. DOI: 10.1109/ACCESS.2023.3243700

Almalki, J., Al Shehri, W., Mehmood, R., Alsaif, K., Alshahrani, S. M., Jannah, N., & Khan, N. A. (2022). Enabling blockchain with IoMT devices for healthcare. *Information (Basel), 13*(10), 448. DOI: 10.3390/info13100448

Alonso, R., Olivadese, R., Ibba, A., & Reforgiato Recupero, D. (2023). Towards the definition of a European Digital Building Logbook: A survey. *Heliyon, 9*(9), e19285. DOI: 10.1016/j.heliyon.2023.e19285

Alowais, S. A., Alghamdi, S. S., Alsuhebany, N., Alqahtani, T., Alshaya, A. I., Almohareb, S. N., Aldairem, A., Alrashed, M., Bin Saleh, K., Badreldin, H. A., Al Yami, M. S., Al Harbi, S., & Albekairy, A. M. (2023). Revolutionizing healthcare: The role of artificial intelligence in clinical practice. *BMC Medical Education*, *23*(1), 689. DOI: 10.1186/s12909-023-04698-z PMID: 37740191

Alqahtani, A., Alsubai, S., & Bhatia, M. (2023). Digital-twin-assisted healthcare framework for adult. *IEEE Internet of Things Journal*, *11*(8), 14963–14970. DOI: 10.1109/JIOT.2023.3345331

Alshammari, K., Beach, T., & Rezgui, Y. (2021). Cybersecurity for digital twins in the built environment: Current research and future directions. *Journal of Information Technology in Construction*, *26*, 159–173. DOI: 10.36680/j.itcon.2021.010

Alzubi, J. A., Alzubi, O. A., Singh, A., & Mahmod Alzubi, T. (2023). A blockchain-enabled security management framework for mobile edge computing. *International Journal of Network Management*, *33*(5), e2240. Advance online publication. DOI: 10.1002/nem.2240

Amofa, S., Xia, Q., Xia, H., Obiri, I. A., Adjei-Arthur, B., Yang, J., & Gao, J. (2024). Blockchain-secure patient Digital Twin in healthcare using smart contracts. *PLoS One*, *19*(2), e0286120. DOI: 10.1371/journal.pone.0286120

Androulaki, E., Barger, A., & Bortnikov, V.. (2018). Hyperledger Fabric: A distributed operating system for permissioned blockchains. *Proceedings of the Thirteenth EuroSys Conference*. DOI: 10.1145/3190508.3190538

Angraal, S., Krumholz, H. M., & Schulz, W. L. (2017). Blockchain technology: Applications in health care. *Circulation: Cardiovascular Quality and Outcomes*, *10*(9), e003800. DOI: 10.1161/CIRCOUTCOMES.117.003800 PMID: 28912202

Anthony, P., & Dada, S. A. (2020). Data-driven optimization of pharmacy operations and patient access through interoperable digital systems. *Int J Multidiscip Res Growth Eval*, *1*(2), 229–244. DOI: 10.54660/.IJMRGE.2020.1.2.229-240

Arbabi, M. S., Lal, C., Veeraragavan, N. R., Marijan, D., Nygård, J. F., & Vitenberg, R. (2022). A survey on blockchain for healthcare: Challenges, benefits, and future directions. *IEEE Communications Surveys and Tutorials*, *25*(1), 386–424. DOI: 10.1109/COMST.2022.3224644

Arigbabu, A. T., Olaniyi, O. O., Adigwe, C. S., Adebiyi, O. O., & Ajayi, S. A. (2024). Data governance in AI-enabled healthcare systems: A case of the project nightingale. *Asian Journal of Research in Computer Science*, *17*(5), 85–107. DOI: 10.9734/ajrcos/2024/v17i5441

Armeni, P., Polat, I., De Rossi, L. M., Diaferia, L., Meregalli, S., & Gatti, A. (2022). Digital twins in healthcare: Is it the beginning of a new era of evidence-based medicine? A critical review. *Journal of Personalized Medicine*, *12*(8), 1255. PMID: 36013204

Arya, S., Aggarwal, S., & Ansar, S. A. (2025). Transforming healthcare with blockchain and digital twins: innovations in IoMT for smart hospitals. In *Blockchain and Digital Twin for Smart Hospitals* (pp. 497–510). Elsevier. DOI: 10.1016/B978-0-443-34226-4.00025-3

Atadoga, A., Elufioye, O. A., Omaghomi, T. T., Akomolafe, O., Odilibe, I. P., & Owolabi, O. R. (2024). Blockchain in healthcare: A comprehensive review of applications and security concerns. *International Journal of Science and Research Archive*, *11*(1), 1605–1613. DOI: 10.30574/ijsra.2024.11.1.0244

Attaran, M. (2022). Blockchain technology in healthcare: Challenges and opportunities. *International Journal of Healthcare Management*, *15*(1), 70–83. DOI: 10.1080/20479700.2020.1843887

Awasthi Ms, N., & Mishra Ms, R. (2025). Leveraging digital twin technology for enhanced patient care and predictive health management. *ANALISTA International Journal of Multidisciplinary Research*, *36*, 36. Advance online publication. DOI: 10.71182/aijmr.2506.0301.4004

Awasthi, M., Raghuvanshi, C. S., Dudhagara, C., & Awasthi, A. (2025). Exploring virtual smart healthcare trends using digital twins. In *Digital twins for smart cities and villages* (pp. 377–406). Elsevier. DOI: 10.1016/B978-0-443-28884-5.00017-8

Azaria, A., Ekblaw, A., Vieira, T., & Lippman, A. (2016, August). Medrec: Using blockchain for medical data access and permission management. In 2016 2nd international conference on open and big data (OBD) (pp. 25-30). IEEE.

Azaria, A., Ekblaw, A., Vieira, T., & Lippman, A. (2016, August). Medrec: Using blockchain for medical data access and permission management. In *2016 2nd international conference on open and big data (OBD)* (pp. 25-30). IEEE.DOI: 10.1109/OBD.2016.21

Azaria, A., Ekblaw, A., Vieira, T., & Lippman, A. (2016). MedRec: Using blockchain for medical data access and permission management. *Proceedings of IEEE Open & Big Data Conference*. DOI: 10.1109/OBD.2016.11

Badakhshan, E., & Ivanov, D. (2025). Integrating digital twin and blockchain for responsive working capital management in supply chains facing financial disruptions. *International Journal of Production Research, 63*(21), 1–35. DOI: 10.1080/00207543.2025.2507112

Balasubramanyam, A., Ramesh, R., Sudheer, R., & Honnavalli, P. B. (2024). Revolutionizing healthcare: A review unveiling the transformative power of digital twins. *IEEE Access : Practical Innovations, Open Solutions, 12*, 69652–69676.

Banoub, R. G., Sanghvi, H., Gill, G. S., Paredes, A. A., Bains, H. K., Patel, A., & Patel, A. (2024). Enhancing ophthalmic care: The transformative potential of digital twins in healthcare. *Cureus, 16*(12). PMID: 39840199

Barati, M., & Rana, O. (2022). Tracking GDPR compliance in cloud-based service delivery. *IEEE Transactions on Services Computing, 15*(3), 1498–1511. DOI: 10.1109/TSC.2020.2999559

Barbaria, S., Jemai, A., Ceylan, H. İ., Muntean, R. I., Dergaa, I., & Boussi Rahmouni, H. (2025). Advancing compliance with HIPAA and GDPR in healthcare: A blockchain-based strategy for secure data exchange in clinical research involving private health information. *Healthcare (Basel), 13*(20), 2594. DOI: 10.3390/healthcare13202594

Barbaria, S., Jemai, A., Ceylan, H. İ., Muntean, R. I., Dergaa, I., & Boussi Rahmouni, H. (2025, October). Advancing compliance with HIPAA and GDPR in healthcare: A blockchain-based strategy for secure data exchange in clinical research involving private health information. [). MDPI.]. *Health Care, 13*(20), 2594. PMID: 41154272

Barricelli, B. R., Casiraghi, E., & Fogli, D. (2019). A survey on digital twin: Definitions, characteristics, applications, and design implications. *IEEE Access : Practical Innovations, Open Solutions, 7*, 167653–167671. DOI: 10.1109/ACCESS.2019.2953499

Bates, D. W., Saria, S., Ohno-Machado, L., Shah, A., & Escobar, G. (2014). Big data in health care: Using analytics to identify and manage high-risk and high-cost patients. *Health Affairs, 33*(7), 1123–1131. DOI: 10.1377/hlthaff.2014.0041 PMID: 25006137

Bathalapalli, V. K. V. V., Mohanty, S. P., Kougianos, E., Iyer, V., & Rout, B. (2024). PUFchain 3.0: Hardware-assisted distributed ledger for robust authentication in healthcare cyber-physical systems. *Sensors (Basel), 24*(3), 938. DOI: 10.3390/s24030938 PMID: 38339656

Batty, M., Axhausen, K. W., Giannotti, F., Pozdnoukhov, A., Bazzani, A., Wachowicz, M., Ouzounis, G., & Portugali, Y. (2012). Smart cities of the future. *The European Physical Journal. Special Topics*, *214*(1), 481–518. DOI: 10.1140/epjst/e2012-01703-3

Baygin, N., Baygin, M., & Karakose, M. (2019, November). Blockchain technology: applications, benefits and challenges. In *2019 1st International Informatics and Software Engineering Conference (UBMYK)* (pp. 1-5). IEEE. DOI: 10.1109/UBMYK48245.2019.8965565

Bell, L., Buchanan, W. J., Cameron, J., & Lo, O. (2018). Applications of blockchain within healthcare. *Blockchain in Healthcare Today*, *1*. Advance online publication. DOI: 10.30953/bhty.v1.8

Bergamini, F., Gallo, G. D., & Micucci, D. (2025). Towards a unified architecture for remote patient monitoring. In *Ambient Intelligence and Smart Environments*. IOS Press., DOI: 10.3233/AISE250009

Bhattacharya, P., Dutta, P. K., Hassan, A., Kundu, N. K., & Verma, J. P. (2024). Quantum computing and supply chain management. In *Advances in logistics, operations and management science book series*. https://doi.org/DOI: 10.4018/979-8-3693-4107-0

Bian, G., Qu, W., & Shao, B. (2023). Blockchain-based trusted federated learning with pre-trained models for COVID-19 detection. *Electronics (Basel)*, *12*(9), 2068. DOI: 10.3390/electronics12092068

Bi, S., Wang, C., Zhang, J., Huang, W., Wu, B., Gong, Y., & Ni, W. (2022). A survey on artificial intelligence aided internet-of-things technologies in emerging smart libraries. *Sensors (Basel)*, *22*(8), 2991. DOI: 10.3390/s22082991 PMID: 35458974

Björnsson, B., Borrebaeck, C., Elander, N., Gasslander, T., Gawel, D. R., Gustafsson, M., Jörnsten, R., Lee, E. J., Li, X., Lilja, S., Martínez-Enguita, D., Matussek, A., Sandström, P., Schäfer, S., Stenmarker, M., Sun, X. F., Sysoev, O., Zhang, H., & Benson, M.Swedish Digital Twin Consortium. (2019). Digital twins to personalize medicine. *Genome Medicine*, *12*(1), 4. DOI: 10.1186/s13073-019-0701-3 PMID: 31892363

Bokolo, A. J. (2022). Exploring interoperability of distributed Ledger and Decentralized Technology adoption in virtual enterprises. *Information Systems and e-Business Management*, *20*(4), 685–718. DOI: 10.1007/s10257-022-00561-8

Boschert, S., & Rosen, R. (2016). Digital twin in industry: State-of-the-art. *Procedia CIRP*, *50*, 1–6. DOI: 10.1016/j.procir.2016.02.114

Boschert, S., & Rosen, R. (2016). Digital twin—the simulation aspect. In Tao, F., & Nee, A. Y. C. (Eds.), *Mechatronic futures* (pp. 59–74). Springer., DOI: 10.1007/978-3-319-32156-1_5

Boussadi, A., & Zapletal, E. (2017). A Fast Healthcare Interoperability Resources (FHIR) layer implemented over i2b2. *BMC Medical Informatics and Decision Making*, *17*(1), 120. Advance online publication. DOI: 10.1186/s12911-017-0513-6

Brogan, J., Baskaran, I., & Ramachandran, N. (2018). Authenticating health activity data using distributed ledger technologies. *Computational and Structural Biotechnology Journal*, *16*, 257–266. DOI: 10.1016/j.csbj.2018.06.004 PMID: 30101004

Bruynseels, K., Santoni de Sio, F., & Van den Hoven, J. (2018). Digital twins in health care: Ethical implications of an emerging engineering paradigm. *Frontiers in Genetics*, *9*, 31. DOI: 10.3389/fgene.2018.00031

Can, O., Dag, T., & Kantarcioglu, M. (2024). A blockchain based hybrid architecture for auditable consent management. *IEEE Access : Practical Innovations, Open Solutions*, *12*, 100419–100445. DOI: 10.1109/ACCESS.2024.3431292

Capece, G., & Lorenzi, F. (2020). Blockchain and Healthcare: Opportunities and Prospects for the EHR. *Sustainability (Basel)*, *12*(22), 9693. DOI: 10.3390/su12229693

Catarinucci, L., De Donno, D., Mainetti, L., Palano, L., Patrono, L., Stefanizzi, M. L., & Tarricone, L. (2015). An IoT-aware architecture for smart healthcare systems. *IEEE Internet of Things Journal*, *2*(6), 515–526. DOI: 10.1109/JIOT.2015.2417684

Cernian, A., Tiganoaia, B., Sacala, I., Pavel, A., & Iftemi, A. (2020). PatientDataChain: A blockchain-based approach to integrate personal health records. *Sensors (Basel)*, *20*(22), 6538. DOI: 10.3390/s20226538 PMID: 33207620

Chakilam, P. K. (2025). Interoperability in healthcare: Leveraging enterprise Integration Architecture for seamless data exchange. *European Modern Studies Journal*, *9*(4), 652–661. DOI: 10.59573/emsj.9(4).2025.63

Chaparro-Cárdenas, S. L., Ramirez-Bautista, J. A., Terven, J., Córdova-Esparza, D. M., Romero-Gonzalez, J. A., Ramírez-Pedraza, A., & Chavez-Urbiola, E. A. (2025, July). A technological review of digital twins and artificial intelligence for personalized and predictive healthcare. [). MDPI.]. *Health Care*, *13*(14), 1763. PMID: 40724790

Chaparro-Cárdenas, S. L., Ramirez-Bautista, J.-A., Terven, J., Córdova-Esparza, D.-M., Romero-Gonzalez, J.-A., Ramírez-Pedraza, A., & Chavez-Urbiola, E. A. (2025). A technological review of Digital Twins and Artificial Intelligence for personalized and predictive healthcare. *Healthcare (Basel), 13*(14), 1763. DOI: 10.3390/healthcare13141763 PMID: 40724790

Chaturvedi, A., Dubey, S., & Sharma, V. (2022). Digital twin applications in healthcare: A review and future directions. *Health Informatics Journal, 28*(1), 146045822210813. DOI: 10.1177/146045822210813

Chaudhry, B., Wang, J., Wu, S., Maglione, M., Mojica, W., Roth, E., Morton, S. C., & Shekelle, P. G. (2006). Systematic review: Impact of health information technology on quality, efficiency, and costs of medical care. *Annals of Internal Medicine, 144*(10), 742–752. DOI: 10.7326/0003-4819-144-10-200605160-00125 PMID: 16702590

Cheng, W., Ou, W., Yin, X., Yan, W., Liu, D., & Liu, C. (2020). A privacy-protection model for patients. *Security and Communication Networks, 2020*, 1–12. DOI: 10.1155/2020/6647562

Chen, H. S., Jarrell, J. T., Carpenter, K. A., Cohen, D. S., & Huang, X. (2019). Blockchain in healthcare: A patient-centered model. *Biomedical Journal of Scientific & Technical Research, 20*(3), 15017. PMID: 31565696

Chen, H., Wei, N., Wang, L., Mobarak, W. F. M., Albahar, M. A., & Shaikh, Z. A. (2024). The role of blockchain in finance beyond cryptocurrency: Trust, data management, and automation. *IEEE Access : Practical Innovations, Open Solutions, 12*, 64861–64885. DOI: 10.1109/ACCESS.2024.3395918

Chhinal, S., Khanal, B., Singh, M., & Ansari, M. S. A. (2025). A blockchain framework for ensuring medical data security in Internet of Medical Things. *Transactions on Emerging Telecommunications Technologies, 36*(10), e70271. Advance online publication. DOI: 10.1002/ett.70271

Choppara, P., & Lokesh, B. (2025). Efficient task scheduling and load balancing in fog computing for crucial healthcare through deep reinforcement learning. *IEEE Access : Practical Innovations, Open Solutions, 13*, 26542–26563. DOI: 10.1109/ACCESS.2025.3539336

Clifton, J., Adair, E., Cheung, M., Torres, C., Andrews, W., Dorsonne, B., & Darnall, B. D. (2024). PROGRESS: A patient-centered engagement infrastructure and multi-level approach to enrich diversity, equity, and inclusion in a national randomized online behavioral pain treatment study. *The Journal of Pain*, •••, 104718. PMID: 39454847

Cocco, L., & Tonelli, R. (2024). A Self-Sovereign Identity–Blockchain-Based Model Proposal for Deep Digital Transformation in the Healthcare Sector. *Future Internet*, *16*(12), 473. DOI: 10.3390/fi16120473

Coorey, G., Figtree, G. A., Fletcher, D. F., Snelson, V. J., Vernon, S. T., Winlaw, D., Grieve, S. M., McEwan, A., Yang, J. Y. H., Qian, P., O'Brien, K., Orchard, J., Kim, J., Patel, S., & Redfern, J. (2022). The health digital twin to tackle cardiovascular disease-a review of an emerging interdisciplinary field. *NPJ Digital Medicine*, *5*(1), 126. DOI: 10.1038/s41746-022-00640-7 PMID: 36028526

Corral-Acero, J., Margara, F., Marciniak, M., Rodero, C., Loncaric, F., Feng, Y., Gilbert, A., Fernandes, J. F., Bukhari, H. A., Wajdan, A., Martinez, M. V., Santos, M. S., Shamohammdi, M., Luo, H., Westphal, P., Leeson, P., DiAchille, P., Gurev, V., Mayr, M., & Lamata, P. (2020). The "Digital Twin" to enable the vision of precision cardiology. *European Heart Journal*, *41*(48), 4556–4564. DOI: 10.1093/eurheartj/ehaa159 PMID: 32128588

Cuff, A. (2023). The evolution of digital health and its continuing challenges. *BMC Digital Health*, *1*(1), 3. DOI: 10.1186/s44247-022-00004-x PMID: 38014367

D'Orsi, L., Capasso, B., Lamacchia, G., Pizzichini, P., Ferranti, S., Liverani, A., & Lo Presti, E. (2024). Recent advances in artificial intelligence to improve immunotherapy and the use of digital twins to identify prognosis of patients with solid tumors. *International Journal of Molecular Sciences*, *25*(21), 11588. PMID: 39519142

Daraghmi, E.-Y., Daraghmi, Y.-A., & Yuan, S.-M. (2019). MedChain: A design of blockchain-based system for medical records access and permissions management. *IEEE Access : Practical Innovations, Open Solutions*, *7*, 164595–164613. DOI: 10.1109/ACCESS.2019.2952942

Darwich, A. S., Polasek, T. M., Aronson, J. K., Ogungbenro, K., Wright, D. F. B., Achour, B., Reny, J.-L., Daali, Y., Eiermann, B., Cook, J., Lesko, L., McLachlan, A. J., & Rostami-Hodjegan, A. (2021). Model-informed precision dosing: Background, requirements, validation, implementation, and forward trajectory of individualizing drug therapy. Annual Review of Pharmacology and Toxicology, 61(1), 225–245. DevOps Engineer/Cloud Solutions Architect USA, S., Adelusi, B. S., Osamika, D., Independent Researcher, O. U. S. A., Chinyeaka Kelvin-Agwu, M., Independent Researcher, L. N., Mustapha, A. Y., Kwara State Ministry of Health, N., Forkuo, A. Y., Independent Researcher, U. S. A., Ikhalea, N., & Independent Researcher USA, T. (2025). A Federated Interoperability Framework for seamless health data exchange using FHIR standards across multi-hospital systems. Engineering and Technology Journal, 10(05). https://doi.org/DOI: 10.1146/annurev-pharmtox-033020-113257

Dean, M. C., Oeding, J. F., Diniz, P., Seil, R., & Samuelsson, K.ESSKA Artificial Intelligence Working Group. (2024). Leveraging digital twins for improved orthopaedic evaluation and treatment. *Journal of Experimental Orthopaedics, 11*(4), e70084. PMID: 39530111

Delerm, F., & Pilottin, A. (2024). Double edged tech: Navigating the public health and legal challenges of digital twin technology. *European Journal of Public Health, 34*(Supplement_3), ckae144–1510.

Dhanushya, J., Ruba, M., Ponkarthika, M., Soundarya, B., Sakthi Priya, V., Dhanushri, S., & Harikrishnan, S. (2025, April). AI-Powered Multipurpose Agrobot for Precision Farming: Crop Health Management, Fertilizer Recommendation and Yield Prediction. In *2025 International Conference on Recent Advances in Electrical, Electronics, Ubiquitous Communication, and Computational Intelligence (RAEEUCCI)* (pp. 1-6). IEEE.

Dimitrov, D. V. (2019). Blockchain applications for healthcare data management. *Healthcare Informatics Research, 25*(1), 51–56. DOI: 10.4258/hir.2019.25.1.51 PMID: 30788182

Diniz, P., Grimm, B., Garcia, F., Fayad, J., Ley, C., Mouton, C., & Seil, R. (2025). Digital twin systems for musculoskeletal applications: A current concepts review. *Knee Surgery, Sports Traumatology, Arthroscopy : Official Journal of the ESSKA, 33*(5), 1892–1910. PMID: 39989345

Dixit, P. (2025). Exploring the Role of Digital Twins in Revolutionizing Healthcare: Opportunities and Challenges. *International Journal of Advanced Research.*

Dong, S., Abbas, K., Li, M., & Kamruzzaman, J. (2023). Blockchain technology and application: An overview. *PeerJ. Computer Science, 9*, e1705. DOI: 10.7717/peerj-cs.1705 PMID: 38077532

Doss, S., Dubey, A., Hanafiah, M. M., & Reddy, C. K. K. (2024). Exploring the advancements and future directions of digital twins in healthcare 6.0. In *Advances in medical technologies and clinical practice book series.* https://doi.org/DOI: 10.4018/979-8-3693-5893-1

Dunphy, P., & Petitcolas, F. A. P. (2018). A first look at identity management schemes on the blockchain. *IEEE Security and Privacy, 16*(4), 20–29. DOI: 10.1109/MSP.2018.3111247

Dwivedi, S. K., Amin, R., & Vollala, S. (2020). Blockchain based secured information sharing protocol in supply chain management system with key distribution mechanism. *Journal of Information Security and Applications*, *54*, 102554. DOI: 10.1016/j.jisa.2020.102554

El Mrabet, A., Alihamidi, I., Tber, A., Benaly, M., Hlou, L., & El Gouri, R. (2025). Proposed architecture for Hospital 4.0: Integrating IoT, edge AI, and blockchain for secure and efficient healthcare systems. [IJOE]. *International Journal of Online and Biomedical Engineering*, *21*(05), 87–102. DOI: 10.3991/ijoe.v21i05.52991

El-Gazzar, R., & Stendal, K. (2020). Blockchain in health care: Hope or hype? *Journal of Medical Internet Research*, *22*(7), e17199. DOI: 10.2196/17199 PMID: 32673219

Ellahi, R. M., Ali, M., Ali Shah, S. A., Qureshi, M. A., Gulzar, S., Wood, L. C., & Ahmed Bekhit, A. E.-D. (2026). Harnessing digital twins: transforming livestock supply chain management: a comprehensive review. *Cogent Food & Agriculture*, *12*(1), 2611196. DOI: 10.1080/23311932.2025.2611196

Elomda, B. M., Abdelaty Abdelbary, T. A., Hassan, H. A., Hamza, K. S., & Kharma, Q. (2025). An enhanced multi-layer blockchain security model for improved latency and scalability. *Information (Basel)*, *16*(3), 241. DOI: 10.3390/info16030241

El-Saleh, A. A., Sheikh, A. M., Albreem, M. A., & Honnurvali, M. S. (2025). The internet of medical things (IoMT): Opportunities and challenges. *Wireless Networks*, *31*(1), 327–344. DOI: 10.1007/s11276-024-03764-8

El-Warrak, L., & de Farias, C. M. (2024). The State of the art of digital twins in health—A quick review of the literature. *Computers*, *13*(9), 228.

Emma, O., & Adams, P. (2025). Revolutionizing Clinical Trials with Blockchain: Strengthening Data Integrity and Building Patient Trust.

Errida, A., & Lotfi, B. (2021). The determinants of organizational change management success: Literature review and case study. *International Journal of Engineering Business Management*, *13*, 18479790211016273. DOI: 10.1177/18479790211016273

European Commission. (2019). Digital economy and society index (DESI) report: Estonia.

European Commission. (2023). eHealth digital maturity assessment of EU member states 2024 report. Publications Office of the European Union.

European Medicines Agency. (2022). Digital transformation of medicines regulation: Strategic reflection.

European Parliament & Council of the European Union. (2016). *Regulation (EU) 2016/679*. General Data Protection Regulation.

Ezz, M., Alaerjan, A. S., & Mostafa, A. M. (2025). Ethical AI in Healthcare: Integrating Zero-Knowledge Proofs and Smart Contracts for Transparent Data Governance. *Bioengineering (Basel, Switzerland)*, *12*(11), 1236. DOI: 10.3390/bioengineering12111236 PMID: 41301192

Fahmy, A. M. (2025). *Exploring the role of AI in predicting chronic disease progression: Diabetes and cardiovascular diseases*. Premier Journal of Public Health., DOI: 10.70389/PJPH.100021

Faisal, S. M., Ishrat, M., & Khan, W. (2025). Digital Twins in Healthcare: Revolutionizing Patient Care and Medical Operations. In *Digital Twins for Smart Cities and Urban Planning* (pp. 69-89). CRC Press.

Fatokun, T., Nag, A., & Sharma, S. (2021). Towards a blockchain assisted patient owned system for electronic health records. *Electronics (Basel)*, *10*(5), 580. DOI: 10.3390/electronics10050580

Fatoum, H., Hanna, S., Halamka, J. D., Sicker, D. C., Spangenberg, P., & Hashmi, S. K. (2021). Blockchain integration with digital technology and the future of health care ecosystems: Systematic review. *Journal of Medical Internet Research*, *23*(11), e19846. DOI: 10.2196/19846 PMID: 34726603

Ferrag, M. A., Derdour, M., Mukherjee, M., Derhab, A., Maglaras, L., & Janicke, H. (2019). Blockchain technologies for the internet of things: Research issues and challenges. *IEEE Internet of Things Journal*, *6*(2), 2188–2204. DOI: 10.1109/JIOT.2018.2882794

Ficili, I., Giacobbe, M., Tricomi, G., & Puliafito, A. (2025). From sensors to data intelligence: Leveraging IoT, cloud, and edge computing with AI. *Sensors (Basel)*, *25*(6), 1763. DOI: 10.3390/s25061763

Finck, M. (2019). Blockchain and the General Data Protection Regulation. *European Data Protection Law Review*, *5*(1), 17–37. DOI: 10.21552/edpl/2018/1/6

Fischer, R.-P., Volpert, A., Antonino, P., & Ahrens, T. D. (2024). Digital Patient Twins for Personalized Therapeutics and Pharmaceutical Manufacturing. *Frontiers in Digital Health*, *5*, 1302338. Advance online publication. DOI: 10.3389/fdgth.2023.1302338 PMID: 38250053

Frempong, D., Benson, C. E., Oyasiji, O., & Okesiji, A. (2024). Blockchain-enabled consent management in healthcare: A framework for enforcing privacy preferences and regulatory compliance. *International Journal of Multidisciplinary Research and Growth Evaluation*, *5*(3), 1059–1068. DOI: 10.54660/.IJMRGE.2024.5.3.1059-1068

Fukawa, N., & Rindfleisch, A. (2023). Enhancing innovation via the digital twin. *Journal of Product Innovation Management*, *40*(4), 391–406. DOI: 10.1111/jpim.12655

Fuller, A., Fan, Z., Day, C., & Barlow, C. (2020). Digital twin: Enabling technologies and future directions. *Computers in Industry*, *119*, 103259. DOI: 10.1016/j.compind.2020.103259

Fuller, A., Fan, Z., Day, C., & Barlow, C. (2020). Digital twin: Enabling technologies, challenges, and open research. *IEEE Access : Practical Innovations, Open Solutions*, *8*, 108952–108971. DOI: 10.1109/ACCESS.2020.2998358

Fuller, A., Fan, Z., Day, C., & Barlow, C. (2020). The implementation of digital twins in predictive maintenance. *Procedia CIRP*, *93*, 169–174. DOI: 10.1016/j.procir.2020.03.065

Fusco, A., Dicuonzo, G., Dell'Atti, V., & Tatullo, M. (2020). Blockchain in healthcare: Insights on COVID-19. *International Journal of Environmental Research and Public Health*, *17*(19), 7167. DOI: 10.3390/ijerph17197167 PMID: 33007951

Gaddapuri, N. S.Naga Srinivasulu Gaddapuri. (2025). Digital Twin Governance: IoT-driven real-time regulatory auditing in smart hospital architectures. *Computer Fraud & Security*, •••, 1462–1470. DOI: 10.52710/cfs.752

Ganesan, M., Sivakumar, N., & Thirumaran, M. (2020). Internet of medical things with cloud-based e-health services for brain tumour detection model using deep convolution neural network. *Electronic Government an International Journal*, *16*(1/2), 69. DOI: 10.1504/EG.2020.105240

Garg, M., Liu, X., Vassilaki, M., Petersen, R. C., Sauver, J. S., & Sohn, S. (2023, December). Navigating Sex-Specific Disease Dynamics in Incident Dementia. In *2023 IEEE International Conference on Bioinformatics and Biomedicine (BIBM)* (pp. 4065-4072). IEEE. DOI: 10.1109/BIBM58861.2023.10385324

Gazerani, P. (2023). Intelligent digital twins for personalized migraine care. *Journal of Personalized Medicine*, *13*(8), 1255. PMID: 37623505

Gebler, R., Reinecke, I., Sedlmayr, M., & Goldammer, M. (2025). Enhancing clinical data infrastructure for AI research: Comparative evaluation of data management architectures. *Journal of Medical Internet Research*, *27*, e74976. DOI: 10.2196/74976

Geetha, B. T., Kafila, K., Ram, S. T., Narkhede, A. P., Ahmad, A. Y. B., & Tiwari, M. (2024, March). Creating resilient digital asset management frameworks in financial operations using blockchain technology. In *2024 International Conference on Trends in Quantum Computing and Emerging Business Technologies (pp.* 1-7*).* IEEE. DOI: 10.1109/TQCEBT59414.2024.10545263

George, B. (2025). Blockchain-Based Land Tenure Systems: A Conceptual Model for Using Decentralized Technologies in Managing Land Rights and Ownership Disputes. *Land Management and Utilization, 1*(2), 32–48. DOI: 10.54963/lmu.v1i2.1527

Ghadi, Y. Y., Mazhar, T., Shahzad, T., Amir khan, M., Abd-Alrazaq, A., Ahmed, A., & Hamam, H. (2024). The role of blockchain to secure internet of medical things. *Scientific Reports, 14*(1), 18422. DOI: 10.1038/s41598-024-68529-x PMID: 39117650

Ghayvat, H., Zuhair, M., Shukla, N., & Kumar, N. (2023). Healthcare-CT: Solid PoD and Blockchain-Enabled Cyber Twin Approach for Healthcare 5.0 Ecosystems. *IEEE Internet of Things Journal, 11*(4), 6119–6130. DOI: 10.1109/JIOT.2023.3312448

Girardi, F., De Gennaro, G., Colizzi, L., & Convertini, N. (2020). Improving the healthcare effectiveness: The possible role of EHR, IoMT and blockchain. *Electronics (Basel), 9*(6), 884. DOI: 10.3390/electronics9060884

Gkintoni, E., & Halkiopoulos, C. (2025). Digital twin cognition: AI-biomarker integration in biomimetic neuropsychology. *Biomimetics (Basel, Switzerland), 10*(10), 640. DOI: 10.3390/biomimetics10100640 PMID: 41149170

Gomes, B., Eisa, S., Matos, D. R., & Pardal, M. L. (2024). Decentralized Storage and Self-Sovereign Identity for Document-Based Claims. *arXiv preprint arXiv:2411.16987.*

Gordon, W. J., & Catalini, C. (2018). Blockchain technology for healthcare: Facilitating the transition to patient-driven interoperability. *Computational and Structural Biotechnology Journal, 16*, 224–230. DOI: 10.1016/j.csbj.2018.06.003 PMID: 30069284

Götz, C. S., Karlsson, P., & Yitmen, I. (2022). Exploring applicability, interoperability and integrability of Blockchain-based digital twins for asset life cycle management. *Smart and Sustainable Built Environment, 11*(3), 532–558. DOI: 10.1108/SASBE-08-2020-0115

Gowthaman, N., Ruba, M., Aswath, S., Hemavarshni, S. N., Bragadeshwaran, R., & Nithish, S. J. (2025, November). Iot Integrated Solution For Smart Vertical Crop Cultivation. In 2025 IEEE 7th International Conference on Computing, Communication and Automation (ICCCA) (pp. 1-6). IEEE.

Grieves, M., & Vickers, J. (2016). Digital twin: Mitigating unpredictable, undesirable emergent behavior in complex systems. In *Transdisciplinary perspectives on complex systems: New findings and approaches* (pp. 85–113). Springer International Publishing.

Grieves, M., & Vickers, J. (2017). Digital twin: Mitigating unpredictable, undesirable emergent behavior in complex systems. In Kahlen, F.-J., Flumerfelt, S., & Alves, A. (Eds.), *Transdisciplinary perspectives on complex systems* (pp. 85–113). Springer., DOI: 10.1007/978-3-319-38756-7_4

Gunjal, P. R., Jondhale, S. R., Mauri, J. L., & Agrawal, K. (2024). Modern Approaches in IoT and Machine Learning for Cyber Security. *Internet of Things : Engineering Cyber Physical Human Systems*. Advance online publication. DOI: 10.1007/978-3-031-09955-7

Gupta, S., Mehra, P., Nandy, B., Mohammed, P. R., Pradhan, P. K., Duseja, S., Sharma, N., & Pujari, P. R. (2025). Blockchain in health care, evolutionary or revolutionary - an evidence-based review. *Journal of Pharmacy & Bioallied Sciences*, *17*(Suppl 1), S63–S65. DOI: 10.4103/jpbs.jpbs_672_24 PMID: 40511197

Habib, G., Sharma, S., Ibrahim, S., Ahmad, I., Qureshi, S., & Ishfaq, M. (2022). Blockchain technology: Benefits, challenges, applications, and integration of blockchain technology with cloud computing. *Future Internet*, *14*(11), 341. DOI: 10.3390/fi14110341

Hanna, M. G., Pantanowitz, L., Dash, R., Harrison, J. H., Deebajah, M., Pantanowitz, J., & Rashidi, H. H. (2025). Future of artificial intelligence (AI)-machine learning (ML) trends in pathology and medicine. *Modern Pathology*, *38*(4), 100705. DOI: 10.1016/j.modpat.2025.100705 PMID: 39761872

Han, T., Ribeiro, I. de L., Magaia, N., Preto, J., Segundo, A. H. F. N., de Macedo, A. R. L., Muhammad, K., & de Albuquerque, V. H. C. (2021). Emerging drone trends for blockchain-based 5G networks: Open issues and future perspectives. *IEEE Network*, *35*(1), 38–43. DOI: 10.1109/MNET.011.2000151

Hariharan, U., Dhanakoti, V., Rajkumar, K., & Jeyavel, J. (2022, March). Safeguarding e-healthcare documents utilizing an infrastructure for advanced keyless signature infrastructure blockchain within the cloud. In *2022 International Conference on Emerging Smart Computing and Informatics (ESCI)* (pp. 1-6). IEEE. DOI: 10.1109/ESCI53509.2022.9758266

Hariyani, D., Hariyani, P., Mishra, S., & Sharma, M. K. (2025). A literature review on transformative impacts of blockchain technology on manufacturing management and industrial engineering practices. *Green Technologies and Sustainability*, *3*(3), 100169. DOI: 10.1016/j.grets.2025.100169

Hasselgren, A., Hanssen Rensaa, J.-A., Kralevska, K., Gligoroski, D., & Faxvaag, A. (2021). Blockchain for increased trust in virtual health care: Proof-of-concept study. *Journal of Medical Internet Research*, *23*(7), e28496. DOI: 10.2196/28496 PMID: 34328437

Health Level Seven International (HL7). (2019). FHIR release 4 (R4) specification.

Hemdan, E. E.-D., El-Shafai, W., & Sayed, A. (2023). Integrating digital twins with IoT-based blockchain: Concept, architecture, challenges, and future scope. *Wireless Personal Communications*, *131*(3), 1–24. DOI: 10.1007/s11277-023-10538-6

Hemdan, E. E.-D., & Sayed, A. (2025). Smart and secure healthcare with digital twins: A deep dive into blockchain, federated learning, and future innovations. *Algorithms*, *18*(7), 401. DOI: 10.3390/a18070401

Hovorushchenko, T., Moskalenko, A., & Osyadlyi, V. (2023). Methods of medical data management based on blockchain technologies. *Journal of Reliable Intelligent Environments*, *9*(1), 5–16. DOI: 10.1007/s40860-022-00178-1 PMID: 35646514

Hughes, J. H., Tong, D. M. H., Burns, V., Daly, B., Razavi, P., Boelens, J. J., Goswami, S., & Keizer, R. J. (2023). Clinical decision support for chemotherapy-induced neutropenia using a hybrid pharmacodynamic/machine learning model. *CPT: Pharmacometrics & Systems Pharmacology*, *12*(11), 1764–1776. DOI: 10.1002/psp4.13019 PMID: 37503916

Hulsen, T. (2024). Applications of the metaverse in medicine and healthcare. *Advances in Laboratory Medicine*, *5*(2), 159–165. DOI: 10.1515/almed-2023-0124 PMID: 38939198

Hussain, S., Rahman, H., Abdulsaheb, G. M., Al-Khawaja, H., & Khalaf, O. I. (2023). A Blockchain-Based Approach for Healthcare Data Interoperability. *International Journal of Advances in Soft Computing & Its Applications*, *15*(2).

Hylock, R. H., & Zeng, X. (2019). A blockchain framework for patient-centered health records and exchange (Health Chain). *Journal of Medical Systems*, *43*(10), 1–9. DOI: 10.1007/s10916-019-1412-5

Iliuţă, M. E., Moisescu, M. A., Pop, E., Ionita, A. D., Caramihai, S. I., & Mitulescu, T. C. (2024). Digital twin—A review of the evolution from concept to technology and its analytical perspectives on applications in various fields. *Applied Sciences (Basel, Switzerland)*, *14*(13), 5454.

Islam, M. M., Rahaman, A., & Islam, M. R. (2020). Development of smart healthcare monitoring system in IoT environment. *SN Computer Science*, *1*(3), 185. DOI: 10.1007/s42979-020-00195-y PMID: 33063046

Islam, M. N., & Kundu, S. (2019). Enabling IC traceability via blockchain pegged to embedded PUF. *ACM Transactions on Design Automation of Electronic Systems*, *24*(3), 1–23. DOI: 10.1145/3315669

Islam, S. M. R., Kwak, D., Kabir, M. H., Hossain, M., & Kwak, K. S. (2015). The Internet of Things for health care: A comprehensive survey. *IEEE Access : Practical Innovations, Open Solutions*, *3*, 678–708. DOI: 10.1109/ACCESS.2015.2437951

Islayem, R., Musamih, A., Salah, K., Jayaraman, R., & Yaqoob, I. (2025). Enhancing medical digital twins within metaverse using blockchain, NFTs and LLMs. *Internet of Things : Engineering Cyber Physical Human Systems*, *32*, 101648. DOI: 10.1016/j.iot.2025.101648

Ismail, L., Materwala, H., & Zeadally, S. (2019). Lightweight blockchain for healthcare. *IEEE Access : Practical Innovations, Open Solutions*, *7*, 149935–149951. DOI: 10.1109/ACCESS.2019.2947613

Jadav, D., Jadav, N. K., Gupta, R., Tanwar, S., Alfarraj, O., Tolba, A., Raboaca, M. S., & Marina, V. (2023). A trustworthy healthcare management framework using amalgamation of AI and blockchain network. *Mathematics*, *11*(3), 637. DOI: 10.3390/math11030637

Jalil, M. S., Arafat, M. S., Islam, R., Rafi, S. S., Jony, M. A. M., & Hossen, F. (2024). AI and Digital Twins in Healthcare: Revolutionizing Remote Patient Monitoring and Precision Medicine.

Jat, A. S., Grønli, T.-M., Ghinea, G., & Assres, G. (2024). Evolving software architecture design in telemedicine: A PRISMA-based systematic review. *Healthcare Informatics Research*, *30*(3), 184–193. DOI: 10.4258/hir.2024.30.3.184 PMID: 39160778

Javed, I. T., Alharbi, F., Bellaj, B., Margaria, T., Crespi, N., & Qureshi, K. N. (2021). Health-id: A blockchain-based decentralized identity management for remote healthcare. Healthcare. 2021; 9: 712. *Cybersecurity and the Digital Health, 175.* Advance online publication. DOI: 10.3390/healthcare9060712 PMID: 34200778

Jimenez, J. I., Jahankhani, H., & Kendzierskyj, S. (2019). Health care in the cyber-space: Medical cyber-physical system and digital twin challenges. In *Digital twin technologies and smart cities* (pp. 79–92). Springer., DOI: 10.1007/978-3-030-18732-3_7

Johnson, Z.. (2024). Digital Twins for Healthcare Using Wearables. *Bioengineering (Basel, Switzerland).* PMID: 38927842

Jones, D., Snider, C., & Hicks, B. (2019). Digital twin-driven smart manufacturing: Case studies and research directions. *Journal of Manufacturing Systems, 53*, 1–14. DOI: 10.1016/j.jmsy.2019.03.003

Jones, D., Snider, C., Nassehi, A., Yon, J., & Hicks, B. J. (2020). Characterizing the digital twin: A systematic literature review. *CIRP Journal of Manufacturing Science and Technology, 29*, 36–52. DOI: 10.1016/j.cirpj.2020.02.002

Joyia, G. J., Liaqat, R. M., Farooq, A., & Rehman, S. (2017). Internet of medical things (IoMT): Applications, benefits and future challenges in healthcare domain. *Journal of Communication, 12*(4), 240–247.

Juanatas, R. A., Almadhor, A., Alsubai, S., Kryvinska, N., Krichen, M., Sampedro, G. A., & Abbas, S. (2025). Securing realistic IoMT environment using Moth-Flame Optimization-based deep learning framework. *Security and Privacy, 8*(5), e70073. Advance online publication. DOI: 10.1002/spy2.70073

Jung, A., Gsell, M. A. F., Augustin, C. M., & Plank, G. (2022). An integrated workflow for building digital twins of cardiac electromechanics-A multi-fidelity approach for personalising active mechanics. *Mathematics, 10*(5), 823. DOI: 10.3390/math10050823 PMID: 35295404

Justinia, T. (2019). Blockchain technologies: Opportunities for solving real-world problems in healthcare and biomedical sciences. *Acta Informatica Medica, 27*(4), 284. DOI: 10.5455/aim.2019.27.284-291 PMID: 32055097

Kalvet, T. (2012). Innovation: A factor explaining e-government success in Estonia. Electronic Government, an International Journal, 9(2), 142–157.

Kamel Boulos, M. N., & Zhang, P. (2021). Digital twins: From personalised medicine to precision public health. *Journal of Personalized Medicine, 11*(8), 745. DOI: 10.3390/jpm11080745 PMID: 34442389

Kamruzzaman, M. M., Yan, B., Sarker, M. N. I., Alruwaili, O., Wu, M., & Alrashdi, I. (2022). Blockchain and fog computing in IoT-driven healthcare services for smart cities. *Journal of Healthcare Engineering*, *9957888*, 1–13. Advance online publication. DOI: 10.1155/2022/9957888 PMID: 35126961

Kang, S. (2026). Blockchain-Secured Multi-Agent Digital Twin Framework for Distributed Manufacturing With Fuzzy PID Control. *IEEE Communications Standards Magazine*, 1–9. DOI: 10.1109/MCOMSTD.2025.3648845

Kantaros, A., Ganetsos, T., Pallis, E., & Papoutsidakis, M. (2025). From Mathematical Modeling and Simulation to Digital Twins: Bridging Theory and Digital Realities in Industry and Emerging Technologies. *Applied Sciences (Basel, Switzerland)*, *15*(16), 9213. DOI: 10.3390/app15169213

Kassab, M., DeFranco, J., Malas, T., Laplante, P., Destefanis, G., & Neto, V. V. G. (2019). Exploring research in blockchain for healthcare and a roadmap for the future. *IEEE Transactions on Emerging Topics in Computing*, *9*(4), 1835–1852. DOI: 10.1109/TETC.2019.2936881

Kasyapa, M. S. B., & Vanmathi, C. (2024). Blockchain integration in healthcare: A comprehensive investigation of use cases, performance issues, and mitigation strategies. *Frontiers in Digital Health*, *6*, 1359858. DOI: 10.3389/fdgth.2024.1359858 PMID: 38736708

Katsoulakis, E., Wang, Q., & Wu, H.. (2024). "Digital Twins for Health: A Scoping Review." *npj. Digital Medicine*, *7*(1), 77. Advance online publication. DOI: 10.1038/s41746-024-01073-0 PMID: 38519626

Katuwal, G. J., Pandey, S., Hennessey, M., & Lamichhane, B. (2018). Applications of blockchain in healthcare: current landscape & challenges. *arXiv preprint arXiv:1812.02776.*

Kaur, A., Sharma, A., Kumar, M., & Bhatia, R. K. (2024). Unleashing the Power of Intelligent Cyber Physical Systems in Healthcare: A Paradigm Shift for the Workforce. In *Intelligent Cyber-Physical Systems for Healthcare Solutions: From Theory to Practice* (pp. 463–483). Springer Nature Singapore. DOI: 10.1007/978-981-97-8983-2_20

Kavinraja, R., & Mithula, S. (2025). *Blockchain-Integrated Drug Tracking System with IoT-Enabled Containers.* Paper presented at the 2025 International Conference on Computational Robotics, Testing and Engineering Evaluation (ICCRTEE).

Kerrison, S., Jusak, J., & Huang, T. (2023). Blockchain-enabled IoT for rural healthcare: Hybrid-channel communication with digital twinning. *Electronics (Basel), 12*(9), 2128. DOI: 10.3390/electronics12092128

Khalifa, F., & Marzouk, M. (2025). Integrated blockchain and Digital Twin framework for sustainable building energy management. *Journal of Industrial Information Integration, 43*, 100747. DOI: 10.1016/j.jii.2024.100747

Khan, A. A., Bourouis, S., Kamruzzaman, M., Hadjouni, M., Shaikh, Z. A., Laghari, A. A., Elmannai, H., & Dhahbi, S. (2023). Data security in healthcare industrial internet of things with blockchain. *IEEE Sensors Journal, 23*(20), 25144–25151. DOI: 10.1109/JSEN.2023.3273851

Khan, M. F., & Abaoud, M. (2023). Blockchain-integrated security for real-time patient monitoring in the Internet of Medical Things using federated learning. *IEEE Access : Practical Innovations, Open Solutions, 11*, 117826–117850. DOI: 10.1109/ACCESS.2023.3326155

Khatoon, A. (2020). A blockchain-based smart contract system for healthcare management. *Electronics (Basel), 9*(1), 94. DOI: 10.3390/electronics9010094

Kherbache, M., Maimour, M., & Rondeau, E. (2021). When digital twin meets network softwarization in the industrial IoT: Real-time requirements case study. *Sensors (Basel), 21*(24), 8194. DOI: 10.3390/s21248194 PMID: 34960288

Khezr, S., Moniruzzaman, M., Yassine, A., & Benlamri, R. (2019). Blockchain technology in healthcare: A comprehensive review and directions for future research. *Applied Sciences (Basel, Switzerland), 9*(9), 1736. DOI: 10.3390/app9091736

Khodaiemehr, H., Bagheri, K., & Feng, C. (2023). Navigating the quantum computing threat landscape for blockchains: A comprehensive survey. Authorea Preprints. DOI: Not available (preprint)

Khosrow-Pour, M. (Ed.). (2015). *Encyclopedia of information science and technology* (3rd ed.). IGI Global.

Kim, H., Park, J., Bennis, M., & Kim, S.-L. (2020). Blockchained on-device federated learning. IEEE Communications Letters: A Publication of the IEEE. *IEEE Communications Letters, 24*(6), 1279–1283. DOI: 10.1109/LCOMM.2019.2921755

Kingdom of Saudi Arabia. (2016). *National Transformation Program 2020*. Government of Saudi Arabia.

Koc, S. (2024). Legal Compliance protocols for Blockchain smart contracts: A new era of regulatory compliance. *Authorea Preprints*. DOI: 10.36227/techrxiv.172954185.58874599/v1

Konopik, J. (2023). The Impact of digital platforms and ecosystems in Healthcare on Value Creation—A Integrative review and Research agenda. *IEEE Access : Practical Innovations, Open Solutions, 11*, 135811–135819. DOI: 10.1109/ACCESS.2023.3336983

Kostkova, P. (2015). Grand challenges in digital health. *Frontiers in Public Health, 3*, 134. DOI: 10.3389/fpubh.2015.00134 PMID: 26000272

Krithika, S., Jayachandran, T., Raghapriya, N. R., Ruba, M., Janani, C., & Sathiyavathi, S. (2025, April). An Effective Denial of Service Texture Features from Malware Grayscale Image. In 2025 3rd International Conference on Artificial Intelligence and Machine Learning Applications Theme: Healthcare and Internet of Things (AIMLA) (pp. 1-7). IEEE. DOI: 10.1109/AIMLA63829.2025.11041501

Kritzinger, W., Karner, M., Traar, G., Henjes, J., & Sihn, W. (2018). Digital twin in manufacturing: A categorical literature review and classification. *IFAC-PapersOnLine, 51*(11), 1016–1022. DOI: 10.1016/j.ifacol.2018.08.474

Kumar, P. R., Meenakshi, S., Shalini, S., Devi, S. R., & Boopathi, S. (2023). Soil Quality Prediction in Context Learning Approaches Using Deep Learning and Blockchain for Smart Agriculture. In Effective AI, Blockchain, and E-Governance Applications for Knowledge Discovery and Management (pp. 1-26). IGI Global. DOI: 10.4018/978-1-6684-9151-5.ch001

Kumar, T., Ramani, V., Ahmad, I., Braeken, A., Harjula, E., & Ylianttila, M. (2018, September). Blockchain utilization in healthcare: Key requirements and challenges. In *2018 IEEE 20th International conference on e-health networking, applications and services (Healthcom) (pp. 1-7). IEEE.* DOI: 10.1109/HealthCom.2018.8531136

Kumar, D. M. (2024). Ethical AI design in blockchain-powered surveillance systems. *Scientific Journal of Artificial Intelligence and Blockchain Technologies, 1*(3). Advance online publication. DOI: 10.63345/sjaibt.v1.i3.103

Kumar, D. S. (2024). GDPR compliance challenges in blockchain-based systems. *Scientific Journal of Artificial Intelligence and Blockchain Technologies, 1*(3). Advance online publication. DOI: 10.63345/sjaibt.v1.i3.104

Kumari, S., Sowmya, K., Sharma, A. K., Kumar, A., & Goel, P. K. (2025). Blockchain and AI in rural healthcare. In *Advances in Computational Intelligence and Robotics* (pp. 191–214). IGI Global., DOI: 10.4018/979-8-3373-3241-3.ch010

Kuo, T. T., Kim, H. E., & Ohno-Machado, L. (2017). Blockchain distributed ledger technologies for biomedical and health care applications. *Journal of the American Medical Informatics Association : JAMIA, 24*(6), 1211–1220. DOI: 10.1093/jamia/ocx068 PMID: 29016974

Kuo, T.-T., & Zhang, P. (2023). Editorial: Blockchain and distributed ledger technology—enabled architectures for improving healthcare. *Frontiers in Blockchain, 6*(1275474), 1275474. Advance online publication. DOI: 10.3389/fbloc.2023.1275474

Kuriakose, S. M., Joseph, J., & Kollinal, R. (2024). The rise of digital twins in healthcare: A mapping of the research landscape. *Cureus, 16*(7). PMID: 39184791

Le Nguyen, T. (2018, August). Blockchain in healthcare: A new technology benefit for both patients and doctors. In *2018 Portland International Conference on Management of Engineering and Technology (PICMET)* (pp. 1-6). IEEE. DOI: 10.23919/PICMET.2018.8481969

Lee, E. A. (2008, May). Cyber physical systems: Design challenges. In *2008 11th IEEE international symposium on object and component-oriented real-time distributed computing (ISORC)* (pp. 363-369). IEEE.

Lee, J., Bagheri, B., & Kao, H. A. (2015). A cyber-physical systems architecture for Industry 4.0-based manufacturing systems. *Manufacturing Letters, 3*, 18–23. DOI: 10.1016/j.mfglet.2014.12.001

Leiva, V., & Castro, C. (2025). Artificial intelligence and blockchain in clinical trials: Enhancing data governance efficiency, integrity, and transparency. *Bioanalysis, 17*(3), 161–176. DOI: 10.1080/17576180.2025.2452774 PMID: 39844748

Leng, J., Tan, R., Liu, Q., Jiang, P., & Xu, K. (2020). Digital twin-based energy-efficient manufacturing. *Journal of Manufacturing Systems, 57*, 234–245. DOI: 10.1016/j.jmsy.2020.04.012

Lilja, S. (2022). *Digital twins : High resolution disease models for optimized diagnosis and treatment*. Linköping University Electronic Press., DOI: 10.3384/9789179292157

Li, T., Shen, Y., Li, Y., Zhang, Y., & Wu, S. (2024). The status quo and future prospects of digital twins for healthcare. *EngMedicine, 1*(3), 100042.

Liu, Y., Cao, X., Chen, T., Jiang, Y., You, J., Wu, M., Wang, X., Feng, M., Jin, Y., & Chen, J. (2025). From screens to scenes: A survey of embodied AI in healthcare. *Information Fusion, 119*, 103033. DOI: 10.1016/j.inffus.2025.103033

Liu, Y., Zhang, L., & Shen, W. (2021). Digital twin for smart cities: Framework, technologies and applications. *Journal of Urban Technology, 28*(1), 3–25. DOI: 10.1080/10630732.2020.1813539

Li, Z. (2022). *Digital-twin Healthcare: A Gateway to Future Medicine*. Preprint.

Lomotey, R. K., Kumi, S., Ray, M., & Deters, R. (2024, June). Synthetic data digital twins and data trusts control for privacy in health data sharing. In *Proceedings of the 2024 ACM Workshop on Secure and Trustworthy Cyber-Physical Systems* (pp. 1-10). DOI: 10.1145/3643650.3658605

Longo, F., Padovano, A., & Umbrello, S. (2020). Value-oriented and ethical design of digital twins. *Computers in Industry, 117*, 103187. DOI: 10.1016/j.compind.2020.103187

Lu, Q., Ye, Z., Fang, Z., Meng, J., Pitt, M., Lin, J., . . . Chen, L. (2021, December). Creating an inter-hospital resilient network for pandemic response based on blockchain and dynamic digital twins. In *2021 winter simulation conference (WSC)* (pp. 1-12). IEEE. DOI: 10.1109/WSC52266.2021.9715517

Lu, J., Sattler, A., Wang, S., Khaki, A. R., Callahan, A., Fleming, S., Fong, R., Ehlert, B., Li, R. C., Shieh, L., Ramchandran, K., Gensheimer, M. F., Chobot, S., Pfohl, S., Li, S., Shum, K., Parikh, N., Desai, P., Seevaratnam, B., & Shah, N. H. (2022). Considerations in the reliability and fairness audits of predictive models for advance care planning. *Frontiers in Digital Health, 4*(943768), 943768. DOI: 10.3389/fdgth.2022.943768

Łukaniszyn, M., Majka, Ł., Grochowicz, B., Mikołajewski, D., & Kawala-Sterniuk, A. (2024). Digital twins generated by artificial intelligence in personalized healthcare. *Applied Sciences (Basel, Switzerland), 14*(20), 9404. DOI: 10.3390/app14209404

Lu, Q., Chen, L., Xie, X., Fang, Z., Ye, Z., & Pitt, M. (2023). Framing blockchain-integrated digital twins for emergent healthcare: A proof of concept. *Proceedings of the Institution of Civil Engineers. Engineering Sustainability, 176*(4), 228–243. DOI: 10.1680/jensu.22.00073

Lu, Y., Xu, X., & Xu, P. (2020). Internet of things (IoT) and digital twin in smart manufacturing: A survey. *Journal of Manufacturing Systems, 57*, 1–14. DOI: 10.1016/j.jmsy.2020.04.009

Maiwada, U. D., Danyaro, K. U., & Sarlan, A. B. (2024). Enhancing 5G energy efficiency through digital twin networks: A comprehensive review. *Digital Twins and Applications, 1*(1), 4–25. DOI: 10.1049/dgt2.12008

Maiwada, U. D., Danyaro, K. U., Sarlan, A., & Alashhab, A. A. (2024). AN IMPROVED 5G MOBILITY HANDOVER EFFICIENT BY CREATING A DIGITAL TWIN NETWORK: A REVIEW. *International Journal of Software Engineering and Computer Systems*, *10*(2), 131–148. DOI: 10.15282/ijsecs.10.2.2024.11.0129

Makhdoom, I., Abolhasan, M., Abbas, H., & Ni, W. (2019). Blockchain's adoption in IoT: The challenges, and a way forward. *Journal of Network and Computer Applications*, *125*, 251–279. DOI: 10.1016/j.jnca.2018.10.019

Mammadova, M. H., & Ahmadova, A. A. (2023). Development of digital twin ecosystem and ontology in medicine. *Technology Transfer Fundamental Principles and Innovative Technical Solutions*, *21–23*, 21–23. Advance online publication. DOI: 10.21303/2585-6847.2023.003203

Mandinyenya, G., & Malele, V. (2025). Post-quantum cryptographic techniques for future-proofing-blockchain-based personal data sharing. *Iraqi Journal for Computers and Informatics*, *51*(2), 109–125. DOI: 10.25195/ijci.v51i2.623

Manteghinejad, A., & Javanmard, S. H. (2021). Challenges and opportunities of digital health in a post-COVID19 world. *Journal of Research in Medical Sciences : the Official Journal of Isfahan University of Medical Sciences*, *26*(1), 11. DOI: 10.4103/jrms.JRMS_1255_20 PMID: 34084190

Margheri, A., Masi, M., Miladi, A., Sassone, V., & Rosenzweig, J. (2020). Decentralised provenance for healthcare data. *International Journal of Medical Informatics*, *141*(104197), 104197. DOI: 10.1016/j.ijmedinf.2020.104197 PMID: 32540775

Market Research Future. (2023). Saudi Arabia digital health and smart hospital market forecast to 2033.

Market Research Future. (2023). Saudi Arabia digital health market forecast to 2033.

Masood, I., Daud, A., Wang, Y., Banjar, A., & Alharbey, R. (2024). A blockchain-based system for patient data privacy and security. *Multimedia Tools and Applications*, *83*(21), 60443–60467. DOI: 10.1007/s11042-023-17941-y

Mazlan, E. M., Sarman, A. M., Kamaruddin, S. S., & Bakar, R. A. (2025). Digital Twin for Dynamic Construction Site Monitoring and Control. *Journal of Technology Management and Business*, *12*(2), 1–13.

Mehra, P., & Kumar, P. (Eds.). (2025). *Incentives and benefits for adopting green entrepreneurship practices*. IGI Global., DOI: 10.4018/979-8-3693-9306-2

Meijer, C., Uh, H. W., & El Bouhaddani, S. (2023). Digital twins in healthcare: Methodological challenges and opportunities. *Journal of Personalized Medicine*, *13*(10), 1522. PMID: 37888133

Mennella, C., Maniscalco, U., De Pietro, G., & Esposito, M. (2024). Ethical and regulatory challenges of AI technologies in healthcare: A narrative review. *Heliyon*, *10*(4), e26297. Advance online publication. DOI: 10.1016/j.heliyon.2024.e26297

Mettler, M. (2016, September). Blockchain technology in healthcare: The revolution starts here. In *2016 IEEE 18th international conference on e-health networking, applications and services (Healthcom)* (pp. 1-3). IEEE.

Miettinen, M., & Lappalainen, P. (2018). Digital twins in healthcare: The promise of predictive and personalized medicine. *Health Informatics Journal*, *24*(2), 152–167. DOI: 10.1177/1460458217726370

Mihai, S., Yaqoob, M., Hung, D. V., Davis, W., Towakel, P., Raza, M., & Nguyen, H. X. (2022). Digital twins: A survey on enabling technologies, challenges, trends and future prospects. *IEEE Communications Surveys and Tutorials*, *24*(4), 2255–2291. DOI: 10.1109/COMST.2022.3208773

Ministry of Health Saudi Arabia. (2022). Seha Virtual Hospital initiative report.

Ministry of Health Saudi Arabia. (2022). Seha Virtual Hospital official report.

Ministry of Health Saudi Arabia. (2023). National e-Health platform overview.

Ministry of Health Saudi Arabia. (2023). National e-Health strategy and digital platforms overview.

Ministry of Health Saudi Arabia. (2024). Health statistical yearbook 2024.

Mishra, D. K., & Mehra, P. S. (2025). Exploring blockchain-based patient-centric healthcare: A comprehensive review. *Concurrency and Computation*, *37*(12–14), e70124. Advance online publication. DOI: 10.1002/cpe.70124

Mittelstadt, B. (2017). Ethics of the algorithm: Key problems and solutions. *Philosophy & Technology*, *30*(4), 1–26. DOI: 10.1007/s13347-016-0229-9

Mittelstadt, B. D., Allo, P., Taddeo, M., Wachter, S., & Floridi, L. (2016). The ethics of algorithms: Mapping the debate. *Big Data & Society*, *3*(2), 2053951716679679. DOI: 10.1177/2053951716679679

Moganti, J., Nookaratnam, P., Venkataramana, G., & Boddeda, B. (2025). Digital twin technology in graft vs host disease. *International Journal of Research in Pharmacy and Allied Science*, *04*(03). Advance online publication. DOI: 10.71431/IJRPAS.2025.4311

Mohammadi, A., Mehrabi, A., & Yousefi, H. (2024). SCALHEALTH: A scalable blockchain-based framework for secure IoT healthcare systems. *arXiv preprint*. https://arxiv.org/abs/2403.08068

Nadeem, M., Kostic, S., Dornhöfer, M., Weber, C., & Fathi, M. (2025). A comprehensive review of digital twin in healthcare in the scope of simulative health-monitoring. *Digital Health*, *11*, 20552076241304078. PMID: 39777066

Nakamoto, S. (2008). Bitcoin: A peer-to-peer electronic cash system.

Narigina, M., Romanovs, A., & Bruzgiene, R. (2024, May). Digital twin technology in healthcare: A literature review. In 2024 IEEE 11th Workshop on Advances in Information, Electronic and Electrical Engineering (AIEEE) (pp. 1-8). IEEE.

Nasir, M. H., Arshad, J., Khan, M. M., Fatima, M., Salah, K., & Jayaraman, R. (2022). Scalable blockchains — A systematic review. *Future Generation Computer Systems*, *126*, 136–162. DOI: 10.1016/j.future.2021.07.035

Ngabo, D., Wang, D., Iwendi, C., Anajemba, J. H., Ajao, L. A., & Biamba, C. (2021). Blockchain-based security mechanism for the medical data at fog computing architecture of internet of things. *Electronics (Basel)*, *10*(17), 2110. DOI: 10.3390/electronics10172110

Nguyen, T. L., Nguyen, L., Hoang, T., Bandara, D., Wang, Q., Lu, Q., Xu, X., Zhu, L., & Chen, S. (2025). Blockchain-empowered trustworthy data sharing: Fundamentals, applications, and challenges. *ACM Computing Surveys*, *57*(8), 1–36. DOI: 10.1145/3718082

Noeikham, P., Buakum, D., & Sirivongpaisal, N. (2024). Architecture designing of digital twin in a healthcare unit. *Health Informatics Journal*, *30*(4), 14604582241296792. Advance online publication. DOI: 10.1177/14604582241296792 PMID: 39447608

O'Donoghue, O., Vazirani, A. A., Brindley, D., & Meinert, E. (2019). Design choices and trade-offs in health care blockchain implementations: Systematic review. *Journal of Medical Internet Research*, *21*(5), e12426. DOI: 10.2196/12426

Obodo, O. R. (2025). Conceptualising blockchain-based consent management in multi-provider healthcare environment. International Journal of Scientific Research and Modern Technology, 116–121. DOI: 10.38124/ijsrmt.v4i9.817

OECD. (2020). Health in the digital age: OECD health policy studies. https://doi.org/DOI: 10.1787/0a5e3f3a-en

OECD. (2023). Health data governance for the digital age.

Ogut, E. (2025). Artificial intelligence in clinical medicine: Challenges across diagnostic imaging, clinical decision support, surgery, pathology, and drug discovery. *Clinics and Practice*, *15*(9), 169. DOI: 10.3390/clinpract15090169 PMID: 41002784

Olatunde, R. V, Gyasiwaa, M. Y., Ayangeakaa, A. S., Usman, M. A., Olorundare, T. O., & Akpughe, O. V. (2025). Digital twin technology in precision medicine and public health: Transforming patient care and epidemiological forecasting. International Journal of Innovative Science and Research Technology, IJISRT25JUN719, 1044–1049. DOI: 10.38124/ijisrt/25jun719

Onwubiko, A., Singh, R., Awan, S., Pervez, Z., & Ramzan, N. (2023). Enabling trust and security in Digital Twin management: A blockchain-based approach with Ethereum and IPFS. *Sensors (Basel)*, *23*(14), 6641. DOI: 10.3390/s23146641 PMID: 37514938

Organisation for Economic Co-operation and Development (OECD). (2025). *Digital government and health data interoperability benchmarking report*. OECD Publishing.

Organisation for Economic Co-operation and Development (OECD). (2025). *Digital health interoperability benchmarking report*. OECD Publishing.

Ostropolets, A., Zhang, L., & Hripcsak, G. (2020). A scoping review of clinical decision support tools that generate new knowledge to support decision making in real time. *Journal of the American Medical Informatics Association : JAMIA*, *27*(12), 1968–1976. DOI: 10.1093/jamia/ocaa200 PMID: 33120430

Ovsianko, D., & Niemkova, E. (2025). Smart contracts as privacy-preserving mechanisms in distributed digital twin systems. Cybersecurity: Education, Science. *Technique*, *1*(29), 107–123. DOI: 10.28925/2663-4023.2025.29.867

Pan, J., Wang, J., Hester, A., Alqerm, I., Liu, Y., & Zhao, Y. (2019). EdgeChain: An edge-IoT framework and prototype based on blockchain and smart contracts. *IEEE Internet of Things Journal*, *6*(3), 4719–4732. DOI: 10.1109/JIOT.2018.2878154

Pantelopoulos, A., & Bourbakis, N. G. (2010). Prognosis—a wearable health-monitoring system for people at risk: Methodology and modeling. *IEEE Transactions on Information Technology in Biomedicine*, *14*(3), 613–621. DOI: 10.1109/TITB.2010.2040085 PMID: 20123575

Papachristou, K., Katsakiori, P. F., Papadimitroulas, P., Strigari, L., & Kagadis, G. C. (2024). Digital Twins' advancements and applications in healthcare, towards precision medicine. *Journal of Personalized Medicine, 14*(11), 1101. DOI: 10.3390/jpm14111101 PMID: 39590593

Park, J., Park, E., Lee, D., Kang, S., Lee, T., Lee, S.-J., Hong, H., Kim, H., Park, Y. R., & Lee, U. (2023). Human digital twins for pervasive healthcare: A scoping review (preprint). *Interactive Journal of Medical Research.* Advance online publication. DOI: 10.2196/46012

Peng, Y., Zhang, M., Yu, F., Xu, J., & Gao, S. (2020). Digital Twin hospital buildings: An exemplary case study through continuous lifecycle integration. *Advances in Civil Engineering, 2020*(1), 1–13. DOI: 10.1155/2020/8846667

Phelan, D., Gottlieb, D., Mandel, J. C., Ignatov, V., Jones, J., Marquard, B., Ellis, A., & Mandl, K. D. (2024). Beyond compliance with the 21st Century Cures Act Rule: A patient controlled electronic health information export application programming interface. *Journal of the American Medical Informatics Association : JAMIA, 31*(4), 901–909. DOI: 10.1093/jamia/ocae013

Pilania, U., Kumar, M., Singh, S., Adhalkha, P., & Satija, T. (2023, December). Securing Confidential Information on WhatsApp with Blockchain Technology. In *International Conference on Advancements in Smart Computing and Information Security* (pp. 53-61). Cham: Springer Nature Switzerland.

Pilania, U., Upadhyay, P., Tanwar, R., & Kumar, M. (2023). A creative domain of blockchain application: NFTs. In *Mobile Radio Communications and 5G Networks: Proceedings of Third MRCN 2022* (pp. 397-406). Singapore: Springer Nature Singapore.

Pilania, U., Kumar, M., Tanwar, R., Upadhyay, P., & Narayan, P. (2024). Music DApp on the Solana Blockchain Platform: Design, Development, and Analysis. In *Quantum and Blockchain-based Next Generation Sustainable Computing* (pp. 121–134). Springer Nature Switzerland. DOI: 10.1007/978-3-031-58068-0_6

Pirtle, C., & Ehrenfeld, J. (2018). Blockchain for healthcare: The next generation of medical records? *Journal of Medical Systems, 42*(9), 172. DOI: 10.1007/s10916-018-1025-3 PMID: 30097733

Pokharel, B. P., Kshetri, N., Sharma, S. R., & Paudel, S. (2025). blockHealthSecure: Integrating Blockchain and Cybersecurity in Post-Pandemic Healthcare Systems. *Information (Basel), 16*(2), 133. DOI: 10.3390/info16020133

Ponkarthika, M. G., A. P., Ruba, M., Kishore, Y. R., M., K., & G. V., M. (2026). Bridging Health Equity in Times of Crisis: Ensuring Inclusive Care During Emergencies and Disasters. In E. Matsumoto, F. Andres, & R. Agrawal (Eds.), Advancing Equity in Global Healthcare Systems (pp. 27-54). IGI Global Scientific Publishing. DOI: 10.4018/979-8-3373-1330-6.ch002

Poovithaa, M., Ruba, M., Ponkarthika, M., Ragul, N., Ragul, V., & Sangeetha, K. (2025, November). IoT Smart Traffic Control System for Hill Roads with Emergency Vehicle Priority. In 2025 IEEE 7th International Conference on Computing, Communication and Automation (ICCCA) (pp. 1-6). IEEE.

Powell, W., Sultanbawa, Y., Thomson, M., Sivakumar, D., Dipu, M. A., Williams, L., Turner-Morris, C., Sigley, G., & He, S. (2024). Blockchain-enabled provenance and supply chain governance for Indigenous foods and botanicals: A design approach study. *Sustainability (Basel)*, *16*(16), 7084. DOI: 10.3390/su16167084

Pradeep, M., Kumari, S., Tyagi, A. K., & Tiwari, S. (2024). Smart hospital in smart cities. In Tyagi, A. K. (Ed.), *Digital twin and blockchain for smart cities*. John Wiley & Sons., DOI: 10.1002/9781394303564.ch24

Prgomet, M., Georgiou, A., & Westbrook, J. I. (2009). The impact of mobile handheld technology on hospital physicians' work practices and patient care: A systematic review. *Journal of the American Medical Informatics Association : JAMIA*, *16*(6), 792–801. DOI: 10.1197/jamia.M3215 PMID: 19717793

Qi, Q., & Tao, F. (2018). Digital twin and big data towards smart manufacturing and Industry 4.0: 360 degree comparison. *IEEE Access : Practical Innovations, Open Solutions*, *6*, 3585–3593. DOI: 10.1109/ACCESS.2018.2793265

Qi, Q., Tao, F., Zuo, Y., Zhao, D., & Nee, A. Y. C. (2020). Digital twin and big data towards smart manufacturing and Industry 4.0: 360 degree comparison. *IEEE Transactions on Industrial Informatics*, *16*(4), 2413–2422. DOI: 10.1109/TII.2019.2947540

Quazi, F., Raju, N., Gorrepati, N., & Abdul Kareem, S. (2024). Blockchain applications in electronic health records (EHRs). International Journal of Global Innovations and Solutions (IJGIS). DOI: 10.21428/e90189c8.5043b7de

Radanović, I., & Likić, R. (2018). Opportunities for use of blockchain technology in medicine. *Journal of Medical Systems*, *42*(8), 152. DOI: 10.1016/j.ijpe.2008.03.010 PMID: 29974270

Raghupathi, W., & Raghupathi, V. (2014). Big data analytics in healthcare: Promise and potential. *Health Information Science and Systems*, *2*(1), 3. DOI: 10.1186/2047-2501-2-3 PMID: 25825667

Rahman, M. H., & Ansar, M. T. (2025). AI-powered QA in healthcare software: Leveraging predictive analytics and digital twins for safe, cost-effective, and agile medical systems. *Journal of Computer Science and Technology Studies*, *7*(9), 619–628. DOI: 10.32996/jcsts.2025.4.1.70

Raja, G. B., Vigneashwaran, R., Rohan, M., Praveen, N., & Vijay, N. (2025). *IoT-based Sewage Atmosphere and Health Monitoring for Sanitation Workers with Alerting System.* Paper presented at the 2025 7th International Conference on Inventive Material Science and Applications (ICIMA). DOI: 10.1109/ICIMA64861.2025.11073919

Rajab, R. M., Abuhmida, M., Wilson, I., & Ward, R. P. (2024). A review of IoMT security and privacy related frameworks. Proceedings of the ... *European Conference on Information Warfare and Security*, 23(1), 733–743. DOI: 10.34190/eccws.23.1.2239

Raja, G. B. (2021). Impact of internet of things, artificial intelligence, and blockchain technology in Industry 4.0. In *Internet of things, artificial intelligence and blockchain technology* (pp. 157–178). Springer. DOI: 10.1007/978-3-030-74150-1_8

Raja, G. B. (2024). Green Communication Technologies and Protocols. In *Artificial Intelligence Techniques for Sustainable Development* (pp. 86–113). CRC Press. DOI: 10.1201/9781003546382-5

Rajput, A. R., Li, Q., Taleby Ahvanooey, M., & Masood, I. (2019). EACMS: Emergency access control management system for personal health record based on blockchain. *IEEE Access : Practical Innovations, Open Solutions*, *7*, 84304–84317. DOI: 10.1109/ACCESS.2019.2917976

Rakic, D. (2018, March). Blockchain Technology in Healthcare. In *ICT4AWE* (pp. 13-20). DOI: 10.5220/0006531600130020

Ramani, R., Mary, A. R., Raja, S. E., & Shunmugam, D. A. (2024). Optimized data management and secured federated learning in the Internet of Medical Things (IoMT) with blockchain technology. *Biomedical Signal Processing and Control*, *93*, 106213. DOI: 10.1016/j.bspc.2024.106213

Rana, S. K., Rana, S. K., Nisar, K., Ag Ibrahim, A. A., Rana, A. K., Goyal, N., & Chawla, P. (2022). Blockchain technology and artificial intelligence based decentralized access control model to enable secure interoperability for healthcare. *Sustainability (Basel)*, *14*(15), 9471. DOI: 10.3390/su14159471

Ranjan, P. R., Yadav, A. S., Verma, A. R., Patil, A., & Gupta, D. P. (2023). Healthcare data management system using blockchain. International Journal of Scientific Research in Computer Science. *Engineering and Information Technology, CSEIT2390250*, 382–387. DOI: 10.32628/CSEIT2390250

Rao, C. B., Suryakanthi, K., Banappagoudar, S. B., Geetha, B. T., Kaur, S., & Kaur, H. (2023, December). Entrepreneurship and innovation in the age of artificial intelligence: A blockchain approach. In *2023 IEEE International Conference on ICT in Business Industry & Government (ICTBIG)* (pp. 1-6). IEEE. DOI: 10.1109/ICTBIG59752.2023.10456198

Rasheed, A., San, O., & Kvamsdal, T. (2020). Digital twin: Values, challenges and future directions. *Simulation Modelling Practice and Theory, 103*, 101–114. DOI: 10.1016/j.simpat.2020.101–114

Rastogi, D., Johri, P., Donelli, M., Agarwal, T., Tiwari, S., & Singh, P. (2025). XAI-BT-EdgeNet: Explainable edge-aware deep learning with squeeze-and-excitation for brain tumor detection and prediction. *Frontiers in Artificial Intelligence, 8*, 1676524. DOI: 10.3389/frai.2025.1676524

Ratta, P., Kaur, A., Sharma, S., Shabaz, M., & Dhiman, G. (2021). Application of Blockchain and Internet of Things in healthcare and medical sector: Applications, challenges, and future perspectives. *Journal of Food Quality, 2021*, 1–20. DOI: 10.1155/2021/7608296

Ravikumar, A. Olimbaevich, I. R., Mashkhura, S., & Musayeva, S. (2025). Transforming Healthcare with Large Language Models and AI agents. In Advances in Computational Intelligence and Robotics (pp. 51–82). IGI Global Scientific Publishing. DOI: 10.4018/979-8-3373-2008-3.ch003

Ravikumar, A. S., Atamuratova, Z., Ashirova, A., Jurayev, K., & Hayitova, M. (2025). Comprehensive evaluation of AI-driven systems in modern hospital environments. In Advances in Computational Intelligence and Robotics (pp. 61–88). IGI Global Scientific Publishing. DOI: 10.4018/979-8-3373-2787-7.ch003

Ravikumar, A. S., Saparbaevich, B. R., Kumar A., S., Jumaniyozova, M., & Toshova, S. (2025). AI-enhanced clinical decision-making through a collaborative approach. In Advances in Computational Intelligence and Robotics (pp. 249–280). IGI Global Scientific Publishing. DOI: 10.4018/979-8-3373-3311-3.ch010

Ravikumar, A. Sapayev, V., Atamuratova, Z., Kholboyev, N., & Sindhuja. (2025). The decentralized diagnostics revolution using federated Learning in medical imaging and beyond. In Advances in Computational Intelligence and Robotics (pp. 353–388). IGI Global Scientific Publishing. DOI: 10.4018/979-8-3373-3306-9.ch013

Ravikumar, R. S., Manujakshi, Aarthi, S., Urazbaeva, Y., & Tamilselvi, S. (2025). Navigating data privacy, security, and regulatory challenges in healthcare AI ensuring fairness, bias mitigation, interpretability, and trust. In Transformative Role of Transformer Models in Healthcare (pp. 25–54). IGI Global Scientific Publishing. DOI: 10.4018/979-8-3373-2038-0.ch002

Ravikumar, R. N., & Aarthi, S. (2025). AI-powered synergistic robotics and IoT ecosystems for predictive and preventive healthcare. In *Robotics and IoT Synergy in Next-Generation Healthcare* (pp. 1–32). IGI Global Scientific Publishing., DOI: 10.4018/979-8-3373-5447-7.ch001

Ravikumar, R. N., Aarthi, S., Kurbanova, S., Polvanov, S., Matchanova, B., & Sathya, K. (2025). Hybrid metaheuristic optimization for neural networks in biomedical imaging. In *Metaheuristic Algorithms and Optimizing Neural Networks for Biomedical Image Processing* (pp. 197–234). IGI Global Scientific Publishing., DOI: 10.4018/979-8-3373-0523-3.ch008

Razdan, S., & Sharma, S. (2022). Internet of medical things (IoMT): Overview, emerging technologies, and case studies. *IETE Technical Review*, *39*(4), 775–788. DOI: 10.1080/02564602.2021.1927863

Rehman, A., Abbas, S., Khan, M. A., Ghazal, T. M., Adnan, K. M., & Mosavi, A. (2022). A secure healthcare 5.0 system based on blockchain technology entangled with federated learning technique. *Computers in Biology and Medicine*, *150*(106019), 106019. DOI: 10.1016/j.compbiomed.2022.106019

Reyna, A., Martín, C., Chen, J., Soler, E., & Díaz, M. (2018). On blockchain and its integration with IoT. *Future Generation Computer Systems*, *88*, 173–190. DOI: 10.1016/j.future.2018.05.046

Riascos, R., Ostrosi, E., Sagot, J.-C., & Stjepandić, J. (2022). Conceptual approach for a Digital Twin of medical devices. In *Advances in Transdisciplinary Engineering*. IOS Press., DOI: 10.3233/ATDE220661

Ricci, A., Croatti, A., Mariani, S., Montagna, S., & Picone, M. (2022). Web of Digital Twins. *ACM Transactions on Internet Technology*, *22*(4), 1–30. DOI: 10.1145/3507909

Roehrs, A., Da Costa, C. A., da Rosa Righi, R., & De Oliveira, K. S. F. (2017). Personal health records: A systematic literature review. *Journal of Medical Internet Research*, *19*(1), e5876. DOI: 10.2196/jmir.5876 PMID: 28062391

Roopa, M. S. (2023). A systematic review: Digital twin in healthcare. *International Journal for Research in Applied Science and Engineering Technology*, *11*(5), 4818–4825.

Roumeliotis, C., Dasygenis, M., Lazaridis, V., & Dossis, M. (2024). Blockchain and digital twins in smart industry 4.0: The use case of supply chain-a review of integration techniques and applications. *Designs*, *8*(6), 105. DOI: 10.3390/designs8060105

Roy, P., Sherazi, S. H. T., Delda, M. J. M., Maqsood, M., & Ahmad, M. (2025). Secure data sharing in healthcare. In *Advances in Healthcare Information Systems and Administration* (pp. 255–286). IGI Global., DOI: 10.4018/979-8-3693-4199-5.ch011

Ruba, M., Ponkarthika, M., Parameshwari, V., Girinath, V. P., Soundarya, B., Janani, M., & Santhini, C. (2025, February). Enhancing underwater tunnel safety through smart inspection: An ROV-based system with AI-powered crack detection using Canny edge detection. In Proceedings of the 2025 3rd International Conference on Intelligent Systems, Advanced Computing and Communication (ISACC) (pp. 1067–1072). IEEE. https://doi.org/DOI: 10.1109/ISACC.2025

Ruba, M., Preetha, D. S., Ponkarthika, M., Gomathi, V., Sudha, E., & Pratheeba, C. (2026c). Smart Pedagogies and Intelligent Campuses: Reimagining Higher Education in the Digital Age. In Harnessing Geospatial Information Systems for Sustainable Economic and Regional Development (pp. 29-54). IGI Global Scientific Publishing.

Ruba, M., Ashwin Prabhu, G., Deka, J., Kavitha, D., Sathiya, S., & Pavithra, S. (2026a). Empowering learners and educators: The transformative role of conversational AI in personalized education and student support. In Assayed, S. (Ed.), *Enhancing student support and learning through conversational AI* (pp. 163–190). IGI Global Scientific Publishing., DOI: 10.4018/979-8-3373-3316-8.ch007

Ruba, M., Ashwin Prabhu, G., Robinson Joel, M., Vishnu Priya, K., Dharshani, L., & Dharani, R. (2026b). Integrating emerging technologies for organizational agility: An interdisciplinary approach to digital transformation. In Roache, D. (Ed.), *High performance leadership for organizational excellence: Innovation, technology, and resilience* (pp. 63–92). IGI Global Scientific Publishing., DOI: 10.4018/979-8-3373-6207-6.ch003

Ruba, M., Girinath, V. P., Ponkarthika, M., Santhini, C., Sakthi Priya, V., & Hemalatha, R. (2023, December). Design and implementation of smart internet-based real-time control of rover with artificial intelligence. In *2023 International Conference on Energy, Materials and Communication Engineering (ICEMCE)* (pp. 1–5). IEEE. https://doi.org/DOI: 10.1109/ICEMCE2023

Sadath, L., Mehrotra, D., & Kumar, A. (2024). Scalability performance analysis of blockchain using hierarchical model in healthcare. *Blockchain in Healthcare Today*, *7*, 10–30953. DOI: 10.30953/bhty.v7.295 PMID: 38715761

Saeed, H., Malik, H., Bashir, U., Ahmad, A., Riaz, S., Ilyas, M., Bukhari, W. A., & Khan, M. I. A. (2022). Blockchain technology in healthcare: A systematic review. *PLoS One*, *17*(4), e0266462. DOI: 10.1371/journal.pone.0266462 PMID: 35404955

Šafran, V., Arioz, U., Sallauka, R., & Mlakar, I. (2025). A scalable and secured HL7 FHIR healthcare platform: Architecture, load testing, and preliminary findings. *International Journal of Education and Information Technologies*, *19*(13), 128–137. DOI: 10.46300/9109.2025.19.13

Saliha, C. B., & Ferhati, K. (2025). Real-world applications of digital twin technology in performance management: Lessons from global healthcare case studies. *International Journal of Innovative Technologies in Social Science*, *1*(45). Advance online publication. DOI: 10.31435/ijitss.1(45).2025.3197

Salunkhe, V., Thumati, P. R. R., Kanchi, P., Chhapola, A., & Goel, O. (2024). EHR Interoperability Challenges Leveraging HL7 FHIR for Seamless Data Exchange in Healthcare. *Darpan International Research Analysis*, *12*(3), 403–419. DOI: 10.36676/dira.v12.i3.98

Sarani Rad, F., Hendawi, R., Yang, X., & Li, J. (2024). Personalized diabetes management with digital twins: A patient-centric knowledge graph approach. *Journal of Personalized Medicine*, *14*(4), 359. DOI: 10.3390/jpm14040359 PMID: 38672986

Saranya, R., & Murugan, A. (2023). A systematic review of enabling blockchain in healthcare system: Analysis, current status, challenges and future direction. *Materials Today: Proceedings*, *80*, 3010–3015. DOI: 10.1016/j.matpr.2021.07.105

Saratkar, S. Y., Langote, M., Kumar, P., Gote, P., Weerarathna, I. N., & Mishra, G. V. (2025). Digital twin for personalized medicine development. *Frontiers in Digital Health*, *7*, 1583466. DOI: 10.3389/fdgth.2025.1583466 PMID: 40851640

Sasitharasarma, S., Alani, N. H. S., & Wisker, Z. L. (2025). Is the healthcare industry ready for Digital Twins? Examining the opportunities and challenges. *Future Internet*, *17*(9), 386. DOI: 10.3390/fi17090386

Satamraju, K. P., & B, M. (2020). Proof of concept of scalable integration of internet of things and blockchain in healthcare. *Sensors (Basel)*, *20*(5), 1389. DOI: 10.3390/s20051389 PMID: 32138380

Saudi Data & AI Authority. (2021). *Personal Data Protection Law*. PDPL.

Saudi Food & Drug Authority. (2022). Digital health and telemedicine regulatory framework.

Saudi Ministry of Health. (2022). National Health Information Exchange (NPHIES) framework.

Saudi Ministry of Health. (2022). National Platform for Health Information Exchange Services (NPHIES) framework.

Saudi Ministry of Health. (2022). NPHIES and national digital health transformation framework.

Schleich, B., Anwer, N., Mathieu, L., & Wartzack, S. (2017). Shaping the digital twin for design and production engineering. *CIRP Annals*, *66*(1), 141–144. DOI: 10.1016/j.cirp.2017.04.040

Sel, K., Osman, D., Zare, F., Masoumi Shahrbabak, S., Brattain, L., Hahn, J. O., & Jafari, R. (2024). Building digital twins for cardiovascular health: From principles to clinical impact. *Journal of the American Heart Association*, *13*(19), e031981. PMID: 39087582

Shahid, J., Ahmad, R., Kiani, A. K., Ahmad, T., Saeed, S., & Almuhaideb, A. M. (2022). Data protection and privacy of the Internet of Healthcare Things (IoHTs). *Applied Sciences (Basel, Switzerland)*, *12*(4), 1927. DOI: 10.3390/app12041927

Shanmugaraja, T., Ruba, M., Priya, V. S., Venkatesh, T., Supriya, M., & Nallamuthu, M. (2023, September). ECG noise elimination using an FPGA version of a modified error normalized LMS adaptive filter. In AIP Conference Proceedings (Vol. 2764, No. 1, p. 060033). AIP Publishing LLC. DOI: 10.1063/5.0144367

Sharma, A., Kaur, S., & Singh, M. (2021). A comprehensive review on blockchain and Internet of Things in healthcare. *Transactions on Emerging Telecommunications Technologies*, *32*(10), e4333. DOI: 10.1002/ett.4333

Sharma, A., Kaur, S., & Singh, M. (2024). A secure blockchain framework for the internet of medical things. *Transactions on Emerging Telecommunications Technologies*, *35*(1), e4917. Advance online publication. DOI: 10.1002/ett.4917

Sharma, M., & Joshi, S. (2021). Barriers to blockchain adoption in health-care industry: An Indian perspective. *Journal of Global Operations and Strategic Sourcing*, *14*(1), 134–169. DOI: 10.1108/JGOSS-06-2020-0026

Sharma, S., Sharma, A., Fuloria, N. K., & Fuloria, S. (2025). Blockchain For Healthcare. *Data Management.*

Shi, W., Cao, J., Zhang, Q., Li, Y., & Xu, L. (2016). Edge computing: Vision and challenges. *IEEE Internet of Things Journal*, *3*(5), 637–646. DOI: 10.1109/JIOT.2016.2579198

Shuvo, S. A., Tabassum, M., Tafannum, N., & Chadni, S. (2025). Machine Learning in Business Intelligence: From Data Mining To Strategic Insights In MIS. *Review of Applied Science and Technology*, *4*(02), 339–369. DOI: 10.63125/drb8py41

Singh, A. P., Pradhan, N. R., Luhach, A. K., Agnihotri, S., Jhanjhi, N. Z., Verma, S., Kavita, , Ghosh, U., & Roy, D. S. (2020). A novel patient-centric architectural framework for blockchain-enabled healthcare applications. *IEEE Transactions on Industrial Informatics*, *17*(8), 5779–5789. DOI: 10.1109/TII.2020.3037889

Singh, M., Fuenmayor, E., Hinchy, E., Qiao, Y., Murray, N., & Devine, D. (2021). Digital Twin: Origin to future. *Applied System Innovation*, *4*(2), 36. DOI: 10.3390/asi4020036

Singh, S. S., Kumar, S., Ahuja, R., & Barua, J. (2025). Fusion of quantum computing and explainable AI: A comprehensive survey on transformative healthcare solutions. *Information Fusion*, *122*, 103217. DOI: 10.1016/j.inffus.2025.103217

Singh, S., Sharma, S. K., Mehrotra, P., Bhatt, P., & Kaurav, M. (2022). Blockchain technology for efficient data management in healthcare system: Opportunity, chal lenges and future perspectives. *Materials Today: Proceedings*, *62*, 5042–5046. DOI: 10.1016/j.matpr.2022.04.998

Singla, D., Kumar, S., Gulzar, Y., Mir, M. S., Gupta, D., Jaziri, W., Sassi, N., & Arora, S. (2024). Designing and implementing a resilient immutability mechanism for enhanced supply chain management in E-healthcare systems. *Frontiers in Sustainable Cities*, *6*, 1403809. Advance online publication. DOI: 10.3389/frsc.2024.1403809

Siyal, A. A., Junejo, A. Z., Zawish, M., Ahmed, K., Khalil, A., & Soursou, G. (2019). Applications of blockchain technology in medicine and healthcare: Challenges and future perspectives. *Cryptography*, *3*(1), 3. DOI: 10.3390/cryptography3010003

SNOMED International. (2022). SNOMED CT global clinical terminology standards.

Sriram, V., Conard, A. M., Rosenberg, I., Kim, D., Saponas, T. S., & Hall, A. K. (2025). Addressing biomedical data challenges and opportunities to inform a large-scale data lifecycle for enhanced data sharing, interoperability, analysis, and collaboration across stakeholders. *Scientific Reports*, *15*(1), 6291. DOI: 10.1038/s41598-025-90453-x PMID: 39984563

tefănigă, S. A., Cordo , A. A., Ivascu, T., Feier, C. V. I., Muntean, C., Stupinean, C. V., & Bolboacă, S. D. (2024). Advancing precision oncology with digital and virtual twins: A scoping review. *Cancers (Basel)*, *16*(22), 3817. PMID: 39594772

Subashini, R.. (2024). Digital Twin - An Innovative Strategy in Healthcare Transformation: An Extensive Review. *Journal of Research in Applied Sciences*.

Suleiman, R., Maradapu Vera Venkata Sai, A., Yu, W., & Wang, C. (2025). Blockchain for Security in Digital Twins. *Future Internet*, *17*(9), 385. DOI: 10.3390/fi17090385

Sun, T., He, X., & Li, Z. (2023). Digital twin in healthcare: Recent updates and challenges. *Digital Health*, *9*, 20552076221149652. DOI: 10.1177/20552076221149651 PMID: 36636729

Sun, T., He, X., Song, X., Shu, L., & Li, Z. (2022). The digital twin in medicine: A key to the future of healthcare? *Frontiers in Medicine*, *9*, 907066. DOI: 10.3389/fmed.2022.907066 PMID: 35911407

Susilo, M. E., Li, C.-C., Gadkar, K., Hernandez, G., Huw, L.-Y., Jin, J. Y., Yin, S., Wei, M. C., Ramanujan, S., & Hosseini, I. (2023). Systems-based digital twins to help characterize clinical dose-response and propose predictive biomarkers in a Phase I study of bispecific antibody, mosunetuzumab, in NHL. *Clinical and Translational Science*, *16*(7), 1134–1148. DOI: 10.1111/cts.13501 PMID: 36908269

Tahar, K., Martin, T., Mou, Y., Verbuecheln, R., Graessner, H., & Krefting, D. (2023). Rare Diseases in hospital information systems-an interoperable methodology for distributed data quality assessments. Methods of Information in Medicine, 62(3–04), 71–89. DOI: 10.1055/a-2006-1018

Taherdoost, H. (2023). Blockchain and healthcare: A critical analysis of progress and challenges in the last five years. *Blockchains*, *1*(2), 73–89. DOI: 10.3390/blockchains1020006

Taherdoost, H. (2023). Privacy and security of blockchain in healthcare: Applications, challenges, and future perspectives. *Sci*, *5*(4), 41. DOI: 10.3390/sci5040041

Taherdoost, H. (2023). The role of blockchain in medical data sharing. *Cryptography*, *7*(3), 36. DOI: 10.3390/cryptography7030036

Taherdoost, H. (2025). Blockchain for security and privacy in the smart healthcare. In *Sensor Networks for Smart Hospitals* (pp. 411–433). Elsevier. DOI: 10.1016/B978-0-443-36370-2.00019-0

Tahir, N. U. A., Rashid, U., Hadi, H. J., Ahmad, N., Cao, Y., Alshara, M. A., & Javed, Y. (2024). Blockchain-based healthcare records management framework: Enhancing security, privacy, and interoperability. *Technologies*, *12*(9), 168. DOI: 10.3390/technologies12090168

Tao, F., Qi, Q., Liu, A., & Kusiak, A. (2018). Data-driven smart manufacturing. *Journal of Manufacturing Systems*, *48*, 157–169. DOI: 10.1016/j.jmsy.2018.01.006

Tao, F., Zhang, H., Liu, A., & Nee, A. Y. C. (2019). Digital twin in industry: State-of-the-art. *IEEE Transactions on Industrial Informatics, 15*(4), 2405–2415. DOI: 10.1109/TII.2018.2873186

Tao, F., Zhang, M., Liu, Y., & Nee, A. Y. C. (2018). *Digital twin driven smart manufacturing*. Academic Press.

Taralunga, D. D., & Florea, B. C. (2021). A blockchain-enabled framework for mHealth systems. *Sensors (Basel), 21*(8), 2828. DOI: 10.3390/s21082828 PMID: 33923842

Thangaraj, P. M., Benson, S. H., Oikonomou, E. K., Asselbergs, F. W., & Khera, R. (2024). Cardiovascular care with digital twin technology in the era of generative artificial intelligence. *European Heart Journal, 45*(45), 4808–4821. DOI: 10.1093/eurheartj/ehae619 PMID: 39322420

Thantharate, P., & Thantharate, A. (2023). ZeroTrustBlock: Enhancing security, privacy, and interoperability of sensitive data through ZeroTrust permissioned blockchain. *Big Data and Cognitive Computing, 7*(4), 165. DOI: 10.3390/bdcc7040165

The Lancet Digital Health. (2023). Representation and fairness in medical AI datasets. The Lancet Digital Health.

Ting, D. S. W., Carin, L., Dzau, V., & Wong, T. Y. (2020). Digital technology and COVID-19. *Nature Medicine, 26*(4), 459–461. DOI: 10.1038/s41591-020-0824-5 PMID: 32284618

Tiwari, K., & Kumar, S. (2025). Accelerating healthcare data access: A blockchain and decentralized indexing approach. *Concurrency and Computation, 37*(15–17), e70172. Advance online publication. DOI: 10.1002/cpe.70172

Tobin, A., & Reed, D. (2017). *The inevitable rise of self-sovereign identity*. Sovrin Foundation.

Topol, E. J. (2019). High-performance medicine: The convergence of human and artificial intelligence. *Nature Medicine, 25*(1), 44–56. DOI: 10.1038/s41591-018-0300-7 PMID: 30617339

Tseng, J. H., Liao, Y. C., Chong, B., & Liao, S. W. (2018). Governance on the drug supply chain via blockchain technology. *International Journal of Environmental Research and Public Health, 15*(6), 1055. DOI: 10.3390/ijerph15061055 PMID: 29882861

Tuli, S., Tuli, S., Wander, G., Wander, P., Gill, S. S., Dustdar, S., Sakellariou, R., & Rana, O. (2020). Next generation technologies for smart healthcare: Challenges, vision, model, trends and future directions. *Internet Technology Letters*, *3*(2), e145. DOI: 10.1002/itl2.145

Turab, M., & Jamil, S. (2023). A comprehensive survey of digital twins in healthcare in the era of metaverse. *BioMedInformatics*, *3*(3), 563–584. DOI: 10.3390/biomedinformatics3030039

Tyagi, A. K. (2024). Blockchain-enabled Internet of Things (IoTs) platforms for IoT-based healthcare and biomedical sectors. In Artificial intelligence-enabled blockchain technology and digital twin for smart hospitals (Chap. 10). Wiley Scrivener. https://doi.org/DOI: 10.1002/9781394287420.ch10

Tyagi, A. K., & Seranmadevi, R. (2024). Blockchain for Enhancing Security and Privacy in the Smart Healthcare. *Digital Twin and Blockchain for Smart Cities*, 343-370.

Tyagi, A. K. (2023). Decentralized everything: A practical use of blockchain technology in future applications. In *Distributed computing to blockchain: Architecture, technology, and applications* (pp. 19–38). Elsevier., DOI: 10.1016/B978-0-323-96146-2.00010-3

Tyagi, A. K. (2024). Dew computing: State of the art, opportunities, and research challenges. In *Machine learning algorithms using Scikit and TensorFlow environments*. IGI Global., DOI: 10.4018/978-1-6684-8531-6.ch017

Tyagi, A. K. (2024). Sensors and digital twin application in healthcare facilities management. In *Artificial intelligence-enabled blockchain technology and digital twin for smart hospitals*. Wiley Scrivener., DOI: 10.1002/9781394287420.ch19

Tyagi, A. K., Balogun, B. F., & Tiwari, S. (2025). Digital twin for blockchain-enabled intelligent transportation systems in smart cities. In Tyagi, A. K., & Tiwari, S. (Eds.), *Human-centric integration of 6G-enabled technologies for modern society*. Academic Press., DOI: 10.1016/B978-0-443-27434-3.00006-4

Tyagi, A. K., Tripathi, K., Tiwari, S., & Kaushik, S. (2025). An efficient technique for privacy preservation, trusted and secure patient-centric services in smart healthcare. In *Proceedings of the 6th International Conference on Recent Trends in Communication & Intelligent Systems (ICRTCIS 2025)* (pp. 31–47).DOI: https://doi.org/DOI: 10.1049/icp.2025.2731

Tyagi, A., Kumari, S., & Tiwari, S. (2024). Internet of Things for smart healthcare: A survey. In Sharma, A. K., Chanderwal, N., Tyagi, S., & Upadhyay, P. (Eds.), *Future of AI in medical imaging*. IGI Global., DOI: 10.4018/979-8-3693-2359-5.ch002

U.S. Department of Health & Human Services. (2013). Summary of the HIPAA privacy rule.

U.S. Food & Drug Administration. (2023). Artificial intelligence/machine learning (AI/ML)-based software as a medical device action plan.

Vallée, A. (2023). Digital twin for healthcare systems. *Frontiers in Digital Health*, *5*, 1253050. DOI: 10.3389/fdgth.2023.1253050

van der Valk, H., Hunker, J., Rabe, M., & Otto, B. (2020, December). Digital twins in simulative applications: A taxonomy. In *2020 Winter Simulation Conference (WSC)* (pp. 2695-2706). IEEE. DOI: 10.1109/WSC48552.2020.9384051

Varriale, V., Michelino, F., & Godinho-Filho, M. (2026). The standalone and integrated value of digital twins and ancillary emerging technologies for enhancing supply chain performance. *Production Planning and Control*, •••, 1–29. DOI: 10.1080/09537287.2025.2608686

Vasiliu-Feltes, I., Mylrea, M., Zhang, C. Y., Wood, T.-C., & Thornley, B. (2023). Impact of blockchain-Digital Twin technology on precision health, pharmaceutical industry, and life sciences: Conference proceedings, Conv2X 2023. *Blockchain in Healthcare Today*, *6*(2). Advance online publication. DOI: 10.30953/bhty.v6.281 PMID: 38187956

Vassil, K. (2016). Estonian e-government ecosystem: Foundation, applications, outcomes.

Vazirani, A. A., O'Donoghue, O., Brindley, D., & Meinert, E. (2020). Blockchain vehicles for efficient Medical Record management. *NPJ Digital Medicine*, *3*(1), 1. DOI: 10.1038/s41746-019-0211-0 PMID: 31934645

Veeramachaneni, V. (2025). Edge computing: Architecture, applications, and future challenges in a decentralized era. *Recent Trends in Computer Graphics and Multimedia Technology*, *7*(1), 8–23. DOI: 10.5281/zenodo.14166793

Velmovitsky, P. E., Bublitz, F. M., Fadrique, L. X., & Morita, P. P. (2021). Blockchain applications in health care and public health: Increased transparency. *JMIR Medical Informatics*, *9*(6), e20713. DOI: 10.2196/20713 PMID: 34100768

Viceconti, A., Geri, T., De Luca, S., Maselli, F., Rossettini, G., Sulli, A., Schenone, A., & Testa, M. (2021). Neuropathic pain and symptoms of potential small-fiber neuropathy in fibromyalgic patients: A national on-line survey. *Joint, Bone, Spine, 88*(4), 105153. DOI: 10.1016/j.jbspin.2021.105153 PMID: 33561533

Villarreal, E. R. D., García-Alonso, J., Moguel, E., & Alegría, J. A. H. (2023). Blockchain for healthcare management systems: A survey on interoperability and security. *IEEE Access : Practical Innovations, Open Solutions, 11*, 5629–5652. DOI: 10.1109/ACCESS.2023.3236505

Vision 2030. (2016). Kingdom of Saudi Arabia Vision 2030.

Wahed, M. A. (2024, November). Real-Time Intrusion Detection and Traffic Analysis Using AI Techniques in IoT Infrastructure. In *2024 1st International Conference on Emerging Technologies for Dependable Internet of Things (ICETI)* (pp. 1-6). IEEE. DOI: 10.1109/ICETI63946.2024.10777213

Wahed, M. A., Alzoubi, A. E., Wahed, S. A., & Kursheva, J. (2025, April). AI-Driven Approach to Predict High-Risk Newborns to Reduce NICU Admission Overcrowding. In *2025 1st International Conference on Computational Intelligence Approaches and Applications (ICCIAA)* (pp. 1-6). IEEE. DOI: 10.1109/ICCIAA65327.2025.11013654

Wahed, M. A., Halasa, A., & Alzboon, M. S. (2025, August). Enhancing Real-Time Detection of Distributed Denial of Service (DDoS) Attacks on IoT Infrastructure. In *2025 5th International Conference on Emerging Smart Technologies and Applications (eSmarTA)* (pp. 1-6). IEEE.

Wahed, M. A., Wahed, S. A., & Alzoubi, A. E. (2025). AI-Driven Cybersecurity for Telemedicine: Enhancing Protection Through Autonomous Defense Systems. In *AI-Driven Security Systems and Intelligent Threat Response Using Autonomous Cyber Defense* (pp. 375-406). IGI Global Scientific Publishing.

Wahed, M. A., & Wahed, S. A. (2025). Autonomous Defense Systems for Surgical Robots Ensuring Cybersecurity in Robotic-Assisted Surgery. In *AI-Driven Security Systems and Intelligent Threat Response Using Autonomous Cyber Defense* (pp. 407–438). IGI Global Scientific Publishing. DOI: 10.4018/979-8-3373-0954-5.ch014

Wahed, S. A. W. A., Shdefat, R. S., & Wahed, M. A. (2025). A Machine Learning Model for Diagnosis and Differentiation of Schizophrenia, Bipolar Disorder and Borderline Personality Disorder. *LatIA, 3*, 133–133. DOI: 10.62486/latia2025133

Wahed, S. A., & Wahed, M. A. (2025). AI-Driven Digital Well-being: Developing Machine Learning Model to Predict and Mitigate Internet Addiction. *LatIA, 3*(3), 73. DOI: 10.62486/latia202573

Wang, D. H. (2020). IoT based Clinical Sensor Data Management and Transfer using Blockchain Technology. *Journal of ISMAC*, *2*(3), 154–159. DOI: 10.36548/jismac.2020.3.003

Wang, E., Tayebi, P., & Song, Y.-T. (2023). Cloud-based digital twins' storage in emergency healthcare. *International Journal of Networked and Distributed Computing*, *11*(2), 75–87. DOI: 10.1007/s44227-023-00011-y

Wang, S., Zhang, Y., & Zhang, Y. (2018). A blockchain-based framework for data sharing with fine-grained access control in decentralized storage systems. *IEEE Access : Practical Innovations, Open Solutions*, *6*, 38437–38450. DOI: 10.1109/ACCESS.2018.2851611

Wang, X. V., Kemény, Z., Váncza, J., & Wang, L. (2017). Human–robot collaborative assembly in cyber-physical production: Classification framework and implementation. *CIRP Annals*, *66*(1), 5–8. DOI: 10.1016/j.cirp.2017.04.101

Wang, Y., Su, Z., Guo, S., Dai, M., Luan, T. H., & Liu, Y. (2023). A survey on digital twins: Architecture, enabling technologies, security and privacy, and future prospects. *IEEE Internet of Things Journal*, *10*(17), 14965–14987. DOI: 10.1109/JIOT.2023.3263909

Weerarathna, I. N., Kumar, P., Verma, P., Raymond, D., Luharia, A., & Mishra, G. (2024, November). Leveraging digital twin technology to combat cardiovascular disease: A comprehensive review. In 2024 2nd DMIHER International Conference on Artificial Intelligence in Healthcare, Education and Industry (IDICAIEI) (pp. 1-6). IEEE.

Wenhua, Z., Qamar, F., Abdali, T. A. N., Hassan, R., Jafri, S. T. A., & Nguyen, Q. N. (2023). Blockchain technology: Security issues, healthcare applications, challenges and future trends. *Electronics (Basel)*, *12*(3), 546. DOI: 10.3390/electronics12030546

White House Office of Science and Technology Policy. (2022). Blueprint for an AI Bill of Rights.

World Bank. (2022). World development indicators: Population data.

World Health Organization (WHO). (2020). *Strengthening the health systems response to COVID-19*. WHO Regional Office for Europe.

World Health Organization. (2019). *International classification of diseases* (11th ed.).

World Health Organization. (2021). *Global strategy on digital health 2020–2025*. WHO.

Wu, D., Xu, X., & Wang, L. (2020). Digital twin-based smart logistics management. *IEEE Access : Practical Innovations, Open Solutions*, *8*, 110807–110817. DOI: 10.1109/ACCESS.2020.3000687

Xue, J., Li, Z., & Zhang, S. (2025). Multi-resource constrained elective surgical scheduling with Nash equilibrium toward smart hospitals. *Scientific Reports*, *15*(1), 3946. DOI: 10.1038/s41598-025-87867-y PMID: 39890977

Xu, M., Chen, X., & Kou, G. (2019). A systematic review of blockchain. *Financial Innovation*, *5*(1), 1–14. DOI: 10.1186/s40854-019-0147-z

Yakubu, B. M., Ali, S. M., Khan, M. I., & Bhattarakosol, P. (2024). PatCen: A blockchain-based patient-centric mechanism for the granular access control of infectious disease-related test records. *PLoS One*, *19*(9), e0310407. DOI: 10.1371/journal.pone.0310407

Yaqoob, I., Salah, K., Jayaraman, R., & Al-Hammadi, Y. (2022). Blockchain for healthcare data management: Opportunities, challenges, and future recommendations. *Neural Computing & Applications*, *34*(14), 11475–11490. DOI: 10.1007/s00521-020-05519-w

Yaqoob, I., Salah, K., Uddin, M., Jayaraman, R., Omar, M., & Imran, M. (2020). Blockchain for digital twins: Recent advances and future research challenges. *IEEE Network*, *34*(5), 290–298. DOI: 10.1109/MNET.001.1900661

Yaqoob, M. M., Alsulami, M., Khan, M. A., Alsadie, D., Saudagar, A. K. J., AlKhathami, M., & Khattak, U. F. (2023). Symmetry in privacy-based healthcare: A review of skin cancer detection and classification using federated learning. *Symmetry*, *15*(7), 1369. DOI: 10.3390/sym15071369

Yaqoob, S., Khan, M. M., Talib, R., Butt, A. D., Saleem, S., Arif, F., & Nadeem, A. (2019). Use of blockchain in healthcare: A systematic literature review. *International Journal of Advanced Computer Science and Applications*, *10*(5). Advance online publication. DOI: 10.14569/IJACSA.2019.0100581

Zaabar, B., Cheikhrouhou, O., Jamil, F., Ammi, M., & Abid, M. (2021). HealthBlock: A secure blockchain-based healthcare data management system. *Computer Networks*, *200*, 108500. DOI: 10.1016/j.comnet.2021.108500

Zhang, P., White, J., Schmidt, D. C., & Lenz, G. (2017, October). Design of blockchain-based apps using familiar software patterns to address interoperability challenges in healthcare. In Proceedings of the PLoP-24th Conference on Pattern Languages of Programs, Vancouver, BC, Canada (pp. 22-25). https://doi.org/ DOI: 10.5555/3290281.3290304

Zhang, Z. (2023). Digital twin: Application and prospect. Theoretical and Natural Science - the Open Access Proceedings Series for Conferences, 12(1), 220–226. DOI: 10.54254/2753-8818/12/20230477

Zhang, K., Zhou, H. Y., Baptista-Hon, D. T., Gao, Y., Liu, X., Oermann, E., Xu, S., Jin, S., Zhang, J., Sun, Z., Yin, Y., Razmi, R. M., Loupy, A., Beck, S., Qu, J., & Wu, J. (2024). Concepts and applications of digital twins in healthcare and medicine. *Patterns (New York, N.Y.)*, *5*(8), 101028. DOI: 10.1016/j.patter.2024.101028 PMID: 39233690

Zhang, P., Kelley, A., Schmidt, D. C., & White, J. (2023). Design pattern recommendations for building decentralized healthcare applications. *Frontiers in Blockchain*, *6*(1006058), 1006058. Advance online publication. DOI: 10.3389/fbloc.2023.1006058

Zhang, P., Schmidt, D. C., White, J., & Lenz, G. (2018). Blockchain technology use cases in healthcare. [). Elsevier.]. *Advances in Computers*, *111*, 1–41. DOI: 10.1016/bs.adcom.2018.03.006

Zhang, P., White, J., Schmidt, D. C., Lenz, G., & Rosenbloom, S. T. (2018). FHIRChain: Applying blockchain to securely and scalably share clinical data. *Computational and Structural Biotechnology Journal*, *16*, 267–278. DOI: 10.1016/j.csbj.2018.07.004

Zhang, Y. F., Gou, L., Tian, Y., Li, T. C., Zhang, M., & Li, J. S. (2016). Design and development of a sharable clinical decision support system based on a semantic web service framework. *Journal of Medical Systems*, *40*(5), 118. DOI: 10.1007/s10916-016-0472-y PMID: 27002818

Zhan, H., Hwang, B., & Krishnankutty, P. (2024). Embracing digital transformation for sustainable development: Barriers to adopting digital twin in asset management within Singapore's energy and chemicals industry. *Sustainable Development (Bradford)*, *33*(2), 2864–2887. DOI: 10.1002/sd.3270

Zhao, T., Song, C., Yu, J., Xing, L., Xu, F., Li, W., & Wang, Z. (2025). Leveraging Immersive Digital Twins and AI-Driven Decision Support Systems for Sustainable Water Reserves Management: A Conceptual Framework. *Sustainability (Basel)*, *17*(8), 3754. DOI: 10.3390/su17083754

Zheng, X., Sun, S., Mukkamala, R. R., Vatrapu, R., & Ordieres-Meré, J. (2019). Accelerating health data sharing: A solution based on the Internet of Things and distributed ledger technologies. *Journal of Medical Internet Research*, *21*(6), e13583. DOI: 10.2196/13583 PMID: 31172963

Zheng, Z., Xie, S., Dai, H. N., Chen, X., & Wang, H. (2018). Blockchain challenges and opportunities: A survey. *International Journal of Web and Grid Services, 14*(4), 352–375. DOI: 10.1504/IJWGS.2018.095647

Zhuang, Y., Shyu, C. R., Hong, S., Li, P., & Zhang, L. (2023). Self-sovereign identity empowered non-fungible patient tokenization for health information exchange using blockchain technology. *Computers in Biology and Medicine, 157*, 106778. DOI: 10.1016/j.compbiomed.2023.106778 PMID: 36934533

Ziegler, V., Schneider, P., Viswanathan, H., Montag, M., Kanugovi, S., & Rezaki, A. (2021). Security and trust in the 6G era. *IEEE Access : Practical Innovations, Open Solutions, 9*, 142314–142327. DOI: 10.1109/ACCESS.2021.3120143

Ziminski, T. B., Demurjian, S. A., Sanzi, E., Baihan, M. S., & Agresta, T. (2020). An Architectural Solution for Health Information Exchange. In *Virtual and Mobile Healthcare* (pp. 283–327). IGI Global., DOI: 10.4018/978-1-5225-9863-3.ch014

About the Contributors

Ben Othman Soufiene is an Assistant Professor of computer science at the Applied College, King Faisal University, Saudi Arabia. He received his Ph.D. degree in computer science from Manouba University in 2016 for his dissertation on "Secure data aggregation in wireless sensor networks. He also holds M.S. degrees from the Monastir University in 2012. My research interests focus on the Internet of Medical Things, Wireless Body Sensor Networks, Wireless Networks, Artificial Intelligence, Machine Learning and Big Data. Dr. Ben Othman has published more than 160 papers at reputed international journals, conferences, and book chapters. He is an Editorial Board Member in the different Journals and Conferences. He serves as an associate editor/academic editor for international journals including IEEE Access, IEEE Sensors, IEEE Internet of Things, Elsevier, Springer, Taylor & Francis, IGI, IET, Telecommunication Computing Electronics and Control, and Wiley. Dr. Ben Othman is a Technical Program Committee Member for more than a dozen of international conferences.

***

Rahmath Nisha A is a dedicated professional with comprehensive, hands-on experience in Human Resource Management (HRM), having successfully managed the entire employee life cycle—from recruitment and onboarding to performance management and employee engagement. She holds an MBA in Human Resource Management, where she was recognized as a Gold Medalist and awarded the title of Best Outgoing Student. Her academic journey began with a Bachelor's degree in Electronics and Communication Engineering, showcasing her diverse educational foundation. Currently serving as an Assistant Professor, she combines industry expertise with academic insight to mentor and inspire the next generation of HR professionals.

Satheeskumar A is serving as an Assistant Professor in the Department of Computer Science and Engineering at Nandha Engineering College. He is actively engaged in teaching, research, and academic mentoring in core areas of computer science. His academic interests include emerging technologies, software development, data analytics, and artificial intelligence. He is committed to fostering innovation-driven learning environments and guiding students in technical projects, research activities, and skill development initiatives. With a strong dedication to academic excellence and professional growth, he continuously contributes to curriculum enhancement, collaborative research, and institutional development activities.

Sharmila A is an Associate Professor at Saveetha School of Management, SIMATS, Chennai, brings 16 years of academic experience with a strong focus on research in human resource management, particularly employee engagement in the IT sector. She is currently guiding three Ph.D. research scholars and serves as a Research Advisory Committee (RAC) member for ten others across various universities. Her scholarly work includes numerous presentations and publications at national and international conferences and in reputed journals. Her research is driven by a commitment to addressing real-world HR challenges, blending academic rigor with practical insight to advance the field meaningfully.

Duggirala Aravind is currently associated with the Department of Aviation, ASET College of Science and Technology, Chennai, India. He previously completed his Bachelor's degree in Electrical and Electronics Engineering at MITS University. His research interests include aviation operations, renewable energy technologies in air transport, Artificial Intelligence, Computer Science, Logistics and Business management. (aravindaset.edu@gmail.com).

Piali Haldar earned her MBA from the Institute of Rural Management Anand and completed her PhD at Birla Institute of Technology, Mesra. Her core areas of specialization include rural marketing, rural development, branding strategy, and consumer behaviour. With over 20 years of experience in academia and research, she has published extensively in renowned journals listed in ABDC and Scopus. She has authored one textbook on Marketing and edited three academic books. Dr. Haldar has presented her research at numerous national and international conferences and has contributed more than 50 papers to reputed journals, edited volumes, and conference proceedings.

Manoj Kumar is presently working as Associate Professor in the Department of Computer Science & Technology, at Manav Rachna University, Faridabad. He has over 16 years of experience including academics, industry & research. He has earned his Ph.D. in the year 2022, in the area of Computer Vision. The title of the thesis work is "Automatic Detection of Moving Object in a Video for smart Surveillance system". His area of expertise is Computer Vision, Artificial Intelligence, Machine Learning, Image Processing, IOT and Blockchain. Dr. Kumar has published many research papers related to moving object detection and tracking in videos and also extracts features moving object/vehicles from video in real-time video surveillance system. Dr. Kumar has published more than 15 papers in SCIE, SCOPUS, WEB OF SCIENCE indexed journals. Dr. Kumar has presented more than 29 papers in various Scopus Indexed International Conferences. The proceedings of the conferences are Scopus indexed and few of them published as a Book chapters. He has published 4 National Patents. He has participated in various workshops & Faculty development programs.

Felista Lizy is employed as an Assistant Professor in the PG Department of Computer Science at A.P.C. Mahalaxmi College for Women, Thoothukudi, Tamil Nadu, India. With more than 17 years of academic and research experience, she actively engages in research in cryptography, artificial intelligence, cybersecurity, cloud computing, blockchain technologies, and data-driven sustainable systems. She has published extensively in reputed Scopus-indexed, UGC-approved, and international peer-reviewed journals, with notable contributions to the performance enhancement of Elliptic Curve Cryptography (ECC) and RSA using innovative approaches such as Runge–Kutta and Game Theory models for secure digital identity applications. Dr. Felista has authored over 20 academic books spanning Python programming, cloud computing, data science, generative AI, big data technologies, and research methodologies, and has contributed several international book chapters published by Springer, IEEE, and other global publishers in areas including AI-driven sustainability, reinforcement learning, IoT–cloud integration, and smart urban systems. She holds two patents in machine learning–based data security and AR/VR application development. In addition to her research contributions, she serves as a reviewer and editorial board member for international journals and has chaired sessions, delivered invited talks, and coordinated national and international conferences, FDPs, and academic workshops. Her current research focuses on AI-enabled intelligent systems, cybersecurity frameworks for smart environments, and sustainable digital ecosystems.

Radhakrishnan M, Head of Training and Placement at Saveetha School of Management, brings over 20 years of experience in academia and placements. With strong communication and coordination skills, he is committed to enhancing students' learning, career development, and overall well-being. He holds a Doctoral degree in Management and is a Certified Soft Skills Trainer and NLP Practitioner from IATD, with additional training in Design Thinking from Intellect. His expertise includes soft skills development, motivational speaking, life coaching, and conducting workshops across diverse disciplines.

Dev Mandal currently serves as an Assistant Professor in the Department of Management at Brainware University, Kolkata. Before this, he worked at ICRA Analytics Ltd and Shriram Finance Ltd. He holds an MBA in Finance and a Bachelor of Commerce degree from Vidyasagar University. Additionally, he has successfully cleared the UGC NET and WB SET examinations in Management.

Urmila Pilania is an accomplished academician and researcher with over 16 years of experience in teaching, research, and academic administration. She is currently serving as an Associate Professor in the Department of Computer Science & Technology at Manav Rachna University (MRU), Faridabad, where she has been contributing since 2011. Her research interests span across Artificial Intelligence, Machine Learning, Steganography, Blockchain, IoT-enabled Smart Healthcare, and Computer Vision. She has guided and mentored numerous students and is currently supervising 04 PhD scholars in the areas of AI and ML. Dr. Pilania has an extensive research portfolio, including 16 research articles in international/national journals, 26 conference papers, 22 book chapters, 3 published books, 1 book in progress, and 6 patents (5 published, 1 granted). She has also contributed significantly to international conferences as a reviewer, session chair, and editorial board member, reflecting her active involvement in the global research community. She earned her PhD in Computer Science & Engineering from Manav Rachna University (2016-2021), M.Tech (CSE) from Vaish College of Engineering, MDU Rohtak (2007-2009), and B.Tech (CSE) from Guru Jambheshwar University of Science & Technology, Hisar (2003-2007). She is also UGC-NET qualified (2019). Dr. Pilania's contributions have been recognized with several honours, including the Outstanding Research Performer Award (2021–22), Long Service Award for 10 years at MRU, and the Women Researcher Award in Computer Science & Technology by Scientific Laurels.

Pooja R is a dental professional who transitioned into the non-clinical domain to pursue a career in healthcare administration. Drawing on a strong clinical foundation, [he/she/they] is committed to bridging the gap between medical expertise and managerial efficiency to drive sustainable improvements in healthcare delivery. Currently pursuing a Master of Business Administration at Saveetha School of Management, [he/she/they] aspires to contribute to the development of patient-centered and strategically driven healthcare systems through effective leadership and innovative management practices.

Suganya R is associated with the Department of Computer Science and Engineering at the Coimbatore Institute of Technology, located in Coimbatore. She is actively involved in academic activities related to computer science and engineering, contributing to teaching, research, and technical development in emerging areas of computing. Her academic interests include modern computing technologies, software development, and advancements in information technology that support innovation in engineering education and industry applications. Through her academic engagement, she supports student learning, research initiatives, and knowledge dissemination within the engineering community. Her work focuses on strengthening technical competencies among students while encouraging research-driven problem solving and technological innovation.

Ravikumar R. N. is currently a Postdoctoral researcher at Universiti Malaysia Perlis, Malaysia. Also, working as an Associate Professor in the department of Computer Engineering at Marwadi University, Rajkot, Gujarat. He has 12+ years of national and international teaching experience. He completed his PhD at Amity University, Rajasthan, M.E at VMRF Deemed University, B.E at Anna University, Chennai. He is the co-founder of the Research Activities Club at Marwadi University and trains students on research activities, which leads to the publication of 7 Scopus/SCI journals, 85+ Book chapters, 25 Conference papers, and 10 patents. His specialization is ML, DL, Federated Learning, Recommendation Systems, and Optimization Techniques.

Tamilarasi Rajamani serves as an Assistant Professor in the School of Computer Science under the Faculty of Engineering and Technology at Villa College-QI Campus, Maldives. She is actively engaged in teaching, research, and academic mentoring within the domains of computer science and emerging digital technologies. Her academic interests include artificial intelligence, data analytics, software engineering, and applied computing solutions for real-world challenges. She is committed to fostering innovative learning environments that encourage critical thinking, problem-solving, and research-driven inquiry among students. Dr. Tamilarasi contributes to curriculum development, project supervision, and interdisciplinary collaboration, supporting the advancement of technology education in the region. She has participated in scholarly initiatives, academic workshops, and knowledge-sharing platforms that strengthen research culture and institutional growth. Through her dedication to academic excellence and student development, she continues to contribute meaningfully to the technological and educational landscape in the Maldives.

Aarthi S is a dedicated Assistant Professor in Computer Science with over six years of teaching experience. She is currently pursuing her Ph.D. at Marwadi University, Gujarat, and holds an M.Phil. and MCA from Bharathiar University, Tamil Nadu. Throughout her academic career, Aarthi has specialized in programming languages such as C++, Java, and C, and contributed to research in recommender systems and AI-related data privacy. She has published journal articles, contributed to book chapters, and actively participated in technical workshops. Known for her student mentorship and engagement in academic events, Aarthi remains committed to fostering innovation and excellence in computer science education.

Kavitha Bharathi S is working as Associate Professor in Computer Technology, Kongu Engineering College, and Perundurai. She has industrial experience and 20 years of experience in Teaching. She completed her UG degree in Computer Science, MCA from Vellalar College for Women, M.phil degree from Bharathiar University, Coimbatore and Ph.D from Anna University, Chennai.Her area of interest in Mobile Grid Computing and Internet of Things. She has published more than 30 papers in National and International Journals, Presented more than 15 papers in national and International conferences, Completed two Projects for academics and organized various funded programs, Seminars and Workshops, Published 2 books. Guided more than 100 UG, PG projects in various emerging trends in technology such as Internet of Things, Mobile Application Development, Augmented and Virtual Reality.

Tamilselvi S is an Assistant Professor in the Department of Computer Technology at Kongu Engineering College, Perundurai. With 9 years of teaching experience, she brings a strong academic background, holding an M.C.A., M.Phil., and Ph.D., from Bharathiar University. Her areas of specialization include Advanced Networking and Cloud Computing, where she actively contributes through teaching and academic research.

Shreha S A is associated with the Department of Clinical Psychology at PSG College of Arts and Science. She demonstrates a strong academic and professional interest in understanding human behavior, emotional functioning, and psychological well-being across diverse populations. Her focus lies in the scientific study of mental health, clinical assessment, and evidence-based psychological interventions. Shreha is particularly interested in exploring the psychological factors that influence individual resilience, coping mechanisms, and mental health outcomes. She values ethical practice, empathy, and cultural sensitivity as core components of effective psychological care. Through continuous learning and engagement with contemporary psychological research, she seeks to strengthen her understanding of clinical frameworks and therapeutic approaches. Shreha aspires to contribute to mental health awareness, early identification of psychological concerns, and the promotion of psychological well-being at both individual and community levels. Her long-term goal is to support evidence-driven, compassionate mental health practices that address emerging psychological challenges in society.

Jogen Sharma is a Ph.D. Research Scholar in Library and Information Science at KIIT Deemed to be University, Bhubaneswar, Odisha, India and Assistant Librarian at the India International Centre (IIC), New Delhi, India. His academic and professional work centers on bibliometric research, digital transformation, and sustainable library practices. He has contributed widely through publications in reputed journals, edited volumes and conferences. His expertise includes implementing advanced technologies to modernize academic libraries and supporting institutional research needs. He is actively involved in professional associations and is committed to advancing innovation and sustainability in Library and Information Science.

Shrikant Tiwari (Senior Member, IEEE) received his Ph.D. in the Department of Computer Science & Engineering (CSE) from the Indian Institute of Technology (Banaras Hindu University), Varanasi (India) in 2012 and M. Tech. in Computer Science and Technology from University of Mysore (India) in 2009. Currently, he is working as a Professor in the Department of Computer Science & Engineering (CSE) School of Computing Science and Engineering (SCSE) at Galgotias University, Greater Noida, Uttar Pradesh (India). He has authored or co-authored more than 35 national and international journal publications, book chapters, and conference articles. He has five patents filed to his credit. His research interests include machine learning, deep learning, computer vision, medical image analysis, pattern recognition, and biometrics. Dr. Tiwari is a member of ACM, IET, FIETE, CSI, ISTE, IAENG, SCIEI. He is also a guest editorial board member and a reviewer for many international journals of repute.

Amit Kumar Tyagi is working as an Assistant Professor, at National Forensic Sciences University, Gandhinagar, Gujarat, India. He received his Ph.D. Degree (Full-Time) in 2018 from Pondicherry Central University, 605014, Puducherry, India. About his academic experience, he has worked as an assistant professor at several institutes like Lord Krishna College of Engineering (LKCE), Ghaziabad (for the periods of July 2009- July 2010, and October 2012- October 2013), Lingaya's Vidyapeeth (formerly known as Lingaya's University), Faridabad (September 2018- May 2019), VIT Chennai (June 2019- November 2022) and NIFT New Delhi (November 2022- September 2025). His supervision experience includes more than

10 Masters' dissertations and one PhD thesis. He has contributed to several projects such as "AARIN" and "P3- Block" to address some of the open issues related to the privacy breaches in Vehicular Applications (such as Parking) and Medical Cyber Physical Systems (MCPS). He has published over 350 research articles in refereed high impact journals, conferences and books, and some of his articles has been awarded as best paper awards.

Srinivasan Vasan is an Assistant Professor in the Department of Humanities and Social Sciences at Graphic Era (Deemed to be University), with 16 years of teaching and field expertise. He has served in the Ministry of Health and Family Welfare, as a Guest Faculty, and as a Mobilization Training Specialist with the State Government. Recently, he contributed to a tuberculosis project funded by GFATM and USAID. He has published 90 papers, with more under peer review in UGC-CARE and SCOPUS journals.

Index

A

B

C

D

E

G

H

I

M

P

V

www.ingramcontent.com/pod-product-compliance
Lightning Source LLC
LaVergne TN
LVHW062337300926
849161LV00007B/1721